Statistical Meta-Analysis
With Applications

Statistical Meta-Analysis With Applications

Joachim Hartung
Dortmund University of Technology

Guido Knapp
Dortmund University of Technology

Bimal K. Sinha
University of Maryland, Baltimore County

WILEY

A JOHN WILEY & SONS, INC., PUBLICATION

Published by John Wiley & Sons, Inc., Hoboken, New Jersey.
Published simultaneously in Canada.

For general information on our other products and services or for technical support, please contact our Customer Care Department within the United States at (800) 762-2974, outside the United States at (317) 572-3993 or fax (317) 572-4002.

Wiley also publishes its books in a variety of electronic formats. Some content that appears in print may not be available in electronic format. For information about Wiley products, visit our web site at www.wiley.com.

Library of Congress Cataloging-in-Publication Data:

Hartung, Joachim, Prof. Dr.
  Statistical meta-analysis with applications / Joachim Hartung, Guido Knapp, Bimal K. Sinha.
    p. cm.
  Includes bibliographical references and index.
  ISBN 978-0-470-29089-7 (cloth)
  1. Statistical hypothesis testing. 2. Meta-analysis. I. Knapp, Guido. II. Sinha, Bimal K., 1946– III. Title.
  QA277.H373 2008
  519.5'6—dc22   2008009435

Printed in the United States of America.

10 9 8 7 6 5 4 3 2 1

To my wife Bärbel and my children Carola, Lisa, Jan, and Jörn

To my parents Magdalena and Wilhelm

In memory of Professor Shailes Bhusan Chaudhuri for his excellent academic training in statistics and parental love during my Ashutosh College years

CONTENTS

PREFACE

Statistical Meta-Analysis with Applications combines our experiences on the topic and brings out a wealth of new information relevant for meta-analysis. Meta-analysis, a term coined by Glass (1976), and also known under different names such as research synthesis, research integration, and pooling of evidence, deals with *the statistical analysis of a large collection of analysis results from individual studies for the purpose of integrating the findings.*

It is a common phenomenon that many studies are carried out over time and space on some important global issues with a common target or goal. As an example, we can cite the 19 studies carried out in the context of effects of second-hand smoking on women! Sometimes the studies may correspond to different experiment settings with one objective in mind. The main reason that many studies on a research topic are carried out rather than a single study is to strengthen the overall conclusion about a certain hypothesis or to negate it with a stronger conviction. When the results of these component studies, either in full or in summary form, are available, it is desirable that we combine the results of these studies in a meaningful way so as to arrive at a valid conclusion about the target parameter. The main object of statistical meta-analysis is precisely to provide methods to meaningfully combine the results from component studies.

There are many aspects of statistical meta-analysis which must be addressed in a book. Most of the concern arises from the nature of the underlying studies, the nature of information available from these studies, and also the nature of assumptions about the distributions of random variables arising in the studies. We have provided a complete treatment of all these aspects in this book.

Several new features of this book are worth mentioning. We have indicated a wide variety of applications of statistical meta-analysis ranging from business to education to environment to health sciences in both univariate and multivariate cases. Our treatment of the statistical meta-analysis about (1) the common mean of several univariate normal populations, (2) tests of homogeneity, (3) one-way random effects model, (4) categorical data, (5) recovery of interblock information, and (6) combination of polls is entirely new, based on many recent results by us and others on these topics. Other topics such as meta-regression, multivariate meta-analysis, and Bayesian meta-analysis also appear in completely new forms in our book. Another special feature of the book is the incorporation of a detailed discussion about computational aspects and related softwares to carry out statistical meta-analysis in practice. Readers will find many extra useful features in this book compared to the existing books on this subject. Our book complements the statistical methods and results described in an excellent Academic Press text *Statistical Methods for Meta-Analysis* by Hedges and Olkin (1985). We put it on record our indebtedness to this book and also to the excellent edited volume *The Handbook of Research Synthesis* by Cooper and Hedges (1994) for many ideas on statistical meta-analysis. We have freely used some of the data sets and basic ideas from these two sources, and indirectly we owe a lot to Professors Harris Cooper, Larry Hedges, and Ingram Olkin!

Although some topics and chapters covered in this book require the knowledge of advanced statistical theory and methods, most of the meta-analysis methods described in the book can be understood and applied with a *solid* master's level background in statistics. Parts of the book can also be used as a graduate text on this topic. We believe that practitioners of statistical meta-analysis will benefit a lot from this book owing to a host of worked-out examples from various contexts. The example data sets and the program code may be downloaded from G.K.'s website at http://www.statistik.uni-dortmund.de/~knapp. Given that the possible application areas of meta-analysis are fairly broad, we have limited ourselves to a selected few applications depending on our own interest and expertise.

Financial support from the Dortmund University of Technology, Dortmund, Germany, and University of Maryland, Baltimore County, Maryland, are thankfully acknowledged. We are also grateful to Professors Leon Glaser, Satish Iyenger, and Neil Timm from the University of Pittsburgh for providing us with reprints of their papers on many aspects of multivariate meta-analysis. We are thankful to Professor Anirban Dasgupta of Purdue University for giving us his kind permission to include his work on *combination of polls* in this book. This certainly adds a new dimension! This book grew out of many lectures delivered on some of the topics of statistical meta-analysis at the University of Hong Kong (B.K.S.), Tunghai University (B.K.S.) (Taichung, Taiwan), University of South Australia (B.K.S), University of Tampere, Finland (G.K. and B.K.S.), University of Turku, Finland (G.K. and B.K.S.), United States Environmental Protection Agency (G.K. and B.K.S.) and the U.S. National Center for Health Statistics (G.K. and B.K.S.), and, of course, at our host institutions

(B.K.S. at the University of Maryland, Baltimore County, J.H. and G.K. at Dortmund University of Technology).

We mention with great pleasure the invitations received from all these places and the many comments we received from the audience, including our own students, which helped us to improve the contents and the presentations. We very much appreciate the excellent academic atmosphere at Dortmund University of Technology and University of Maryland, Baltimore County, where most of the book was written.

Last but not least, we express our sincere thanks to our understanding family members who occasionally had to put up with our changing moods due to the tremendous pressure in writing this book with as much information and accuracy as possible.

JOACHIM HARTUNG
GUIDO KNAPP
BIMAL K. SINHA

Dortmund, Germany
Baltimore, Maryland
June 2008

CHAPTER 1

INTRODUCTION

Meta-analysis, a term coined by Glass (1976), is intended to provide *the statistical analysis of a large collection of analysis results from individual studies for the purpose of integrating the findings.*

Meta-analysis, or research synthesis, or research integration is precisely a scientific method to accomplish this goal by applying sound statistical procedures, and indeed it has a long and old history. The very invention of least squares by Legendre (1805) and Gauss (1809) is an attempt to solve just a unique problem of meta-analysis: use of astronomical observations collected at several observatories to estimate the orbit of comets and to determine meridian arcs in geodesy (Stigler, 1986). In order to determine the relationship between mortality and inoculation with a vaccine for enteric fever, Pearson (1904) used data from five small independent samples and computed a pooled estimate of correlation between mortality and inoculation in order to evaluate the efficacy of the vaccine. As an early application of meta-analysis in the physical sciences, Birge (1932) combined estimates across experiments at different laboratories to establish reference values for some fundamental constants in physics. Early works of Cochran (1937), Yates and Cochran (1938), Tippett (1931), and Fisher (1932) dealt with combining information across experiments in the agricultural sciences in order to derive estimates of treatment effects and test their significance. Likewise, there

Statistical Meta-Analysis with Applications. By Joachim Hartung, Guido Knapp, Bimal K. Sinha
Copyright © 2008 John Wiley & Sons, Inc.

are plenty of applications of meta-analysis in the fields of education, medicine, and social sciences, some of which are briefly described below.

In the field of education, meta-analysis is useful in combining studies about coaching effectiveness to improve Scholastic Aptitude Test (SAT) scores in verbal and math (Rubin, 1981; DerSimonian and Laird, 1983), in studying the effect of open education on (i) attitude of students toward school and (ii) student independence and self-reliance, and in combining studies about the relationship between teacher indirectness and student achievement (Hedges and Olkin, 1985). In social science, there is a need to combine several studies of gender differences in separate categories of quantitative ability, verbal ability, and visual-spatial ability (Hedges and Olkin, 1985). For some novel applications of meta-analysis in the field of medicine, we refer to Pauler and Wakefield (2000) for three applications involving dentrifice data, antihypertension data, and preeclampsia data, to Berry (2000) for questions about benefits and risks of mammography of women based on six studies, to Brophy and Joseph (2000) for meta-analysis involving three studies to compare streptokinase and tissue-plasminogen activator to reduce mortality following an acute myocardial infarction, and lastly to Dominici and Parmigiani (2000) for an application of meta-analysis involving studies in which outcomes are reported on continuous variables for some medical outcomes in some studies and on binary variables on similar medical outcomes in some other studies. Of course, there are numerous other diverse applications of meta-analysis in many other fields. We mention several applications below.

A: Business applications. In the context of business management and administration, one often encounters several studies with a common effect, and the problem then is of drawing suitable inference about the common effect based on the information from all the studies. Here are some examples. In the context of studying price elasticity, Tellis (1988) reports results from 42 studies! Sethuraman (1995) performed meta-analysis of national brand and store brand cross-promotional price elasticities. Lodish et al. (1995) reported results of 389 real world split cable TV advertising experiments: How TV advertising works? Churchill et al. (1985) reported meta-analysis of the determinants of salesperson performance. Farley and Lehmann (1986, 2001) and Farley, Lehmann, and Sawyer (1995) emphasized the important role of meta-analysis in international research in marketing. A current major thrust in marketing has been an attempt to create global products and brands while retaining local requirements: think global, act local. Deciding which elements of which products can be produced globally and which locally requires meta-analysis of each of the elements.

B: Environmental applications. In the context of environmental problems, there are several situations where the meta-analysis methods can be successfully applied. Here is a partial list of such applications.

Evaluation of superfund cleanup technologies (Sinha, O'Brien, and Smith, 1991; Sinha and Sinha, 1995). Cleaning up of superfund waste sites (nuclear/chemical/biological) at the National Priorities List (NPL), based on an index comprising four measures, air, groundwater, soil, and surface water, often requires innovative/extremely expensive technology. A critical study of performance of the suggested technologies after a certain amount of time is highly desirable. If found useful, the technologies can be encouraged to continue at the same site. If otherwise, this should be determined as soon as possible so that suitable corrective measures can be taken. Towards this end, a common procedure is to study a preremediation baseline sample and an interim sample taken after a certain period of operation of the technology and test if a desirable percentage of the total contaminant has been removed. Comparison of a few such technologies can be based on several studies, and a data synthesis or pooling of evidence is very natural here in order to determine the final ranking of the technologies.

Assessment of gasoline quality (Yu, Sun, and Sinha, 2002). The U.S. Environmental Protection Agency (EPA) evaluates/regulates gasoline quality based on what is known as Reid vapor pressure (RVP). Samples of gasoline are taken from various pumps and RVPs are measured in two ways: on-site at the field level (cheap and quick) and also off-site at the laboratory level (expensive/higher precision). This usually results in two types of data: field data and lab data. Gasoline quality based on RVP can then be determined combining the evidence in both the data sets—a clear application of meta-analysis!

Water quality in Hillsdale Lake (Li, Nussbaum, and Sinha, 2000). Hillsdale Lake, a large federal reservoir located about 30 miles from the Kansas City metropolitan area, was authorized by the U.S. Congress in 1954 as part of a comprehensive flood control plan for the Osage and Missouri River Basins. The lake is a major recreational resource— over 500,000 visitors annually—and is also a significant source of drinking water. It is therefore essential that the water quality in this lake, as measured by Secchi depth, be regulated regularly. To achieve this, typically data from a survey of lake users in the various categories of swimming, fishing, boating, skiing, and water sports can be collected and analyzed in order to establish what level of water clarity users perceive as good. Again, it is quite possible that several studies are conducted for this purpose, and there is a need to pool the evidence from such studies to arrive at an overall conclusion about the water clarity level.

A comparison of CMW and DPW for groundwater monitoring (Li, 2000). Long-term monitoring of contamination of groundwater at former military land sites is performed by boring wells into the ground at predetermined locations and then assessing trace amounts of certain chemicals. There are two well-known methods for this purpose: an expensive traditional method of conventionally monitored wells (CMWs) and a relatively cheaper new methodology of direct push wells (DPWs). In order to compare these two methods, a joint study was conducted by the United States Air Force with the EPA to evaluate the assessment of pollutants. The former Hanscom Air Force Base (HAFB) located in Middlesex County, Massachusetts, and straddling the towns of Bedford, Concord, Lexington, and Lincoln was selected as the study site, and groundwater samples were collected for an assessment of long-term monitoring with both CMWs and DPWs based on 31 paired well locations. Data were collected on nine volatile organic carbons (VOCs): vinyl chloride, 1,1-DCA, benzene, toluene,

o-xylene, *trans*-1,2-DCE, TCE, and 1,4-DCA—labeled as VOC1, VOC2, VOC3, VOC4, VOC5, VOC6, VOC7, VOC8, and VOC9. The site was divided into three regions, and data were collected separately in each region. It is then in the spirit of meta-analysis that we combine the results of the three regions and decide if the two methods perform equally or there is a significant difference.

Effect of second-hand smoking on women. This of course is a vital environmental issue with a potential for adverse health effects. Several studies were conducted in many parts of the world to determine if second-hand smoking is harmful for women, and it is absolutely essential that we carry out a meta-analysis, pooling the evidence from all the studies, in order to find out the underlying state of the matter. The relevant data set is reported in Section 18.6. We should mention that based on a suitable meta-analysis of the collected information, an advisory committee of the EPA designated environmental tobacco smoke as a carcinogen.

C: Health sciences applications. In the context of medicine or health science problems, there are several situations where the meta-analysis methods can be successfully applied. Here is a partial list of such applications.

Antiplatelet drug for patients with ischemic attacks. In 1988, the question of whether to prescribe an antiplatelet drug for patients with transient ischemic attacks to prevent stroke was controversial. At that time, many randomized trials of antiplatelet drugs to treat patients with cerebrovascular disease have been completed, but the studies were variable in question and their results were contradictory. A meta-analysis of these studies by the Antiplatelet Trialist' Collaboration (1988) found a highly significant 22% reduction in the estimated relative risk of stroke, myocardial infarction, and vascular death in patients with cerebrovascular disease who were treated with an antiplatelet drug.

Functional dyspepsia (Allescher et al., 2001). Nonulcer dyspepsia is characterized by a variety of upper abdominal symptoms in the absence of organic disease. Within the general population, dyspepsia is very common, and as a result, empirical therapy without prior diagnostic procedures has been recommended for the management of these patients. Both acid-suppressive substances such as histamine H_2-receptor antagonists (H_2-RAs) and gastroprokinetics have been suggested as first-line, empirical therapy. Clinical trials of H_2-RAs have yielded somewhat contradictory results and benefit seems largely confined to refluxlike or ulcerlike dyspepsia subgroups. All these findings came out of an appropriate meta-analysis study.

Dentifrice (Johnson, 1993). In a series of nine randomized controlled clinical trials, sodium monofluorophosphate (SMFP) was compared to sodium fluoride (NaF) dentifrice in the prevention of caries development. The data consist of treatment differences, $NaF_i - SMFP_i$, where NAF_i is the change from baseline in the decayed/missing (due to caries)/filled-surface dental index at three years follow-up for regular use of NaF and $SMFP_i$ is defined similarly for $i = 1, \ldots, 9$. A statistical meta-analysis is in order here.

Recovery time after aneasthesia (Whitehead, 2002). A multicenter study with nine centers was undertaken to compare two anaesthetic agents undergoing short surgical procedures, where rapid recovery is important. The response of interest is the recovery time [time from when the anaesthetic gases are turned off until the patients open their eyes (in minutes)]. A meta-analysis would be quite appropriate in this context. Incidentally, a logarithmic transformation of the underlying data produces almost normal data.

As the scope of meta-analysis grew over the years, several terminologies also came into existence, such as quantitative research synthesis, pooling of evidence, or creating an overview. While most of the early works, including Mosteller and Bush (1954), provided a logical foundation for meta-analysis, the appearance of several books, notably Glass, McGaw, and Smith (1981), Hunter, Schmidt, and Jackson (1982), Rosenthal (1984), Hedges and Olkin (1985), and the edited volume by Cooper and Hedges (1994), and literally thousands of meta-analytic papers during the last 20 years or so, primarily covering applications in health sciences and education, has made the subject to have a very special role in diverse fields of applications.

The essential character of meta-analysis is that it is the statistical analysis of the summary findings of many empirical studies, which are called primary analyses, all targeted towards a common goal. However, differences among the constituent studies due to sampling designs, presence of different covariates, and so on, can and do exist while sharing a common objective. A fundamental assumption behind conducting a meta-analysis or pooling of evidence or information or data across studies in order to obtain an average effect across all studies is that the size of the effect (basic parameter of interest) reported in each study is an estimate of a common effect size of the whole population of studies. It is therefore essential to test for homogeneity of population effect sizes across studies before conducting a meta-analysis if obtaining an estimate of average effect or its test is the primary goal of the meta-analysis.

The notion of effect size is central to many meta-analysis studies which often deal with comparing two treatments, control and experimental, in an effort to find out if there is a significant difference between the two. In the case of continuous measurements, a standardized mean difference plays an important role to measure such a difference. In the case of qualitative attributes, the difference or ratio of two proportions, odds ratio, and φ coefficient are used to capture such differences. Again, when the objective is to study the relationship between two variables, an obvious choice is the usual correlation coefficient.

Recent meta-analytic work, however, concentrates on discovering and explaining variations in effect sizes rather than assuming that they remain the same across studies, which is perhaps rarely the case owing to uncontrollable differences in study contexts, designs, treatments, and subjects. When results of several scientific studies of the same phenomena exist and more or less agree, by conducting an appropriate test of homogeneity and accepting the hypothesis of homogeneity, the case for summarizing results of all studies with a single average effect size can be strengthened and defended. If, however, this hypothesis is rejected, no single number can adequately account for the variety of reported results. Thus, if the results from various studies differ either significantly or even marginally, we should make an attempt to investigate methods to account for the variability by further work. This is precisely the spirit of some recent research in meta-analysis using random and mixed effects models, allowing inclusion of trial-specific covariates which may explain a part of the observed heterogeneity. In other words, a set of conflicting findings from different studies is looked upon as an opportunity for learning and discovering the sources of variation among the reported outcomes rather than a cause for dismay.

While most common meta-analysis applications involve comparison of just one variable (experimental) with another (control), multivariate data can also arise in meta-analysis due to several reasons. First, the primary studies themselves can be multivariate in nature because these studies may measure multiple outcomes for each subject and are typically known as multiple-endpoint studies. It should, however, be noted that not all studies in a review would have the same set of outcomes. For example, studies of SAT do not all report math and verbal scores. In fact, only about half of the studies dealt with in Becker (1990) provided coaching results for both math and verbal! Secondly, multivariate data may arise when primary studies involve several comparisons among groups based on a single outcome. As an example, Ryan, Blakeslee, and Furst (1986) studied the effects of practice on motor skill levels on the basis of a five-group design, four different kinds of practice groups and one no-practice group, thus leading to comparisons of multivariate data. These kinds of studies are usually known as multiple-treatment studies.

As mentioned earlier, although most statistical methods of meta-analysis focus on deriving and studying properties of a common estimated effect which is supposed to exist across all studies, when heterogeneity across studies is believed to exist, a meta-analyst must estimate the extent and sources of heterogeneity among studies if the hypothesis of homogeneity is not found to be tenable. While fixed effects models discussed in this book under the assumption of homogeneous effects sizes continue to be the most common method of meta-analysis, the assumption of homogeneity given variability among studies due to varying research and evaluation protocols may be unrealistic. In such cases, a random effects model which avoids the homogeneity assumption and models effects as random and coming from a distribution is recommended. The various study effects are believed to arise from a population, and random effects models borrow strength across studies in providing estimates of both study-specific effects and underlying population effect.

Whether a fixed effects model or a random effects model, a Bayesian approach considers all parameters (population effect sizes for fixed effects models, in particular) as random and coming from a superpopulation with its own parameters. There are several advantages for a Bayesian approach to meta-analysis. The Bayesian paradigm provides in a very natural way a method for data synthesis from all studies by incorporating model and parameter uncertainty. Moreover, a predictive distribution for future observations coming from any study, which may be a quantity of central interest to some decision makers, can be easily developed based on what have been already observed. The use of Bayesian hierarchical models often leads to more appropriate estimates of parameters compared to the asymptotic ones arising from maximum likelihood, especially in the case of small sample sizes of component studies, which is typical in meta-analysis.

There are at least two other vital issues with meta-analysis procedures. Although it is true that most of the primary studies to be included in a meta-analysis provide a complete background of the problem being considered along with relevant entire or summary data, it also happens sometimes that some studies report only the ultimate finding in terms of the sign of the estimated underlying effect size being positive or negative or in terms of the significance or nonsignificance of the test for the absence of an effect size. It then poses a challenge for the statisticians to develop suitable statistical procedures to take into account this kind of incomplete or scanty information to carry out meta-analysis. Fortunately, there are techniques under the category of vote counting procedures to effectively deal with such situations.

The problem of selection or publication bias is rather crucial in the context of meta-analysis since the reported studies on which meta-analysis is typically based tend to be mostly significant and there could be many potential nonsignificant studies which are not reported at all simply because of their nonsignificant findings and hence these studies are not amenable to meta-analysis considerations. Such a situation is bound to happen in almost any meta-analysis scenario in spite of one's best attempt to get hold of all relevant studies, and statistically valid corrective measures should be developed and followed to deal with such a serious publication bias issue. Again, fortunately, there are some valid statistical procedures to tackle this vital problem.

We now point out that in the context of statistical meta-analysis, there are four important stages of research synthesis:

(i) **problem formulation** stage

(ii) **data collection** stage

(iii) **data evaluation** stage

(iv) **data analysis and interpretation** stage.

We describe these four stages below.

At the formulation stage of the research synthesis problem, we clearly spell out the universe to which generalizations are made (fixed effects model and random effects model) and the nature of the effect size parameters to be inferred upon (Hedges, 1994). Since research synthesis extends our knowledge through the combination and comparison of primary studies, it is important for us to indicate the perspective of the fixed effects model where the universe to which generalizations are made consists of ensembles of studies identical to those in the study sample. On the other hand, the random effects model perspective is relevant when the universe to which generalizations are made consists of a population of studies from which the study sample is drawn. Objectively and clearly defining the nature of the effect size parameter to be estimated or tested in a meta-analysis problem is also fundamental. One instance about the inference of an effect size is to ascertain the relationship between two variables X and Y in terms of either (a) estimation of the magnitude of the relationship (effect size) along with an indication of the accuracy or the reliability of the estimated effect size (standard error or confidence interval) or (b) a test of significance of the difference between the realized effect size and the effect size expected under the null hypothesis of no relation between X and Y. Some other common effect size measures are given by the standardized difference of two means, standardized difference of two proportions, difference of two correlations, ratio of proportions, odds ratio, risk ratio, and so on. We have elaborated on all these measures in Chapter 2.

The data collection or literature search stage in research synthesis is indeed very challenging. This is of course different from primary analysis of studies. There are usually five major modes of searching for sources of primary research, namely, manual and computer search of subject indexes from abstract databases, footnote chasing (references in review/nonreview papers and books), consultation (formal/informal requests, conferences), browsing through library shelves, and manual and computer citation searches (White, 1994). While it is hoped that these search procedures, in addition to reviewing books/book chapters, research/technical reports, conference papers, and other possible sources, would lead to an exhaustive collection of relevant literature for the problem under study, sometimes we also need to use special ways and means to retrieve what are known as fugitive literature and information appearing in unpublished papers/technical reports, unpublished dissertations/master's theses, and the like. In this context, publication bias is quite relevant while doing the research synthesis, bearing in mind the fact that often research leading to nonsignificant conclusions are not reported at all or rarely so (the well known file-drawer problem). We have addressed this important issue in Chapter 13.

Not all studies available for meta-analysis may qualify for inclusion due to various reasons. The data evaluation stage consists of carefully checking the nature and sources of primary research data, missing observations in primary data, and sources of potential bias in the primary data, all in an attempt to assign suitable weights to the various primary data sources at the time of carrying out meta-analysis or data synthesis.

Finally, the data analysis stage, which is the main purpose of this book, deals with statistically describing and combining various primary studies. Naturally what we need here is a wide collection of sound statistical methods depending on the nature of the underlying problem. We describe ways to combine various measures of effect sizes either for estimation or test or confidence interval and also ways to deal with missing values in primary studies as well as publication bias. In the sequel, we need statistical procedures for univariate and multivariate cases, discrete and continuous cases, and also frequentist and Bayesian methods.

Given the above broad spectrum of topics that can be covered under the umbrella of a book on meta-analysis, our goal in writing this book is primarily concerned with some statistical aspects of meta-analysis. As already mentioned, the heart of the enterprise of carrying out meta-analysis or synthesizing research consists of comparing and combining the results of individual primary studies of a particular, focused research question, and the emphasis is essentially on two types of statistical analysis: combining results of tests of significance of effect size and combining estimates of effect size. The effect size, as explained earlier, is a generic term referring to the magnitude of an effect or more generally the size of the relation between two variables.

Moreover, in case of diverse research findings from comparable studies, an attempt must be made to understand and point out reasons for such differences.

Keeping the above general points in mind, the outline of the book is as follows.

Chapter 2 describes various standard measures of effect size based on means, proportions, φ coefficient, odds ratio, and correlations. Some illustrative examples to explain the related computations and concepts are included.

Chapter 3 deals with methods of combining individual tests based on primary research with plenty of applications. This chapter is exclusively based on combination of P-values mainly because the studies which are meant for meta-analysis more often report their P-values than other details of the study. The methods described here are exact and also appear in standard textbooks on meta-analysis. It should be mentioned that there are other methods based on suitably combining often independent component test statistics. However, the sampling distributions of the combination of such test statistics may not be readily available. We discuss these aspects in detail in Chapter 5 in the context of inference about a common mean of several univariate normal populations.

Chapter 4 describes methods of combining individual estimates of effect sizes based on primary research to efficiently estimate the common effect size parameter as well as to construct its confidence interval. The methods suggested in this chapter are mainly asymptotic in nature and again are quite routine.

Chapter 5 is devoted to a detailed analysis of a special kind of meta-analysis problem, namely, inference about the common mean of several univariate normal populations with unknown and unequal variances. This problem has a long and rich history and is very significant in applications. Most of the results presented here are new and have not appeared in any textbook before. Two classic data sets are used throughout to explain the concepts.

Chapter 6 describes various tests of the important hypothesis of the homogeneity of population effect sizes in some particular models. In the context of statistical meta-analysis, one should carry out these tests of homogeneity of effect sizes before applying tools of combining the effect sizes. The results presented here are based on the review papers by Hartung and his students.

One-way random effects models, useful when the basic hypothesis of homogeneity of effect sizes does not hold, is taken up in Chapter 7. There is a huge literature on this topic and we have made an attempt to present all the important results in this connection. Typically, there are two scenarios: error variances are all equal (homogeneous case) and error variances are not equal (heterogeneous case). We have dealt with both cases. The reader will find a variety of new and novel solutions in this chapter.

Chapter 8 extends the results of the previous three chapters to the meta-analysis of comparative trials with normal outcome. Results in the fixed effects as well as in the random effects model are provided for the effect sizes difference of means, standardized difference of means, and ratio of means.

Meta-analysis procedures to analyze categorical data of both binary and ordinal nature are presented in Chapter 9. We have provided fixed effects as well as random effects results with motivating examples. This is another nice feature of the book.

Meta-regression, multivariate meta-analysis, and Bayesian meta-analysis are, respectively, presented in three subsequent chapters—10, 11, and 12. In Chapter 10, we describe meta-analysis regression procedures with one and more than one covariate with illustrations. In Chapter 11, we describe both aspects of multiple-endpoint and multiple-treatment studies. We have provided a unified Bayesian approach to meta-analysis with some examples in Chapter 12. All these three chapters provide unique features to our book.

The important concepts of publication bias and vote counting procedures, which also appear in standard textbooks, are taken up in Chapters 13 and 16. As mentioned earlier, these problems arise when we do not have access to all the literature on the subject under study and also when there is not enough evidence in the studies which are indeed available.

We describe in Chapter 14 the statistical methods for recovery of interblock information. One of the earliest applications of statistical meta-analysis (Yates, 1939, 1940; Rao, 1947) consists of combining what are known as intrablock and interblock estimates of treatment effects in the presence of random block effects in two-way mixed effects models. Early tests of significance of treatment effects in this context were based on combining the P-values using Fisher's method. Since this method does not take into account the underlying statistical structure, methods to improve it were suggested in several papers (Feingold, 1985, 1988; Cohen and Sackrowitz, 1989; Mathew, Sinha, and Zhou, 1993; Zhou and Mathew; 1993). We describe all these procedures in detail in this chapter, which is a new and novel contribution to the vast literature on statistical meta-analysis.

A different kind of meta-analysis dealing with a combination of polls is presented in Chapter 15. This particular topic has applications in market research and is completely new. This is based on a technical report by Dasgupta and Sinha (2006).

There are many computational aspects of statistical meta-analysis which are taken up in Chapter 17 using the general statistical software packages SAS and R. Sample programs for both softwares are explained with examples.

Finally, sample data sets which are analyzed throughout the book are included in the final section of the book, Chapter 18. The References section at the end contains a long list of papers referred to in this book.

We conclude this introductory chapter with two observations. First, although we have described a variety of diverse scenarios where meta-analysis methods can be successfully applied, we have not made an attempt to do so. Our illustrations of the methods are naturally limited to our judgment and own experiences. Second, except in some chapters, virtually all of the statistical methods described in this book are based on standard large sample results for the (asymptotic) distributions of sample means, sample proportions, sample correlations, and so on, and hence due caution should be exercised when using these methods. Some of the frequently quoted results are listed below for ready reference (see Rao, 1973; Rohatgi, 1976):

1. $X_1, \ldots, X_n$ are independently and identically distributed (iid) with mean μ and variance σ^2. Then, for large n,

$$\bar{X} = \frac{1}{n} \sum_{i=1}^{n} X_i \sim N\left(\mu, \frac{\sigma^2}{n}\right),$$

that is,

$$\frac{\sqrt{n}\,(\bar{X} - \mu)}{\sigma} \sim N(0, 1).$$

This is a standard version of the celebrated central limit theorem (CLT).

2. $X_1, \ldots, X_n$ are iid with mean μ and variance σ^2. Then, for large n,

$$\frac{\sqrt{n}\,(\bar{X} - \mu)}{S} \sim N(0, 1),$$

where $S^2 = \sum_{i-1}^{n}(X_i - \bar{X})^2/(n-1)$. This is an application of CLT coupled with Cramer's theorem (Slutsky's theorem).

3. $X \sim B(n, P)$. Then, for large n,

$$\frac{X - n\,P}{\sqrt{n\,P\,Q}} \sim N(0, 1),$$

where $Q = 1 - P$, that is,

$$\frac{\sqrt{n}(p - P)}{\sqrt{P\,Q}} \sim N(0, 1),$$

where $p = X/n$. This is a standard application of the CLT.

4. $X \sim B(n, P)$. Then, for large n, writing $p = X/n$,

$$\sin^{-1} \sqrt{p} \sim N\left(\sin^{-1} \sqrt{P}, \frac{1}{4n}\right).$$

This is a well-known version of Fisher's variance-stabilizing transformation applied to the binomial proportion.

5. $(X_1, Y_1), \ldots, (X_n, Y_n)$ are iid from a bivariate distribution with means (μ_1, μ_2), variances (σ_1^2, σ_2^2), and correlation ρ. Then, for large n,

$$r \sim N\left(\rho, \frac{(1 - \rho^2)^2}{n - 1}\right),$$

where r is the usual sample correlation defined as

$$r = \frac{\sum_{i=1}^{n}(X_i - \bar{X})(Y_i - \bar{Y})}{\left[\sum_{i=1}^{n}(X_i - \bar{X})^2 \; \sum_{i=1}^{n}(Y_i - \bar{Y})^2\right]^{1/2}}.$$

This is also an application of CLT coupled with Cramer's theorem (Slutsky's theorem; see Rao, 1973).

6. $(X_1, Y_1), \ldots, (X_n, Y_n)$ are iid from a bivariate distribution with means (μ_1, μ_2), variances (σ_1^2, σ_2^2), and correlation ρ. Then, for large n,

$$z \sim N\left(\zeta, \frac{1}{n-3}\right),$$

where

$$z = \frac{1}{2} \ln\left(\frac{1+r}{1-r}\right) \quad \text{and} \quad \zeta = \frac{1}{2} \ln\left(\frac{1+\rho}{1-\rho}\right).$$

This is a well-known version of Fisher's variance-stabilizing transformation applied to the sample correlation coefficient.

CHAPTER 2

VARIOUS MEASURES OF EFFECT SIZE

Quite often the main objective in a study is to compare two treatments: **experimental** and **control**. When these treatments are applied to a set of experimental units, the outcomes can be of two types, qualitative and quantitative, leading to either proportions or means. Accordingly, effect sizes are also essentially of these two types: those based on differences of two means and those based on differences of two proportions. A third type of effect size, namely, correlation, arises when the objective in a study is to ascertain the nature and extent of the relationship between two variables.

2.1 EFFECT SIZE BASED ON MEANS

An effect size based on means is defined as follows. Denote the population means of the two groups (experimental and control) by μ_1 and μ_2 and their variances by σ_1^2 and σ_2^2, respectively. Then the effect size θ based on means is a standardized difference between μ_1 and μ_2 and can be expressed as

$$\theta = \frac{\mu_1 - \mu_2}{\sigma},\tag{2.1}$$

Statistical Meta-Analysis with Applications. By Joachim Hartung, Guido Knapp, Bimal K. Sinha
Copyright © 2008 John Wiley & Sons, Inc.

where σ denotes either the standard deviation σ_2 of the population control group or an average population standard deviation (namely, an average of σ_1 and σ_2).

The above measure of effect size θ can be easily estimated based on sample values, and this is explained below. Suppose we have a random sample of size n_1 from the first population with the sample mean $\bar{X}_1$ and sample variance S_1^2 and also a random sample of size n_2 from the second population with the sample mean $\bar{X}_2$ and sample variance S_2^2. One measure of the effect size θ, known as Cohen's d (Cohen, 1969, 1977, 1988), is then given by

$$d = \frac{\bar{X}_1 - \bar{X}_2}{S}, \tag{2.2}$$

where the standardized quantity S is the pooled sample standard deviation defined as $S = \sqrt{S^2}$ where

$$S^2 = \frac{(n_1 - 1)\, S_1^2 + (n_2 - 1)\, S_2^2}{n_1 + n_2}$$

with

$$(n_1 - 1)\, S_1^2 = \sum_{i=1}^{n_1} (X_{1i} - \bar{X}_1)^2 \quad \text{and} \quad (n_2 - 1)\, S_2^2 = \sum_{i=1}^{n_2} (X_{2i} - \bar{X}_2)^2.$$

A second measure of θ, known as Hedges's g (Hedges, 1981, 1982), is defined as

$$g = \frac{\bar{X}_1 - \bar{X}_2}{S^*}, \tag{2.3}$$

where the standardized quantity S^* is also the pooled sample standard deviation defined as $S^* = \sqrt{S^{*2}}$ with

$$S^{*2} = \frac{(n_1 - 1)\, S_1^2 + (n_2 - 1)\, S_2^2}{n_1 + n_2 - 2}.$$

It can be shown that (see Hedges and Olkin, 1985)

$$\mathrm{E}(g) \approx \theta + \frac{3\,\theta}{4N - 9}, \tag{2.4}$$

$$\sigma^2(g) = \mathrm{Var}(g) \approx \frac{1}{\tilde{n}} + \frac{\theta^2}{2(N - 3.94)}, \tag{2.5}$$

where

$$N = n_1 + n_2, \quad \tilde{n} = \frac{n_1\, n_2}{n_1 + n_2}.$$

In case the population variances are identical in both groups, under the assumption of normality of the data, Hedges (1981) shows that $\sqrt{\tilde{n}}\, g$ follows a noncentral t distribution with noncentrality parameter $\sqrt{\tilde{n}}\, \theta$ and $n_1 + n_2 - 2$ degrees of freedom. Consequently, the exact mean and variance of Hedges's g are given by

$$\mathrm{E}(g) = \sqrt{\frac{N - 2}{2}}\, \frac{\Gamma\left[(N - 3)/2\right]}{\Gamma\left[(N - 2)/2\right]}\, \theta, \tag{2.6}$$

$$\sigma^2(g) = \mathrm{Var}(g) = \frac{N - 2}{N - 4}\,(1 + \theta^2) - \theta^2\, \frac{N - 2}{2}\, \frac{\{\Gamma\left[(N - 3)/2\right]\}^2}{\{\Gamma\left[(N - 2)/2\right]\}^2} \tag{2.7}$$

and $\Gamma(\cdot)$ denotes the gamma function. As Cohen's d is proportional to Hedges's g, the results in Eq. (2.6) can be easily transferred providing the mean and variance of Cohen's d. The exact mean in Eq. (2.6) is well approximated by Eq. (2.4) so that an approximately unbiased standardized mean difference g^* is given as

$$g^* = \left(1 - \frac{3}{4N - 9}\right) g. \tag{2.8}$$

Finally, a third measure of θ, known as Glass's Δ (Glass, McGaw, and Smith, 1981), is defined as

$$\Delta = \frac{\bar{X}_1 - \bar{X}_2}{S_2}, \tag{2.9}$$

where the standardized quantity is just S_2, the sample standard deviation based on the control group alone. This is typically justified on the ground that the control group is in existence for a longer period than the experimental group and is likely to provide a more stable estimate of the common variance. Again under the assumption of normality of the data, Hedges (1981) shows that $\sqrt{\tilde{n}}\,\Delta$ follows a noncentral t distribution with noncentrality parameter $\sqrt{\tilde{n}}\,\theta$ and $n_2 - 1$ degrees of freedom.

The variances of the above estimates of θ, in large samples, are given by the following:

$$\sigma^2(d) = \text{Var}(d) \approx \left[\frac{n_1 + n_2}{n_1\, n_2} + \frac{\theta^2}{2\,(n_1 + n_2 - 2)}\right] \left[\frac{n_1 + n_2}{n_1 + n_2 - 2}\right],$$

$$\sigma^2(g) = \text{Var}(g) \approx \frac{n_1 + n_2}{n_1\, n_2} + \frac{\theta^2}{2\,(n_1 + n_2 - 2)},$$

$$\sigma^2(\Delta) = \text{Var}(\Delta) \approx \frac{n_1 + n_2}{n_1\, n_2} + \frac{\theta^2}{2\,(n_2 - 1)}.$$

The estimated variances are then obtained by replacing θ in the above expressions by the respective estimates of θ, namely, d, g, and Δ. These are given below:

$$\hat{\sigma}^2(d) = \widehat{\text{Var}}(d) = \left[\frac{n_1 + n_2}{n_1\, n_2} + \frac{d^2}{2\,(n_1 + n_2 - 2)}\right] \left[\frac{n_1 + n_2}{n_1 + n_2 - 2}\right],$$

$$\hat{\sigma}^2(g) = \widehat{\text{Var}}(g) = \frac{n_1 + n_2}{n_1\, n_2} + \frac{g^2}{2\,(n_1 + n_2 - 2)},$$

$$\hat{\sigma}^2(\Delta) = \widehat{\text{Var}}(\Delta) = \frac{n_1 + n_2}{n_1\, n_2} + \frac{\Delta^2}{2\,(n_2 - 1)}.$$

Large sample tests for $H_0 : \theta = 0$ versus $H_1 : \theta \neq 0$ are typically based on the standardized normal statistics

$$Z = \frac{\hat{\theta}}{\hat{\sigma}(\hat{\theta})}, \tag{2.10}$$

where $\hat{\theta}$ is an estimate of θ defined above with $\hat{\sigma}(\hat{\theta})$ as its estimated standard error and H_0 is rejected if $|Z|$ exceeds $z_{\alpha/2}$, the upper $\alpha/2$ cut-off point of the standard normal distribution. Of course, if the alternative is one-sided, namely, $H_2 : \theta > 0$, then H_0 is rejected if Z exceeds z_α, the upper α cut-off point of the standard normal distribution. Again, if one is interested in constructing confidence intervals for θ, it is evident that, in large samples, the individual confidence intervals are given by

$$1 - \alpha \approx \Pr\left[\hat{\theta} - z_{\alpha/2}\,\hat{\sigma}(\hat{\theta}) \le \theta \le \hat{\theta} + z_{\alpha/2}\,\hat{\sigma}(\hat{\theta})\right]. \tag{2.11}$$

Example 2.1. We use a data set from Hedges and Olkin (1985, p. 17) where a set of seven studies deals with sex differences in cognitive abilities. Originally, studies on sex differences in four cognitive abilities (quantitative, verbal, visual-spatial, and field articulation) were considered. We use only the effect size estimates derived from studies with quantitative ability. The relevant data are basically reproduced in Table 2.1 and include the total sample size (N) of each study, estimates of Hedges's g, and unbiased effect size estimates g^*. For further information about the studies let us refer to Hedges and Olkin (1985).

Table 2.1   Studies of gender difference in quantitative ability

Study	Total sample size (N)	Standardized mean difference (g)	Unbiased standardized mean difference (g^*)	95% CI on θ
1	76	0.72	0.71	$[\ 0.256, 1.184]$
2	6, 167	0.06	0.06	$[\ 0.010, 0.110]$
3	355	0.59	0.59	$[\ 0.377, 0.803]$
4	1, 050	0.43	0.43	$[\ 0.308, 0.552]$
5	136	0.27	0.27	$[-0.068, 0.608]$
6	2, 925	0.89	0.89	$[\ 0.814, 0.966]$
7	45, 222	0.35	0.35	$[\ 0.331, 0.369]$

For each study above, we can carry out the test for $H_0 : \theta = 0$ versus $H_1 : \theta \ne 0$ as well as construct a confidence interval for θ based on the above discussion. Thus, for study 1, using the standardized mean difference g (Hedges's g) = 0.72 and assuming $n_1 = n_2 = 38$, we get

$$Z = \frac{g}{\left[\dfrac{n_1 + n_2}{n_1\,n_2} + \dfrac{g^2}{2\,(n_1 + n_2 - 2)}\right]^{1/2}} = \frac{0.72}{0.2369} = 3.039$$

and hence reject H_0 with $\alpha = 0.05$. Moreover, based on Eq. (2.11), the 95% confidence interval (CI) for θ is obtained as $[0.256\ ,\ 1.184]$. It may be noted that the conclusions based on $g^* = 0.71$ are the same. All the 95% confidence intervals for the seven studies are summarized in the last column of Table 2.1.

When the analysis is to be carried out on the original metric, the difference of μ_1 and μ_2, sometimes called the absolute difference between means, is the appropriate measure. The difference between means may be easier to interpret than the dimensionless standardized mean difference. The difference of the sample means, $\bar{X}_1 - \bar{X}_2$, is an unbiased estimator of the parameter of interest in this situation with variance $\sigma_1^2/n_1 + \sigma_2^2/n_2$. By plugging in the sample variances, the estimated variance of $\bar{X}_1 - \bar{X}_2$ is $S_1^2/n_1 + S_2^2/n_2$.

2.2   EFFECT SIZE BASED ON PROPORTIONS

An effect size θ based on proportions is derived as follows. Denote the population proportions of the two groups (experimental and control) by π_1 and π_2. One measure θ_1 of the effect size θ is then given by

$$\theta_1 = \pi_1 - \pi_2 \tag{2.12}$$

which is simply the difference between the two population proportions.

A second measure θ_2 of θ based on Fisher's variance-stabilizing transformation (of a sample proportion) is defined as

$$\theta_2 = \sin^{-1}\sqrt{\pi_1} - \sin^{-1}\sqrt{\pi_2}. \tag{2.13}$$

A third measure θ_3 of θ, commonly known as the rate ratio, also called relative risk or risk ratio, is given by

$$\theta_3 = \frac{\pi_1}{\pi_2}. \tag{2.14}$$

The measures θ_1 and θ_2 are such that the value 0 indicates no difference, while for the measure θ_3, the value 1 indicates no difference. Often $\theta_3^* = \ln \theta_3$, which is the natural logarithm of θ_3, is used so that the same value 0 indicates no difference in all three cases. The above measures of θ can be easily estimated. Suppose a random sample of size n_1 from the first population yields a count of X_1 for the attribute under study while a random sample of size n_2 from the second population yields a count of X_2. Then, if $p_1 = X_1/n_1$ and $p_2 = X_2/n_2$ denote the two sample proportions, estimates of θ are obtained as

$$\begin{aligned}
\hat{\theta}_1 &= p_1 - p_2, \\
\hat{\theta}_2 &= \sin^{-1}\sqrt{p_1} - \sin^{-1}\sqrt{p_2}, \\
\hat{\theta}_3^* &= \ln\frac{p_1}{p_2},
\end{aligned}$$

with the respective variances as

$$\sigma^2(\hat{\theta}_1) = \mathrm{Var}(\hat{\theta}_1) = \frac{\pi_1\,(1-\pi_1)}{n_1} + \frac{\pi_2\,(1-\pi_2)}{n_2},$$

$$\sigma^2(\hat{\theta}_2) = \mathrm{Var}(\hat{\theta}_2) \approx \frac{1}{4\,n_1} + \frac{1}{4\,n_2},$$

$$\sigma^2(\hat{\theta}_3^*) = \mathrm{Var}(\hat{\theta}_3^*) \approx \frac{1-\pi_1}{n_1\,\pi_1} + \frac{1-\pi_2}{n_2\,\pi_2}.$$

As before, large sample tests for $H_0 : \theta = 0$ versus $H_1 : \theta \neq 0$ are typically based on the standardized normal statistics

$$Z = \frac{\hat{\theta}}{\hat{\sigma}(\hat{\theta})}, \tag{2.15}$$

where $\hat{\sigma}(\hat{\theta})$ is the estimated standard error of $\hat{\theta}$ and H_0 is rejected if $|Z|$ exceeds $z_{\alpha/2}$, the upper $\alpha/2$ cut-off point of the standard normal distribution. Of course, if the alternative is one-sided, namely, $H_2 : \theta > 0$, then H_0 is rejected if Z exceeds z_α, the upper α cut-off point of the standard normal distribution. Again, if one is interested in constructing confidence intervals for θ, it is evident that, in large samples, the individual confidence intervals are given by

$$1 - \alpha \approx \Pr\left[\hat{\theta} - z_{\alpha/2}\,\hat{\sigma}(\hat{\theta}) \leq \theta \leq \hat{\theta} + z_{\alpha/2}\,\hat{\sigma}(\hat{\theta})\right]. \tag{2.16}$$

Example 2.2. Consider a comparative study in which the experimental treatment is applied to a random sample of $n_1 = 80$ subjects and the control treatment is applied to a random sample of $n_2 = 70$ subjects. If the unimproved proportions are $p_1 = 0.60$ and $p_2 = 0.80$, the value of $\hat{\theta}_1$ is -0.20 and its estimated standard error is

$$\hat{\sigma}(\hat{\theta}_1) = \left(\frac{0.60 \times 0.40}{80} + \frac{0.80 \times 0.20}{70}\right)^{1/2} = 0.0727.$$

An approximate 95% confidence interval for θ_1 is $\hat{\theta}_1 \pm 1.96 \times \hat{\sigma}(\hat{\theta}_1)$, which turns out to be the interval

$$-0.20 \pm 1.96 \times 0.0727,$$

or the interval from -0.34 to -0.06. Incidentally, since this interval does not contain 0, we reject the null hypothesis $H_0 : \theta_1 = 0$.

For the same data, an estimate of θ_2 is given by $\hat{\theta}_2 = 0.8861 - 1.1071 = -0.2211$ with $\widehat{\text{Var}}(\hat{\theta}_2) = 0.006696$, resulting in $Z = -2.702$. We therefore reject $H_0 : \theta_2 = 0$. A 95% confidence interval for θ_2 is easily obtained as

$$\left[\hat{\theta}_2 - 1.96\,\sigma(\hat{\theta}_2), \hat{\theta}_2 + 1.96\,\sigma(\hat{\theta}_2)\right] = [-0.501, -0.074].$$

Finally, again for the same data, the estimated rate ratio is $\hat{\theta}_3 = 0.60/0.80 = 0.75$, so group 1 is estimated to be at a risk that is 25% less than group 2's risk. To construct a confidence interval for θ_3, one first obtains the value $\hat{\theta}_3^* = \ln \hat{\theta}_3 = -0.2877$ and then obtains the value of its estimated standard error as

$$\hat{\sigma}(\hat{\theta}_3^*) = \left(\frac{0.40}{80 \times 0.60} + \frac{0.20}{70 \times 0.80}\right)^{1/2} = (0.0119)^{1/2} = 0.1091.$$

An approximate 95% confidence interval for θ_3^* has as its lower limit

$$\ln(\theta_{3L}^*) = -0.2877 - 1.96 \times 0.1091 = -0.5015$$

and as its upper limit

$$\ln(\theta^*_{3U}) = -0.2877 + 1.96 \times 0.1091 = -0.0739.$$

The resulting interval for θ_3 extends from $\exp(-0.5015) = 0.61$ to $\exp(-0.0739) = 0.93$.

2.3 EFFECT SIZE BASED ON φ COEFFICIENT AND ODDS RATIO

This section is patterned after Fleiss (1994). Consider a cross-sectional study in which measurements are made on a pair of binary random variables, X and Y, and their association is of primary interest. Examples include studies of attitudes or opinions (agree/disagree), case-control studies in epidemiology (exposed/not exposed), and intervention studies (improved/not improved).

Table 2.2 presents notation for the underlying parameters and Table 2.3 presents notation for the observed frequencies in the 2×2 table cross-classifying subjects' categories on the two variables X and Y, the levels of both labeled as 0 or 1.

Table 2.2   Probabilities associated with two binary characteristics

	Y		
X	Positive	Negative	Total
Positive	Π_{11}	Π_{12}	$\Pi_{1.}$
Negative	Π_{21}	Π_{22}	$\Pi_{2.}$
Total	$\Pi_{.1}$	$\Pi_{.2}$	1

Table 2.3   Observed frequencies on two binary characteristics

	Y		
X	Positive	Negative	Total
Positive	n_{11}	n_{12}	$n_{1.}$
Negative	n_{21}	n_{22}	$n_{2.}$
Total	$n_{.1}$	$n_{.2}$	$n_{..}$

Then one measure of association between X and Y can be described as the product moment correlation coefficient between the two numerically coded variables and is equal to

$$\varphi = \frac{\Pi_{11}\,\Pi_{22} - \Pi_{12}\,\Pi_{21}}{\sqrt{\Pi_{1.}\,\Pi_{2.}\,\Pi_{.1}\,\Pi_{.2}}}. \tag{2.17}$$

Based on the data shown in Table 2.3, the maximum likelihood estimator of φ is equal to

$$\hat{\varphi} = \frac{n_{11}\, n_{22} - n_{12}\, n_{21}}{\sqrt{n_{1.}\, n_{2.}\, n_{.1}\, n_{.2}}}, \tag{2.18}$$

which is closely related to the classical chi-square statistic for testing for association in a fourfold table: $\chi^2 = n_{..}\, \hat{\varphi}^2$. The large sample estimated standard error of $\hat{\varphi}$ is given by (Bishop, Fienberg, and Holland, 1975, pp. 381–382)

$$\hat{\sigma}(\hat{\varphi}) = \frac{1}{\sqrt{n_{..}}} \left[1 - \hat{\varphi}^2 + \hat{\varphi} \left(1 + \frac{\hat{\varphi}^2}{2} \right) \frac{(p_{1.} - p_{2.})(p_{.1} - p_{.2})}{\sqrt{p_{1.}\, p_{.1}\, p_{2.}\, p_{.2}}} \right.$$
$$\left. - \frac{3}{4} \hat{\varphi}^2 \left(\frac{(p_{1.} - p_{2.})^2}{p_{1.}\, p_{2.}} + \frac{(p_{.1} - p_{.2})^2}{p_{.1}\, p_{.2}} \right) \right]^{1/2}. \tag{2.19}$$

A second measure of the association between X and Y is provided by the odds ratio (sometimes referred to as the cross-product ratio) defined as

$$\omega = \frac{\Pi_{11}\, \Pi_{22}}{\Pi_{12}\, \Pi_{21}}. \tag{2.20}$$

If the observed multinomial frequencies are as displayed in Table 2.3, the maximum likelihood estimator of ω is

$$\hat{\omega} = \frac{n_{11}\, n_{22}}{n_{12}\, n_{21}}. \tag{2.21}$$

The motivation for using ω as a measure of association between two binary variables stems from the following observation. Suppose that the study calls for $n_{1.}$ units to be sampled from the population which are positive on X and for $n_{2.}$ units to be sampled from the population which are negative on X. Then $\Pi_{11}/\Pi_{1.}$ represents the conditional probability that Y is positive given that X is positive, namely, $\Pr(Y+ \mid X+)$, and hence the odds for Y being positive, conditional on X being positive, is equal to

$$
\begin{aligned}
\text{odds}(Y+\mid X+) &= \frac{\Pr(Y+\mid X+)}{\Pr(Y-\mid X+)} \\
&= \frac{\Pi_{11}/\Pi_{1.}}{\Pi_{12}/\Pi_{1.}} = \frac{\Pi_{11}}{\Pi_{12}}.
\end{aligned}
$$

Analogously, the odds for Y being positive, conditional on X being negative, is equal to

$$
\begin{aligned}
\text{odds}(Y+\mid X-) &= \frac{\Pr(Y+\mid X-)}{\Pr(Y-\mid X-)} \\
&= \frac{\Pi_{21}/\Pi_{2.}}{\Pi_{22}/\Pi_{2.}} = \frac{\Pi_{21}}{\Pi_{22}}.
\end{aligned}
$$

The odds ratio w is simply defined as the ratio of these two odds values, leading to

$$w = \frac{\text{odds}(Y+|X+)}{\text{odds}(Y+|X-)} = \frac{\Pi_{11}/\Pi_{12}}{\Pi_{21}/\Pi_{22}} = \frac{\Pi_{11}\,\Pi_{22}}{\Pi_{12}\,\Pi_{21}}. \tag{2.22}$$

A value of 1 for w represents no association between X and Y while values more than 1 (less than 1) mean positive (negative) association. In practice, it is customary to use $w^* = \ln w$, the natural logarithm of the odds ratio, and its sample analogue $\hat{w}^* = \ln \hat{w}$, rather than the odds ratio directly. The large sample standard error of $\hat{w}^*$ (Woolf, 1955) is given by the equation

$$\hat{\sigma}(\hat{w}^*) = \left(\frac{1}{n_{11}} + \frac{1}{n_{12}} + \frac{1}{n_{21}} + \frac{1}{n_{22}} \right)^{1/2} \tag{2.23}$$

which can be readily used to test hypotheses for w and also to construct a confidence interval for w.

Example 2.3. Consider a hypothetical study with the data as shown in Table 2.4.

Table 2.4   Hypothetical frequencies in a fourfold table

X	Y		Total
	Positive	Negative	
Positive	135	15	150
Negative	40	10	50
Total	175	25	200

The value of $\hat{\varphi}$ for the above frequencies is easily computed as

$$\hat{\varphi} = \frac{135 \times 10 - 15 \times 40}{\sqrt{150 \times 50 \times 175 \times 25}} = 0.130931,$$

which represents a modest association. Its estimated standard error, based on formula (2.19), is obtained as

$$\hat{\sigma}(\hat{\varphi}) = \frac{1}{\sqrt{200}}\,(1.245388)^{1/2} = 0.079.$$

Similarly, we compute $\hat{w} = 2.25$ and hence $\hat{w}^* = \ln \hat{w} = 0.811$ with $\hat{\sigma}(w^*) = 0.4462$.

We can test the null hypothesis of no association, that is, $H_0 : \varphi = 0$ versus $H_1 : \varphi \neq 0$ based on

$$Z = \frac{\hat{\varphi}}{\hat{\sigma}(\hat{\varphi})} = 1.66$$

which leads to acceptance of H_0 with $\alpha = 0.05$. Also, a 95% confidence interval for φ is obtained as

$$\text{LB} = \hat{\varphi} - 1.96\,\hat{\sigma}(\hat{\varphi}) = -0.024, \quad \text{UB} = \hat{\varphi} + 1.96\,\hat{\sigma}(\hat{\varphi}) = 0.286.$$

Likewise, we can also test the null hypothesis of no association, that is, $H_0 : \omega^* = 0$ versus $H_1 : \omega^* \neq 0$ based on

$$Z = \frac{\hat{\omega}^*}{\hat{\sigma}(\hat{\omega}^*)} = 1.82$$

which leads to acceptance of H_0 with $\alpha = 0.05$. Also, a 95% confidence interval for ω^* is obtained as

$$\text{LB} = \hat{\omega}^* - 1.96\,\hat{\sigma}(\hat{\omega}^*) = -0.063, \quad \text{UB} = \hat{\omega}^* + 1.96\,\hat{\sigma}(\hat{\omega}^*) = 1.685$$

which yields $[0.939, 5.395]$ as the confidence interval for ω.

2.4 EFFECT SIZE BASED ON CORRELATION

Finally, an effect size based on correlation is directly taken as the value of the correlation ρ itself, or its well known ζ-value, based on Fisher's variance-stabilizing transformation (of r), given by

$$\zeta = \frac{1}{2}\left[\ln \frac{1+\rho}{1-\rho}\right]. \tag{2.24}$$

These measures are readily estimated by the sample correlation r (for ρ) or its transformed version z (for ζ) given by

$$z = \frac{1}{2}\left[\ln \frac{1+r}{1-r}\right] \tag{2.25}$$

with respective approximate variances as (see Rao, 1973)

$$\text{Var}(r) \approx \frac{(1-\rho^2)^2}{n-1},$$

$$\text{Var}(z) \approx \frac{1}{n-3}.$$

Large sample tests for $H_0 : \rho = 0$ versus $H_1 : \rho \neq 0$ are typically based on the standardized normal statistics

$$Z_1 = \frac{r\sqrt{n-1}}{1-r^2},$$

$$Z_2 = z\sqrt{n-3}$$

and H_0 is rejected if $|Z_1|$ (or $|Z_2|$) exceeds $z_{\alpha/2}$, the upper $\alpha/2$ cut-off point of the standard normal distribution. Of course, if the alternative is one-sided, namely, $H_2 : \rho > 0$, then H_0 is rejected if Z_1 or Z_2 exceeds z_α, the upper α cut-off point of the standard normal distribution. Again, if one is interested in constructing confidence

Table 2.5   Studies of the relationship between an observation measure
of teacher indirectness and student achievement

Study	No. of teachers	Correlation coefficient r	95% CI on ρ	95 % CI on ζ	95 % CI on ρ (retransformed)
1	15	-0.073	$[-0.594, 0.448]$	$[-0.639, 0.493]$	$[-0.564, 0.456]$
2	16	0.308	$[-0.150, 0.766]$	$[-0.225, 0.862]$	$[-0.222, 0.697]$
3	15	0.481	$[\ \ 0.078, 0.884]$	$[-0.042, 1.090]$	$[-0.041, 0.797]$
4	16	0.428	$[\ \ 0.015, 0.841]$	$[-0.086, 1.001]$	$[-0.086, 0.762]$
5	15	0.180	$[-0.327, 0.687]$	$[-0.384, 0.748]$	$[-0.366, 0.634]$
6	17	0.290	$[-0.159, 0.739]$	$[-0.225, 0.822]$	$[-0.222, 0.676]$
7	15	0.400	$[-0.040, 0.840]$	$[-0.142, 0.989]$	$[-0.141, 0.757]$

intervals for ρ, it is evident that, in large samples, the individual confidence intervals
based on r for ρ and z for ζ are given by

$$1 - \alpha \quad \approx \quad \Pr\left[r - \frac{z_{\alpha/2}\,(1 - r^2)}{\sqrt{n-1}} \leq \rho \leq r + \frac{z_{\alpha/2}\,(1 - r^2)}{\sqrt{n-1}} \right], \quad (2.26)$$

$$1 - \alpha \quad \approx \quad \Pr\left[z - \frac{z_{\alpha/2}}{\sqrt{n-3}} \leq \zeta \leq z + \frac{z_{\alpha/2}}{\sqrt{n-3}} \right]. \quad (2.27)$$

Clearly, the second equation above can be used to provide a confidence interval for ρ
using the relation between ρ and ζ.

Example 2.4. Let us consider the data set from Hedges and Olkin (1985, p. 25),
which is reproduced in the second and third columns of Table 2.5. Several studies
reported correlations between an observational measure of teacher indirectness and
student achievement. In these data the sample size is the number of teachers. The
correlation coefficient reflects the relationship between a score on teacher indirectness
from an observational measure and mean class achievement.

For the first study, we can test $H_0 : \rho = 0$ versus $H_1 : \rho \neq 0$ based on both Z_1
and Z_2. A direct computation gives

$$Z_1 = -0.275, \quad z = -0.073, \quad Z_2 = -0.253.$$

Taking $\alpha = 0.05$, which means $z_{\alpha/2} = 1.96$, we accept H_0. To construct a confidence
interval for ρ with confidence level 0.95, we can use Eq. (2.26) or (2.27). The first
equation gives $[-0.594, 0.448]$ as the confidence interval for ρ. On the other hand,
the second equation yields $[-0.639, 0.493]$ as the confidence interval for ζ. Using
Eq. (2.24), we convert this to the interval for ρ as $[-0.564, 0.456]$. A similar analysis
can be carried out for all the other studies. The results are given in Table 2.5.

CHAPTER 3

COMBINING INDEPENDENT TESTS

3.1 INTRODUCTION

Methodology for combining findings from repeated research studies did in fact begin with the idea of combining independent tests back in the 1930s (Tippett, 1931; Fisher, 1932; Pearson, 1933). Here we provide a comprehensive review of the so-called omnibus or nonparametric statistical methods for testing the significance of combined results. The presentation here is quite routine and standard, and the methods discussed here appear in other textbooks as well. The main results do not depend on the form of the underlying distribution, except for the assumption that the relevant test statistics follow continuous distributions. It should be noted that all the measures of effect size discussed in Chapter 2 behave normally in large samples, implying thereby that this crucial assumption is indeed satisfied when the sample size is large.

All the methods of combining tests depend on what is popularly known as a P-value. A key point is that the observed P-values derived from continuous test statistics follow a uniform distribution under the null hypothesis regardless of the form of the test statistic, the underlying testing problem, and the nature of the parent population from which samples are drawn. This is indeed a robust result. Quite generally, suppose $X_1, \ldots, X_n$ is a random sample from a certain population indexed by the

Statistical Meta-Analysis with Applications. By Joachim Hartung, Guido Knapp, Bimal K. Sinha
Copyright © 2008 John Wiley & Sons, Inc.

parameter θ and $T(X_1, \ldots, X_n)$ is a test statistic for testing $H_0 : \theta = \theta_0$ against $H_1 : \theta > \theta_0$, where θ_0 is a null value, and suppose also that H_0 is rejected for large values of $T(x_1, \ldots, x_n)$. Then if the (continuous) null distribution of $T(X_1, \ldots, X_n)$ is denoted by $g(t)$, the P-value based on $T(X_1, \ldots, X_n)$ is defined as

$$P = \int_{T(x_1,\ldots,x_n)}^{\infty} g(t) \, dt = \Pr[T(X_1, \ldots, X_n) > T(x_1, \ldots, x_n)|H_0], \qquad (3.1)$$

which stands for the probability of observing as extreme a value of $T(X_1, \ldots, X_n)$ as the observed one $T(x_1, \ldots, x_n)$ under the null hypothesis. Here $x_1, \ldots, x_n$ denote the observed realizations of the X_i's. Since the null hypothesis H_0 is rejected for large values of $T(x_1, \ldots, x_n)$, this is equivalent to rejecting H_0 for small values of P.

In most meta-analysis applications, the P-values are computed from the approximate normal distribution of the relevant test statistics. Thus, if $T(X_1, \ldots, X_n)$ is approximately normally distributed with mean $\mu(\theta)$ and variance $\sigma^2(\theta, n)$, the P-value is computed as

$$
\begin{aligned}
P &= \Pr[T(X_1, \ldots, X_n) > T(x_1, \ldots, x_n)|H_0] \\
&= \Pr\left[N(0, 1) > \frac{T(x_1, \ldots, x_n) - \mu(\theta_0)}{\sigma(\theta_0, n)}\right]. \qquad (3.2)
\end{aligned}
$$

In cases where the alternative hypothesis is both-sided, namely, $H_2 : \theta \neq \theta_0$, we consider the test based on

$$\chi_1 = \frac{|T(X_1, \ldots, X_n) - \mu(\theta_0)|}{\sigma(\theta_0, n)}, \qquad (3.3)$$

which follows a chi distribution with 1 degree of freedom (df) under the null hypothesis. The P-value is then computed as

$$P = \Pr\left[\chi_1 > \frac{|T(x_1, \ldots, x_n) - \mu(\theta_0)|}{\sigma(\theta_0, n)}\right]. \qquad (3.4)$$

Alternatively, we can also consider the test based on

$$\chi_1^2 = \left[\frac{|T(X_1, \ldots, X_n) - \mu(\theta_0)|}{\sigma(\theta_0, n)}\right]^2, \qquad (3.5)$$

which follows a chi-square distribution with 1 df under H_0, and the P-value is then computed as

$$P = \Pr\left[\chi_1^2 > \left\{\frac{|T(x_1, \ldots, x_n) - \mu(\theta_0)|}{\sigma(\theta_0, n)}\right\}^2\right]. \qquad (3.6)$$

Obviously, Eqs. (3.4) and (3.6) provide equivalent formulations, and in any event, H_0 is always rejected for small values of P.

The general principle of combining test statistics is as follows: Consider k different studies in which test problems H_{0i} versus H_{1i} are considered, $i = 1, \ldots, k$. A combined test procedure tests the global null hypothesis

$$H_0 : \text{ All } H_{0i} \text{ true}, \ i = 1, \ldots, k,$$

versus the alternative

$$H_1 : \text{ Some of the } H_{1i} \text{ true}.$$

The problem of selecting a test for H_0 is complicated by the fact that there are many different ways in which the omnibus null hypothesis H_0 can be false.

Two general properties a combined test procedure should fulfill are admissibility and monotonicity:

- A combined test procedure is said to be admissible if it provides a (not necessarily the only) most powerful test against some alternative hypothesis for combining some collection of tests.

- A combined test procedure is said to be monotone if the combined test procedure rejects the null hypothesis H_0 for one set of P-values and it must also reject the hypothesis for any set of componentwise smaller P-values.

Birnbaum (1954) showed that every monotone combined test procedure is admissible and therefore optimal for some testing situation.

3.2 DESCRIPTION OF COMBINED TESTS

We are now ready to describe the methods for summarizing significance values based on repeated tests. The basic scenario is that we have carried out independent tests for the same effect size parameter θ and of course for the same null hypothesis H_0 against a given alternative (either one-sided like H_1 or both-sided like H_2) on a number of occasions, say k, resulting in the P-values $P_1, \ldots, P_k$. Note that these P-values are usually computed on the basis of Eq. (3.2) or (3.4) or (3.6), depending on the nature of the alternative hypothesis (one-sided or both-sided). It is quite possible that some of these tests lead to the nonrejection of H_0 while others lead to its rejection when the tests are carried out independently and separately at a given level of significance. What we are interested in is a combined test of H_0 at an overall level of significance α.

There are two broad classes of combined tests based on the P-values: one based on uniform distribution methods and the other based on probability transformation methods. There are three main combined tests under the former case, namely, Tippett's method, Wilkinson's method, and the one based on the mean of the P_i's. Likewise, there are four main combined tests under the latter case, namely, Stouffer's method (also known as inverse normal method), a modified (weighted) Stouffer's method, Fisher's method, and the logit method. All these methods are described below with examples. Each of the methods described below satisfies the monotonicity principle and is therefore optimal for some testing situation. For details on the other summaries, see Becker (1994), Hedges and Olkin (1985), and Rosenthal (1978).

Minimum P Method. Tippett's (1931) minimum P test rejects the null hypothesis H_0 if any of the k P-values is less than α^*, where $\alpha^* = 1 - (1 - \alpha)^{1/k}$. In other words, we reject H_0 if

$$\min(P_1, \ldots, P_k) = P_{[1]} < \alpha^* = 1 - (1 - \alpha)^{1/k}. \tag{3.7}$$

The rejection region for this test is thus explicitly defined as the union of the rejection regions from all k separate studies. This method is a special case of Wilkinson's (1951) method.

Example 3.1. Consider the following set of probabilities, which are ordered as 0.015, 0.077, 0.025, 0.045, 0.079. The minimum P-value is $P_{[1]} = 0.015$. If we desire an error rate of $\alpha = 0.05$ for the combined significance test, we reject H_0 if $P_{[1]}$ is less than $\alpha^* = 1 - (1 - 0.05)^{1/5} = 1 - 0.9898 = 0.0102$. Since $P_{[1]} = 0.015 > \alpha^* = 0.0102$, the minimum P test fails to reject H_0 for this set of data.

Wilkinson's method. This method, due to Wilkinson (1951), rejects H_0 if the rth smallest P-value, $P_{[r]}$, is small, that is, less than some c for some fixed r. Since under H_0, $P_{[r]}$ follows a beta distribution with the parameters r and $k - r + 1$, it is easy to determine the cut-off point c for this test from the following equation:

$$\alpha = \int_0^c \frac{u^{r-1}(1 - u)^{k-r}}{B(r, k - r + 1)} \, du, \tag{3.8}$$

where $B(\cdot)$ is the usual beta function.

Example 3.2. Consider the same set of probabilities as in Example 3.1, namely, 0.015, 0.077, 0.025, 0.045, 0.079. Taking $r = 2$, a direct computation shows $c = 0.077$. Since $P_{[2]} = 0.025$, we reject H_0. Similarly, we can get $c = 0.1892$ for $r = 3$ and $c = 0.3425$ for $r = 4$, and since $P_{[3]} = 0.045$ and $P_{[4]} = 0.077$, we reject H_0 in all these cases.

Test based on mean of P_i's. Another test based on the mean of the P_i-values is also possible, and the test rejects H_0 when the mean is small. However, the null distribution of the mean is not simple for small values of k, and so this test is rarely used. On the other hand, for a large value of k, one can use the central limit theorem to approximate the distribution of the mean of P_i's by a suitable normal distribution.

Stouffer's method. This method, due to Stouffer and his colleagues (1949), also known as the inverse normal method, is widely used in the social sciences and is highly recommended in this context (Mosteller and Bush, 1954). It is based on the fact that the z-value based on the P-value, defined as

$$z = \Phi^{-1}(P), \tag{3.9}$$

is a standard normal variable under the null hypothesis H_0, where $\Phi(\cdot)$ is the standard normal cumulative distribution function (cdf). Thus, when the P-values $P_1, \ldots, P_k$ are converted to the z-values $z_1, \ldots, z_k$, we have iid standard normal variables under H_0. The combined significance test is essentially based on the sum of these z-values, which has a normal distribution under the null hypothesis with mean 0 and variance k. The test statistic

$$Z = \sum_{i=1}^{k} \frac{z(P_i)}{\sqrt{k}} \qquad (3.10)$$

is thus a standard normal variable under H_0 and hence can be compared with the critical values in the standard normal table. Since small P-values correspond to small (in fact, negative) z-values, the combined test rejects H_0 when Z is less than $-z_\alpha$, or, equivalently, $|Z| > z_\alpha$.

Some authors suggest to compute the z scores from the P-values by using the formula

$$z = \Phi^{-1}(1 - P). \qquad (3.11)$$

If this is done, the resulting z-value, say Z^*, will be large for small values of P, implying thereby that H_0 is rejected when Z^* is large.

Example 3.3. We can compute the value of the sum-of-z's test for our small data set given above in Example 3.1. First, we obtain the standard normal deviates for the five P-values, namely,

$$z(0.015) = -2.1701, \quad z(0.077) = -1.4257, \quad z(0.025) = -1.9601,$$

$$z(0.045) = -1.6961, \quad z(0.079) = -1.4257.$$

The z-values are summed, giving $z(P_i) = -8.6637$. The sum is divided by the square root of $k = 5$, leading to the normal test statistic $Z = -3.8745$. The absolute value $|Z|$ is compared with the critical value z_α for a one-tailed test at $\alpha = 0.05$, which is 1.645. Thus, the sum-of-z's test also rejects H_0 for this data set.

Fisher's method. This method, which is a special case of the inverse chi-square transform, was described by Fisher (1932), and is widely used in meta-analysis. The method is based on the fact that the variable $-2 \ln P$ is distributed as a chi-square variable with 2 degrees of freedom under the null hypothesis whenever P has a uniform distribution. The sum of k of these values is therefore a chi-square variable with $2k$ degrees of freedom under H_0. The test thus rejects H_0 when $-2 \sum_{i=1}^{k} \ln P_i$ exceeds the $100(1 - \alpha)\%$ critical value of the chi-square distribution with $2k$ degrees of freedom.

Example 3.4. We compute the sum-of-logs statistic for the sample data set given above. First, we compute the natural logarithm of each P-value:

$$\ln(0.015) = -4.1997, \quad \ln(0.077) = -2.5639, \quad \ln(0.025) = -3.6888,$$

$$\ln(0.045) = -3.1011, \quad \ln(0.079) = -2.5383.$$

These values are summed and multiplied by -2. The value of the test statistic is $-2 \times (-16.0919) = 32.1839$. We compare this value with $\alpha = 0.05$ upper-tail critical value, which is 18.307 for the chi-square distribution with 10 degrees of freedom. Therefore, we reject H_0 using Fisher's procedure. This test suggests that at least one population has a parameter θ that is nonzero.

Logit Method. George (1977) proposed this method using the statistic

$$G = -\sum_{i=1}^{k} \ln \left[\frac{P_i}{1 - P_i} \right] \left[\frac{k\pi^2(5k + 2)}{3(5k + 4)} \right]^{-1/2} \tag{3.12}$$

as another combined significance technique. The argument is that the logit, that is, $\ln[P/(1 - P)]$, is distributed as a logistic variable under H_0 and further that the distribution of the sum of the logits, suitably normalized, is close to the t distribution. There are usually two approximations of the null distribution of G which can be used. First, we can approximate the null distribution of G with the t distribution based on $5k + 4$ degrees of freedom. The test based on this approximation rejects H_0 if G exceeds the $100(1 - \alpha)\%$ critical value of the t distribution with $5k + 4$ degrees of freedom. Another approximation is based on the observation that, under H_0, $\ln[P_i/(1 - P_i)]$ could be viewed as approximately normal with a zero mean and variance of $\pi^2/3$. The test based on this approximation therefore rejects H_0 when

$$G^* = -\sum_{i=1}^{k} \ln \left(\frac{P_i}{1 - P_i} \right) \left(\frac{3}{k\pi^2} \right)^{1/2} \tag{3.13}$$

exceeds z_α.

Example 3.5. We apply the logit test for the same data set as above. We first compute the natural logarithm of $P/(1 - P)$ for each P-value. The values are

$$\ln(0.015/0.985) = -4.1846, \quad \ln(0.077/0.923) = -2.4838,$$

$$\ln(0.025/0.075) = -3.6636, \quad \ln(0.045/0.955) = -3.0550,$$

$$\ln(0.079/0.921) = -2.4560.$$

These values are summed, which gives $\sum_{i=1}^{5} \ln[P_i/(1 - P_i)] = -15.843$. The sum is multiplied by $-[5\pi^2(27)/(3 \times 29)]^{-1/2}$ or -0.2555. The resultant test statistic is 4.048, which is compared with the $100(1 - \alpha)$ percentile point of the t distribution with 29 degrees of freedom. The critical value being 1.699 for $\alpha = 0.05$, we reject H_0 on the basis of the logit method.

We now provide one example of practical applications of combinations of P-values.

Example 3.6. We refer to the data set in Section 18.6, which is reproduced in Table 3.1. Given the estimated relative risks (here: odds ratios) and the corresponding 95% confidence intervals, the one-sided P-values in Table 3.1 are calculated as follows:

taking the natural logarithm of the upper and lower bound of the confidence interval, the standard error of the estimate is the length of the transformed confidence interval divided by 3.92. According to large-sample theory, the estimate divided by the standard error is standard normally distributed under the null hypothesis of no difference between the groups. Thus, $P = 1 - \Phi\left[\hat{\theta}/\hat{\sigma}(\theta)\right]$ because large values of the estimate are in favor of the alternative.

Table 3.1   Studies on second-hand smoking

Study	Estimated relative risk	95% CI	P	Study	Estimated relative risk	95% CI	P
1	1.52	$[0.88, 2.63]$	0.0669	11	0.79	$[0.25, 2.45]$	0.6572
2	1.52	$[0.39, 5.99]$	0.2740	12	1.55	$[0.90, 2.67]$	0.0571
3	0.81	$[0.34, 1.90]$	0.6844	13	1.65	$[1.16, 2.35]$	0.0027
4	0.75	$[0.43, 1.30]$	0.8460	14	2.01	$[1.09, 3.71]$	0.0127
5	2.07	$[0.82, 5.25]$	0.0623	15	1.03	$[0.41, 2.55]$	0.4747
6	1.19	$[0.82, 1.73]$	0.1805	16	1.28	$[0.76, 2.15]$	0.1760
7	1.31	$[0.87, 1.98]$	0.0990	17	1.26	$[0.57, 2.82]$	0.2855
8	2.16	$[1.08, 4.29]$	0.0143	18	2.13	$[1.19, 3.83]$	0.0056
9	2.34	$[0.81, 6.75]$	0.0580	19	1.41	$[0.54, 3.67]$	0.2411
10	2.55	$[0.74, 8.78]$	0.0690				

Table 3.2 shows the transformed P-values according to Fisher's method, inverse normal method, and logit method.

The smallest P-value is 0.0027 from study 13, and the critical value is also 0.0027 with $\alpha = 0.05$ in the minimum P method. Based on the accuracy of the reported confidence intervals in this example, we cannot reject H_0.

The value of the test statistic in Fisher's method is 90.0237, and we reject H_0 as 53.3835 is the critical value from a chi-square distribution with 38 degrees of freedom.

The absolute value of the test statistic in Stouffer's method, $|Z| = 20.57/\sqrt{(19)} = 4.7191$, exceeds the critical value 1.645. Thus, the sum-of-z's test rejects H_0 at $\alpha = 0.05$.

The sum of the logit values is -38.4852. This sum is multiplied by -0.1278 and the resultant test statistic is 4.9184. The critical value being 1.6604, we reject H_0 on the basis of the logit method.

There is no general recommendation for the choice of the combination method. All the combination methods are optimal for some testing situations. Hedges and Olkin (1985) summarize some results on the performance of the various combination methods given above in Table 3.3 considering such criteria as admissibility, monotonicity, and Bahadur efficiency. They conclude that Fisher's test is perhaps the best one to use if there is no indication of particular alternatives. For more details, we refer to Hedges and Olkin (1985). Marden (1991) introduced the notions of sensitivity and sturdiness to compare the performance of combination test procedures.   Based on five combination methods, namely minimum P, maximum P (Wilkinson's test with

Table 3.2   Transformed P-values of studies on second-hand smoking

Study	P	$-2\ln(P)$	$z(P)$	$\ln[P/(1-P)]$
1	0.0669	5.4088	−1.4992	−2.6351
2	0.2740	2.5895	−0.6009	−0.9746
3	0.6844	0.7584	0.4801	0.7741
4	0.8460	0.3345	1.0193	1.7034
5	0.0623	5.5529	−1.5361	−2.7121
6	0.1805	3.4238	−0.9134	−1.5128
7	0.0990	4.6249	−1.2872	−2.2082
8	0.0143	8.4933	−2.1886	−4.2322
9	0.0580	5.6946	−1.5718	−2.7876
10	0.0690	5.3480	−1.4835	−2.6025
11	0.6572	0.8395	0.4049	0.6509
12	0.0571	5.7268	−1.5798	−2.8046
13	0.0027	11.8190	−2.7805	−5.9068
14	0.0127	8.7273	−2.2343	−4.3508
15	0.4747	1.4900	−0.0634	−0.1012
16	0.1760	3.4741	−0.9306	−1.5434
17	0.2855	2.5071	−0.5666	−0.9174
18	0.0056	10.3659	−2.5357	−5.1773
19	0.2411	2.8452	−0.7028	−1.1467
Sums		90.0237	−20.5700	−38.4852

Table 3.3   Methods for summarizing significance values

Uniform distribution methods	Probability transformation methods
Wilkinson	Sum of z's (Stouffer)
Minimum P	Weighted sum of z's
Mean P	Sum of logs (Fisher)
	Logit

largest P-value), sum of P's, sum of logs, and sum of z's, again Fisher's test turns out to be best.

Draper et al. (1992) pointed out that combining P-values can lead to incorrect conclusions because

- acceptance or rejection can depend more on the choice of the statistic than on the data and

- the information in a highly informative experiment can be masked and thereby largely disregarded.

A P-value itself is not as informative as the estimate and standard error on which it is based. If this more complete summary information about a study is available, it makes good sense to use it and avoid P-values altogether. However, methods that combine P-values have their place when such precise information is unavailable.

An important assumption in the just described combination methods is the independence of the P-values of the various trials. Hartung (1999a) argues that, due to restrictions in randomization in the trials, for instance by the usually nonrandom choice of the positioning of the trials, a possible correlation structure between the study results might be present. Hartung (1999a) presents a method for combining dependent P-values, thereby proposing an extension of the weighted inverse normal method, where the dependence of the results is parameterized by a single correlation coefficient. Instead of the inverse normal method, Makambi (2003) suggests a similar approach using Fisher's inverse chi-square method.

CHAPTER 4

METHODS OF COMBINING EFFECT SIZES

In this chapter we describe the standard methods of combining effect sizes from various independent studies for both point estimation as well as confidence interval estimation. We refer to Hedges and Olkin (1985) and Rosenthal (1994) for further reading.

The general principle is the following. Consider k independent studies with the ith study resulting in the estimated effect size T_i, which is an estimate of the population effect size θ_i, and suppose $\hat{\sigma}^2(T_i)$ is the estimated variance of T_i, $i = 1, \ldots, k$. Usually, T_i is based on a random sample of size n_i from the ith population or study, and, in large samples, T_i has an approximate normal distribution with mean θ_i and variance $\sigma^2(T_i) = \sigma^2_{(\theta_i; n_i)}$. In most cases the variance $\sigma^2_{(\theta_i; n_i)}$ indeed depends on θ_i so that it is unknown, and $\hat{\sigma}^2(T_i)$ represents an estimate of $\sigma^2_{(\theta_i; n_i)}$. In some cases, T_i may be stochastically independent of $\hat{\sigma}^2(T_i)$ (see Chapter 7).

We assume that (popularly known as the homogeneity assumption)

$$\theta_1 = \cdots = \theta_k = \theta, \tag{4.1}$$

where θ denotes the common population effect size.

Statistical Meta-Analysis with Applications. By Joachim Hartung, Guido Knapp, Bimal K. Sinha   **35**
Copyright © 2008 John Wiley & Sons, Inc.

This leads to

$$\tilde{\theta} = \frac{\sum_{i=1}^{20} T_i/\hat{\sigma}^2(T_i)}{\sum_{i=1}^{20} 1/\hat{\sigma}^2(T_i)} = 0.3978$$

and

$$\widehat{\mathrm{Var}}(\tilde{\theta}) \approx \left[\sum_{i=1}^{20} \frac{1}{\hat{\sigma}^2(T_i)} \right]^{-1} = 0.00118.$$

Moreover, taking $\alpha = 0.05$, we get

$$\mathrm{LB} \approx \tilde{\theta} - 1.96\sqrt{\widehat{\mathrm{Var}}(\tilde{\theta})} = 0.3305, \quad \mathrm{UB} \approx \tilde{\theta} + 1.96\sqrt{\widehat{\mathrm{Var}}(\tilde{\theta})} = 0.4651.$$

For testing $H_0 : \theta = 0$, we compute $|Z| = 11.58$, which implies we reject H_0 at level 0.05. Finally, the test for homogeneity of the θ_i's is carried out by computing $\chi^2 = 25.65$, which when compared with the table value 30.14 of χ^2 with 19 degrees of freedom leads to acceptance of the assumption (4.1).

Using Fisher's z transformation for this data set, that is,

$$z_i = 0.5 \ln \left(\frac{1 + r_i}{1 - r_i} \right)$$

and recalling that $\widehat{\mathrm{Var}}(z_i) = v_i = 1/(n_i - 3)$, we obtain

$$\sum_{i=1}^{20} \frac{z_i}{v_i} = 201.3513, \quad \sum_{i=1}^{20} \frac{1}{v_i} = 530,$$

and

$$\sum_{i=1}^{20} \frac{z_i^2}{v_i} = 97.4695.$$

This leads to

$$\tilde{\zeta} = \frac{\sum_{i=1}^{20} z_i/v_i}{\sum_{i=1}^{20} 1/v_i} = 0.3799$$

and

$$\widehat{\mathrm{Var}}(\tilde{\zeta}) \approx \left[\sum_{i=1}^{20} \frac{1}{v_i} \right]^{-1} = 0.00189.$$

Moreover, taking $\alpha = 0.05$, we get

$$\mathrm{LB} \approx \tilde{\zeta} - 1.96\sqrt{\widehat{\mathrm{Var}}(\tilde{\zeta})} = 0.2948, \quad \mathrm{UB} \approx \tilde{\zeta} + 1.96\sqrt{\widehat{\mathrm{Var}}(\tilde{\zeta})} = 0.4650.$$

For testing $H_0 : \zeta = 0$, we compute $|Z| = 8.74$, which implies we reject H_0 at level 0.05. Finally, the test for homogeneity of the ζ_i's is carried out by computing $\chi^2 = 20.97$, which when compared with the table value 30.14 of χ^2 with 19 df leads to acceptance of the assumption (4.1). Converting results to the metric of the correlation coefficient we obtain $\tilde{\theta} = 0.3626$ with 95% confidence interval $[0.2865, 0.4342]$.

Table 4.2 Percentage of albumin in plasma protein

Experiment	n_i	Mean	Variance s_i^2	95% CI on mean
A	12	62.3	12.986	[60.0104, 64.5896]
B	15	60.3	7.840	[58.7494, 61.8506]
C	7	59.5	33.433	[54.1524, 64.8476]
D	16	61.5	18.513	[59.2073, 63.7927]

Example 4.2. Here we examine the data reported in Meier (1953) about the percentage of albumin in plasma protein in human subjects. The data set is given in Table 4.2.

For this data set, using the mean as T_i and the variance of T_i as $\hat{\sigma}^2(T_i) = s_i^2/n_i$, we obtain

$$\sum_{i=1}^{4} \frac{T_i}{\hat{\sigma}^2(T_i)} = 238.5492, \quad \sum_{i=1}^{4} \frac{1}{\hat{\sigma}^2(T_i)} = 3.9110,$$

and

$$\sum_{i=1}^{4} \frac{T_i^2}{\hat{\sigma}^2(T_i)} = 14553.47.$$

This leads to

$$\tilde{\theta} = \frac{\sum_{i=1}^{4} T_i/\hat{\sigma}^2(T_i)}{\sum_{i=1}^{4} 1/\hat{\sigma}^2(T_i)} = 60.9949$$

and

$$\widehat{\mathrm{Var}}(\tilde{\theta}) \approx \left[\sum_{i=1}^{4} \frac{1}{\hat{\sigma}^2(T_i)} \right]^{-1} = 0.2557.$$

Moreover, taking $\alpha = 0.05$, we get

$$\mathrm{LB} \approx \tilde{\theta} - 1.96\sqrt{\hat{\sigma}^2(\tilde{\theta})} = 60.0038, \quad \mathrm{UB} \approx \tilde{\theta} + 1.96\sqrt{\hat{\sigma}^2(\tilde{\theta})} = 61.9860.$$

Finally, the test for homogeneity of the θ_i's is carried out by computing $\chi^2 = 3.1862$, which when compared with the table value 7.815 of χ^2 with 3 df leads to acceptance of the assumption (4.1).

Example 4.3. These data are quoted from Eberhardt, Reeve, and Spiegelman (1989) and deal with the problem of estimation of mean selenium in nonfat milk powder by combining the results of four methods. The data are given in Table 4.3.

For this data set, using the mean as T_i and the variance as $\hat{\sigma}^2(T_i) = s_i^2/n_i$, we obtain

$$\sum_{i=1}^{4} \frac{T_i}{\hat{\sigma}^2(T_i)} = 661.9528, \quad \sum_{i=1}^{4} \frac{1}{\hat{\sigma}^2(T_i)} = 6.0396,$$

Table 4.3   Selenium in nonfat milk powder

Methods	n_i	Mean	Variance s_i^2	95% CI on mean
Atomic absorption spectrometry	8	105.0	85.711	$[\ 97.2601, 112.7399]$
Neutron activation:				
1. Instrumental	12	109.75	20.748	$[106.8559, 112.6441]$
2. Radiochemical	14	109.5	2.729	$[108.5462, 110.4538]$
Isotope dilution mass spectrometry	8	113.25	33.640	$[108.4011, 118.0989]$

and

$$\sum_{i=1}^{4} \frac{T_i^2}{\hat{\sigma}^2(T_i)} = 72556.6.$$

This leads to

$$\tilde{\theta} = \frac{\sum_{i=1}^{4} T_i/\hat{\sigma}^2(T_i)}{\sum_{i=1}^{4} 1/\hat{\sigma}^2(T_i)} = 109.6021$$

and

$$\widehat{\mathrm{Var}}(\tilde{\theta}) \approx \left[\sum_{i=1}^{4} \frac{1}{\hat{\sigma}^2(T_i)}\right]^{-1} = 0.1656.$$

Moreover, taking $\alpha = 0.05$, we get

$$\mathrm{LB} \approx \tilde{\theta} - 1.96\sqrt{\hat{\sigma}^2(\tilde{\theta})} = 108.8045, \quad \mathrm{UB} \approx \tilde{\theta} + 1.96\sqrt{\hat{\sigma}^2(\tilde{\theta})} = 110.3996.$$

Finally, the test for homogeneity of the θ_i's is carried out by computing $\chi^2 = 5.2076$, which when compared with the table value 7.815 of χ^2 with 3 df leads to acceptance of the assumption (4.1).

Example 4.4. The results of nine randomized controlled trials comparing SMFP to NaF dentifrices (toothpastes) in the prevention of caries development have been reanalyzed in Abrams and Sanso (1998). Let us consider the difference of means as the parameter of interest. Then, Table 4.4 contains the observed differences of means and corresponding standard errors for the nine studies. More details on this data set can be found in Section 18.3.

For this data set, using the difference of means as T_i and the variance as the squared standard error, we obtain

$$\sum_{i=1}^{9} \frac{T_i}{\hat{\sigma}^2(T_i)} = 33.2037, \quad \sum_{i=1}^{9} \frac{1}{\hat{\sigma}^2(T_i)} = 117.2006,$$

and

$$\sum_{i=1}^{9} \frac{T_i^2}{\hat{\sigma}^2(T_i)} = 14.7873.$$

Table 4.4 Nine randomized trials comparing SMFP to NaF
dentifrices in the prevention of caries development

Study	Difference SMFP − NaF	Standard error
1	0.86	0.5756
2	0.33	0.5610
3	0.47	0.3507
4	0.50	0.2511
5	−0.28	0.5404
6	0.04	0.2751
7	0.80	0.7826
8	0.19	0.1228
9	0.49	0.2784

This leads to

$$\tilde{\theta} = \frac{\sum_{i=1}^{9} T_i/\hat{\sigma}^2(T_i)}{\sum_{i=1}^{9} 1/\hat{\sigma}^2(T_i)} = 0.2833$$

and

$$\widehat{\mathrm{Var}}(\tilde{\theta}) = \left[\sum_{i=1}^{9} \frac{1}{\hat{\sigma}^2(T_i)}\right]^{-1} = 0.0085.$$

Moreover, taking $\alpha = 0.05$, we get

$$\mathrm{LB} = \tilde{\theta} - 1.96\sqrt{\widehat{\mathrm{Var}}(\tilde{\theta})} = 0.1022, \quad \mathrm{UB} = \tilde{\theta} + 1.96\sqrt{\widehat{\mathrm{Var}}(\tilde{\theta})} = 0.4644.$$

Finally, the test for homogeneity of the θ_i's is carried out by computing $\chi^2 = 5.38$, which when compared with the table value 15.51 of χ^2 with 8 df leads to acceptance of the assumption (4.1).

CHAPTER 5

INFERENCE ABOUT A COMMON MEAN OF SEVERAL UNIVARIATE NORMAL POPULATIONS

In this chapter we consider a very special kind of meta-analysis problem, namely, statistical inference about the common mean of several univariate normal populations with unknown and possibly unequal variances, and provide a review of this rich literature.

One of the oldest and interesting problems in statistical meta-analysis is inference about a common mean of several univariate normal populations with unknown and possibly unequal variances. The motivation of this problem comes from a balanced incomplete block design (BIBD) with uncorrelated random block effects and fixed treatment effects. In this set-up, one has two estimates—namely, the intrablock estimate $\hat{\tau}$ and the interblock estimate $\tilde{\tau}$ of the vector τ of treatment contrasts. Under the usual assumption of normality and independence, $\hat{\tau}$ and $\tilde{\tau}$ are independent, following normal distributions with a common mean vector τ but unknown and unequal intrablock and interblock variances (see Montgomery, 1991, pp. 184–186). The problem thus is to derive an estimate of τ on the basis of $\hat{\tau}$ and $\tilde{\tau}$ and also to provide some tests for hypotheses concerning this common vector of treatment contrasts. This, of course, is a multivariate version of the standard univariate common mean problem, which is the subject of discussion of this chapter. The special case of two populations with equal sample sizes is treated with some detail.

Statistical Meta-Analysis with Applications. By Joachim Hartung, Guido Knapp, Bimal K. Sinha
Copyright © 2008 John Wiley & Sons, Inc.

and a standard conditional argument yields

$$
\begin{aligned}
\mathrm{Var}(\hat{\mu}_{\mathrm{GD}}) &= \mathrm{E}\left\{\mathrm{Var}(\hat{\mu}_{\mathrm{GD}}|S_1,\ldots,S_k)\right\} + \mathrm{Var}\left\{\mathrm{E}(\hat{\mu}_{\mathrm{GD}}|S_1,\ldots,S_k)\right\} \\
&= \mathrm{E}\left[\left\{\sum_{i=1}^{k}\frac{n_i\,\sigma_i^2}{S_i^4}\right\} \Big/ \left\{\sum_{i=1}^{k}\frac{n_i}{S_i^2}\right\}^2\right].
\end{aligned} \tag{5.6}
$$

The exact variance expression of $\hat{\mu}_{\mathrm{GD}}$, the expectation in Eq. (5.6), is not easy to get. However, Khatri and Shah (1974) derived this exact variance for $k = 2$ in an infinite series form involving hypergeometric functions. Unfortunately, this infinite series form has little use when one wants to compare $\mathrm{Var}(\hat{\mu}_{\mathrm{GD}})$ against individual sample mean variances $(\sigma_i^2/n_i, 1 \le i \le k)$. For the two-population case $(k = 2)$, Graybill and Deal (1959) were the first to derive necessary and sufficient conditions such that

$$
\mathrm{Var}(\hat{\mu}_{\mathrm{GD}}) \le \frac{\sigma_i^2}{n_i}, \quad 1 \le i \le k \qquad \text{and for all } \sigma_1^2,\ldots,\sigma_k^2. \tag{5.7}
$$

The following result is due to Graybill and Deal (1959).

Proposition 5.1. For $k = 2$, the inequality (5.7) holds if and only if $n_i \ge 11, i = 1, 2$.

The implication of the above result is far reaching. If either n_1 or n_2 is less than 11, then $\hat{\mu}_{\mathrm{GD}}$ does not have a uniformly smaller variance than $\bar{X}_1$ or $\bar{X}_2$, that is, $\bar{X}_1$ or $\bar{X}_2$ can sometimes be better than $\hat{\mu}_{\mathrm{GD}}$ in terms of having smaller variances. This was later extended by Norwood and Hinkelmann (1977) for k populations, which is stated below.

Proposition 5.2. The inequality (5.7) holds if and only if
(a) $n_i \ge 11 \ \forall i$ or
(b) $n_i = 10$ for some i and $n_j \ge 19 \ \forall j \ne i$.

It is possible to generalize Proposition 5.2 further by considering a more general common mean estimator of μ of the form

$$
\hat{\mu}_c = \left\{\sum_{i=1}^{k}\frac{c_i\, n_i}{S_i^2}\bar{X}_i\right\} \Big/ \left\{\sum_{i=1}^{k}\frac{c_i\, n_i}{S_i^2}\right\} \tag{5.8}
$$

where $c = (c_1,\ldots,c_k)'$ is a vector of nonnegative real constants. Obviously $c = (1,\ldots,1)'$ produces the estimator $\hat{\mu}_{\mathrm{GD}}$. The following result, which is an extension of Proposition 5.2, is due to Khatri and Shah (1974) (for $k = 2$) and Shinozaki (1978) (for general k).

Proposition 5.3. The estimator $\hat{\mu}_c$ in Eq. (5.8) has a uniformly smaller variance than each $\bar{X}_i$ if and only if

$$
\text{(a)} \qquad \frac{c_j}{c_i} \le 2\,\frac{(n_i-1)(n_j-5)}{(n_i+1)(n_j-1)} \qquad \forall i \ne j;
$$

$$
\text{(b)} \qquad n_i \ge 8 \qquad \forall i; \qquad \text{and}
$$

$$
\text{(c)} \qquad (n_i-7)(n_j-7) \ge 16 \ \ \forall i \ne j.
$$

Even though the estimators (5.8) are more general than $\hat{\mu}_{GD}$, for all practical purposes $\hat{\mu}_{GD}$ seems to be the most natural choice in this class. This is more obvious when the sample sizes are all equal, that is, when $n_1 = \cdots = n_k = n$ (say), because then Proposition 5.3 implies that $\mathrm{Var}(\hat{\mu}_{GD}) \leq \sigma_i^2/n, 1 \leq i \leq k$, if and only if $n \geq 11$.

A question which arises naturally is: Is it possible to improve over $\bar{X}_i$ ($1 \leq i \leq k$) for smaller sample sizes by using estimators other than $\hat{\mu}_{GD}$? Investigation on unbiased estimators other than $\hat{\mu}_{GD}$ was stimulated by the works of Cohen and Sackrowitz (1974) and Brown and Cohen (1974).

Cohen and Sackrowitz (1974) considered the simple case of $k = 2$ and $n_1 = n_2 = n$. Define $T = S_2^2/S_1^2$ and

$$
\begin{aligned}
G_n(T) &= {}_2F_1\left(1, \frac{3-n}{2}; \frac{n-1}{2}; T\right) && \text{for } 0 \leq T \leq 1; \\
&= \left(\frac{n-3}{n-1}\right) T^{-1} {}_2F_1\left(1, \frac{5-n}{2}; \frac{n+1}{2}; T^{-1}\right) && \text{for } T > 1.
\end{aligned}
$$

$$(5.9)$$

where ${}_2F_1$ is a hypergeometric function.

Proposition 5.4. For $k = 2$ and $n_1 = n_2 = n$, consider the common mean estimator

$$
\hat{\mu}(a_n) = [1 - a_n G_n(T)]\bar{X}_1 + a_n G_n(T)\bar{X}_2, \tag{5.10}
$$

where $a_n = (n-3)^2/[(n+1)(n-1)]$ for n odd and $a_n = (n-4)/(n+2)$ for n even. The estimator $\hat{\mu}(a_n)$ is unbiased and minimax for all $n \geq 5$. Also, the estimator $\hat{\mu}(1)$ (i.e., replace a_n by 1) is better than both $\bar{X}_1$ and $\bar{X}_2$ for $n \geq 10$.

As $n \to \infty$, $G_n(T) \to (1+T)^{-1}$ and $a_n \to 1$. Therefore, the weights given to the sample means in Eq. (5.10) are converging strongly to the optimal weights in the case where the variances are known. Hence, for large values of n, the estimator $\hat{\mu}(a_n)$ is essentially the same as the estimator $\hat{\mu}_{GD}$. Note that $\hat{\mu}(a_n)$ is better than $\bar{X}_1$ for $n \geq 5$, whereas $\hat{\mu}_{GD}$ is not better than either $\bar{X}_1$ or $\bar{X}_2$ for $n < 11$. For $n = 10$, $\hat{\mu}(1)$ has a smaller variance than $\bar{X}_i (i = 1, 2)$ and this is clearly an advantage over $\hat{\mu}_{GD}$. Cohen and Sackrowitz (1974) also provided some other type of unbiased estimators which are better than $\bar{X}_1$ only for $n \geq 5$.

Brown and Cohen (1974) considered the case of unequal sample sizes for $k = 2$ and obtained the following result.

Proposition 5.5. Assume $k = 2$ and $n_1, n_2 \geq 2$. The estimator

$$
\hat{\mu}^a = \bar{X}_1 + a(\bar{X}_2 - \bar{X}_1)\left(\frac{S_1^2}{n_1}\right)\bigg/\left\{\frac{S_1^2}{n_1} + \frac{(n_2-1)S_2^2}{n_2(n_2+2)} + \frac{(\bar{X}_1 - \bar{X}_2)^2}{(n_2+2)}\right\} \tag{5.11}
$$

is unbiased and has a smaller variance than $\bar{X}_1$ provided $n_2 \geq 3$ and $0 < a \leq a(n_1, n_2)$ where $a(n_1, n_2) = 2(n_2 + 2)/[n\, \mathrm{E}\{\max(V^{-1}, V^{-2})\}]$, where V has F distribution with $n_2 + 2$ and $n_1 - 1$ degrees of freedom.

Exact values of $a(n_1, n_2)$ are given in Brown and Cohen (1974) for selected values of (n_1, n_2). It was also shown that when $n_2 = 2$ the estimator $\hat{\mu}^a$ in Eq. (5.11) is not better than $\bar{X}_1$ uniformly for any value of a. Brown and Cohen (1974) also considered a slight variation of the estimator (5.11) of the form

$$\hat{\mu}_a = \bar{X}_1 + a(\bar{X}_2 - \bar{X}_1)\left(\frac{S_1}{n_1}\right) \bigg/ \left\{\frac{S_1}{n_1} + \frac{S_2}{n_2}\right\} \tag{5.12}$$

and showed that $\hat{\mu}_a$ has a smaller variance than $\bar{X}_1$ for $n_1 \geq 2$ and $n_2 \geq 6$ whenever $0 < a < a(n_1, n_2 - 3)$.

Unification of all the results presented above appears in an excellent paper by Bhattacharya (1980).

For the two-population equal-sample-size case, Zacks (1966) considered two quite different classes of estimators. Note that in a decision-theoretic set-up under the loss function $(\hat{\mu} - \mu)^2 / \max(\sigma_1^2, \sigma_2^2)$, the grand mean $\bar{X} = (\bar{X}_1 + \bar{X}_2)/2$ is admissible as well as minimax; a more general result is due to Kubokawa (1990). Zacks (1966) combined $\hat{\mu}_{GD}$ and $\bar{X}$ to generate the following two classes of randomized estimators:

$$\hat{\mu}(\tau_o) = I(T, \tau_o)\bar{X} + \{1 - I(T, \tau_o)\}\,\hat{\mu}_{GD} \tag{5.13}$$

and

$$\tilde{\mu}(\tau_o) = I(T, \tau_o)\bar{X} + J_1(T, \tau_o)\bar{X}_1 + J_2(T, \tau_o)\bar{X}_2 \tag{5.14}$$

where

$$I(T, \tau_o) = \begin{cases} 1 & \text{if } \tau_o^{-1} \leq T \leq \tau_o, \\ 0 & \text{otherwise;} \end{cases}$$

$$J_1(T, \tau_o) = \begin{cases} 1 & \text{if } T > \tau_o^{-1}, \\ 0 & \text{otherwise;} \end{cases}$$

$$J_2(T, \tau_o) = \begin{cases} 1 & \text{if } T < \tau_o^{-1}, \\ 0 & \text{otherwise;} \end{cases}$$

and $\tau_o \in [0, \infty)$ is a known constant. The values of τ_o both in $\hat{\mu}(\tau_o)$ and in $\tilde{\mu}(\tau_o)$ are the critical values of the F tests of significance (to compare the variances), according to which one decides whether to apply the estimators $\bar{X}$, $\hat{\mu}_{GD}$, $\bar{X}_1$, or $\bar{X}_2$. Zacks (1966) provided variance and efficiency expressions of $\hat{\mu}(\tau_o)$ and $\tilde{\mu}(\tau_o)$. Somewhat similar classes of estimators have been considered by Mehta and Gurland (1969), but these estimators have very little practical importance.

5.1.2   Properties of $\hat{\mu}_{GD}$

Earlier we have seen the variance expression of the unbiased estimator $\hat{\mu}_{GD}$, see Eq. (5.6). The exact probability distribution of $\hat{\mu}_{GD}$ is somewhat complicated. However, for $k = 2$ and $n_1 = n_2 = n$, Nair (1980) gave an approximate cdf of $\hat{\mu}_{GD}$. But for general k, if we can find an unbiased estimator $\widehat{\text{Var}}(\hat{\mu}_{GD})$ of $\text{Var}(\hat{\mu}_{GD})$, then the studentized version

$$\frac{\hat{\mu}_{GD} - \mu}{\sqrt{\widehat{\text{Var}}(\hat{\mu}_{GD})}}$$

follows $N(0,1)$ asymptotically (i.e., as $\min_{1 \le i \le k} n_i \to \infty$). This can be used for testing as well as interval estimation of μ at least in large samples.

Finding an unbiased estimator $\widehat{\text{Var}}(\hat{\mu}_{GD})$ of $\text{Var}(\hat{\mu}_{GD})$ is not an easy task. From expression (5.6), it is enough to define real-valued functions $\psi_i = \psi_i(S_1^2, \ldots, S_k^2), 1 \le i \le k$, such that

$$E(\psi_i) = \sigma_i^2 \, E\left[\left\{ S_i^2 \sum_{j=1}^{k} \frac{n_j}{S_j^2} \right\}^{-2} \right]$$

so that an unbiased estimator of $\text{Var}(\hat{\mu}_{GD})$ is obtained as

$$\widehat{\text{Var}}(\hat{\mu}_{GD}) = \sum_{i=1}^{k} n_i \psi_i. \tag{5.15}$$

Making use of Haff's (1979) Wishart identity for the univariate case, Sinha (1985) derived the expression for ψ_i with the form

$$\psi_i = \lim_{m \to \infty} \psi_{i,m}, \quad \text{where}$$

$$\psi_{i,m} = \sum_{l=0}^{m-1} \frac{S_i^{2(l+1)} 2^l (l+1)! A_{(-i)}^l}{(n_i+1)^{[l]}(n_i + A_{(-i)} S_i^2)^{l+2}} \, , \quad m \ge l \tag{5.16}$$

with $A_{(-i)} = \sum_{j \ne i} n_j / S_j^2$ and $(n_i+1)^{[l]} = (n_i+1) \cdots (n_i + 2l - 1)$ for $l \ge 1$; $(n_i+1)^{[l]} = 1$ for $l = 0, i = 1, 2, \ldots, k$. The following result, which approximates $\widehat{\text{Var}}(\hat{\mu}_{GD})$, is due to Sinha (1985).

Proposition 5.6. Let $n = \min_{1 \le i \le k}(n_i)$. Then using $\psi_{i,m}$ as in Eq. (5.16),

$$\left| E\left(\sum_{i=1}^{k} n_i \psi_{i,m} \right) - \text{Var}(\hat{\mu}_{GD}) \right| = O(n^{-(m+1)}).$$

Using the above result, we get $(\hat{\mu}_{GD} - \mu)/\sqrt{\sum_{i=1}^{k} n_i \psi_{i,m}} \sim N(0,1)$ as $n \to \infty$. A first-order approximation to $\widehat{\text{Var}}(\hat{\mu}_{GD})$, say $\widehat{\text{Var}}_{(1)}(\hat{\mu}_{GD})$, is obtained as (by taking $m = 1$)

$$\widehat{\text{Var}}_{(1)}(\hat{\mu}_{GD}) =$$
$$\left(\sum_{i=1}^{k} \frac{n_i}{S_i^2} \right)^{-1} \left[1 + \sum_{i=1}^{k} \frac{4}{n_i+1} \left(\frac{n_i / S_i^2}{\sum_{j=1}^{k} n_j / S_j^2} - \frac{n_i^2 / S_i^4}{\left(\sum_{j=1}^{k} n_j / S_j^2 \right)^2} \right) \right]$$
$$\tag{5.17}$$

which is comparable to the approximation

$$\widehat{\text{Var}}(\hat{\mu}_{\text{GD}}) \approx$$

$$\left(\sum_{i=1}^{k} \frac{n_i}{S_i^2} \right)^{-1} \left[1 + \sum_{i=1}^{k} \frac{4}{n_i - 1} \left(\frac{n_i / S_i^2}{\sum_{j=1}^{k} n_j / S_j^2} - \frac{n_i^2 / S_i^4}{\left(\sum_{j=1}^{k} n_j / S_j^2 \right)^2} \right) \right]$$

$$(5.18)$$

due to Meier (1953). Incidentally, Rukhin (2007) used similar ideas to derive an unbiased estimate of the variance of the characteristic $\bar{X}_i - \hat{\mu}_{\text{GD}}$, known as degree of equivalence of the ith study.

Decision-theoretic estimation of the common mean has been addressed by several authors. Zacks (1966) pointed out for $k = 2$ and $n_1 = n_2$ that, while $\bar{X}_1$ is minimax under the loss function $(\hat{\mu} - \mu)^2 / \sigma_1^2$, a minimax estimator for the loss $(\hat{\mu} - \mu)^2 / \max(\sigma_1^2, \sigma_1^2)$ is not $\bar{X}_1$ but $\bar{X} = (\bar{X}_1 + \bar{X}_2)/2$. Kubokawa (1990) extended this result for general k and showed the minimaxity as well as admissibility of the grand mean $\bar{X} = \sum_{i=1}^{k} \bar{X}_i / k$ under the loss function $(\hat{\mu} - \mu)^2 / (\max_{1 \leq i \leq k} \sigma_i^2)$. Zacks (1970) also derived Bayes and fiducial equivariant estimators for $k = 2$ and gave their variance expressions.

It may be mentioned that, under the standard squared error loss function $(\hat{\mu} - \mu)^2$, the exact admissibility (or otherwise) of $\hat{\mu}_{\text{GD}}$ is still an open problem. Minimax estimation under the loss $(\hat{\mu} - \mu)^2$ is not meaningful since estimators have unbounded risks under this loss.

Sinha and Mouqadem (1982) considered the special case $k = 2$ and $n_1 = n_2 = n$ and obtained some restricted admissibility results for $\hat{\mu}_{\text{GD}}$. Note that $\hat{\mu}_{\text{GD}}$ can be written as (with $k = 2$ and $n_1 = n_2 = n$)

$$\hat{\mu}_{\text{GD}} = \bar{X}_1 + (\bar{X}_2 - \bar{X}_2) \left(\frac{S_1^2}{S_1^2 + S_2^2} \right) \qquad (5.19)$$

which is affine equivariant, that is, equivariant under the group of transformations

$$(\bar{X}_1, \bar{X}_2, S_1^2, S_2^2) \rightarrow (a\bar{X}_1 + b, a\bar{X}_2 + b, a^2 S_1^2, a^2 S_2^2), \ a > 0, \ b \in \mathbb{R}.$$

Let $D = (\bar{X}_2 - \bar{X}_1)$ and define the following four classes of estimators:

$$\mathcal{C}_0 = \left\{ \hat{\mu} \mid \hat{\mu} = \bar{X}_1 + D\phi_0, \ 0 \leq \phi_0(S_2^2/S_1^2) \leq 1 \right\}; \qquad (5.20)$$

$$\mathcal{C}_1 = \left\{ \hat{\mu} \mid \hat{\mu} = \bar{X}_1 + D\phi_1, \ 0 \leq \phi_1(S_1^2, S_2^2) \leq 1 \right\}; \qquad (5.21)$$

$$\mathcal{C}_2 = \left\{ \hat{\mu} \mid \hat{\mu} = \bar{X}_1 + D\phi_2, \ 0 \leq \phi_2(S_1^2/D^2, S_2^2/D^2) \leq 1 \right\}; \qquad (5.22)$$

$$\mathcal{C} = \left\{ \hat{\mu} \mid \hat{\mu} = \bar{X}_1 + D\phi, \ 0 \leq \phi(S_1^2, S_2^2, D^2) \leq 1 \right\}. \qquad (5.23)$$

Clearly, $\mathcal{C}_0 \subset \mathcal{C}_1 \subset \mathcal{C}$ and $\mathcal{C}_0 \subset \mathcal{C}_2 \subset \mathcal{C}$. The classes $\mathcal{C}_0$ and $\mathcal{C}_2$ are equivariant under affine transformations whereas the estimators in $\mathcal{C}_1$ and $\mathcal{C}$ are equivariant under location transformations only. The following result is due to Sinha and Mouqadem (1982).

Proposition 5.7.

(a) The estimator $\hat{\mu}_{\mathrm{GD}}$ is admissible in $\mathcal{C}_0$ and $\mathcal{C}_2$.

(b) The estimator $\hat{\mu}_{\mathrm{GD}}$ is extended admissible in $\mathcal{C}$ for $n \geq 5$, that is, there does not exist any $\hat{\mu}$ such that $\mathrm{E}(\hat{\mu} - \mu)^2 \leq \mathrm{Var}(\hat{\mu}_{\mathrm{GD}}) - \epsilon$ for all σ_1^2, σ_2^2 and for any $\epsilon > 0$.

(c) An estimator of the form

$$\hat{\mu} = \bar{X}_1 + D \left(\frac{S_1^2 + c_1}{S_1^2 + S_2^2 + c_1 + c_2} \right)$$

is admissible in $\mathcal{C}_1$ for any $c_1, c_2 > 0$.

Extended admissibility of $\hat{\mu}_{\mathrm{GD}}$ in $\mathcal{C}$ is a strong indication of the true admissibility of $\hat{\mu}_{\mathrm{GD}}$ in $\mathcal{C}$, although this is still open. Incidentally, any estimator $\hat{\mu} \in \mathcal{C}$ has variance given by

$$\mathrm{Var}(\hat{\mu}) = \frac{\sigma_1^2 \sigma_2^2}{n(\sigma_1^2 + \sigma_2^2)} + \mathrm{E}\left\{ D^2 \left(\phi - \frac{\sigma_1^2}{\sigma_1^2 + \sigma_2^2} \right)^2 \right\}. \tag{5.24}$$

If we impose the condition that D is independent of ϕ, then $\hat{\mu} \in \mathcal{C}$ becomes an unbiased estimator of μ with variance

$$\mathrm{Var}(\hat{\mu}) = \frac{\sigma_1^2 \sigma_2^2}{n(\sigma_1^2 + \sigma_2^2)} + \frac{\sigma_1^2 + \sigma_2^2}{n} \mathrm{E}\left\{ \left(\phi - \frac{\sigma_1^2}{\sigma_1^2 + \sigma_2^2} \right)^2 \right\}. \tag{5.25}$$

Therefore, in this context performance of an unbiased estimator $\hat{\mu} \in \mathcal{C}$ can be judged by the performance of an estimator ϕ of $\sigma_1^2/(\sigma_1^2 + \sigma_2^2)$, which is a rather interesting observation. It is clear from the previous discussion that quite generally we can characterize the unbiased estimators of μ as

$$\hat{\mu}(h_1, h_2) = \bar{X}_1 + D h_1(D) \phi \left[S_1^2, S_2^2, h_2(D) \right] \tag{5.26}$$

where $h_i(D), i = 1, 2$, are any two even functions. Variance of $\hat{\mu}(h_1, h_2)$ is given as

$$\mathrm{Var}[\hat{\mu}(h_1, h_2)] = \frac{\sigma_1^2 \sigma_2^2}{n(\sigma_1^2 + \sigma_2^2)} + \mathrm{E}\left[D^2 \left\{ h_1 \phi - \frac{\sigma_1^2}{\sigma_1^2 + \sigma_2^2} \right\}^2 \right]. \tag{5.27}$$

Even though the admissibility of $\hat{\mu}_{\mathrm{GD}}$ seems a near certainty when there is no a priori information about the population variances, strangely enough this popular estimator becomes inadmissible if we have some prior knowledge about the unknown variances. Consider the simple case of $k = 2$ and $n_1 = n_2 = n$. If it is found out (after data collection) that $\sigma_1^2 \leq \sigma_2^2$ (which can be checked through a suitable hypothesis testing); then one can construct a better estimator of μ as shown by Sinha (1979).

Proposition 5.8. Assume $\sigma_1^2 \leq \sigma_2^2$. For $k = 2$ and $n_1 = n_2 = n$, define

$$\hat{\mu}^* = \bar{X}_1 + (\bar{X}_2 - \bar{X}_1) \min \left\{ \frac{1}{2}, \frac{S_1^2}{S_1^2 + S_2^2} \right\}.$$

Then $\hat{\mu}^*$ is an unbiased estimator of μ and $\mathrm{Var}(\hat{\mu}^*) \leq \mathrm{Var}(\hat{\mu}_{\mathrm{GD}}) \ \forall \sigma_1^2 \leq \sigma_2^2$.

For unequal sample sizes n_1 and n_2 one can have a similar result provided $\sigma_1^2/n_1 \leq \sigma_2^2/n_2$.

5.2   ASYMPTOTIC COMPARISON OF SOME ESTIMATES OF COMMON MEAN FOR $k = 2$ POPULATIONS

In this section we present some recent results due to Mitra and Sinha (2007) on an asymptotic comparison of some selected estimates of the common mean μ for $k = 2$ and $n_1 = n_2 = n$.

Let $\mathcal{C}_u$ be the general class of unbiased estimates of μ, defined as

$$\mathcal{C}_u = \{\hat{\mu}_\phi : \hat{\mu} = \bar{x}_1 + D\phi(s_1^2, s_2^2, D^2)\}$$

where $D = \bar{x}_2 - \bar{x}_1$. Note that $\mathrm{E}[D|D^2] = 0$ (Khuri, Mathew, and Sinha, 1998, Lemma 7.5.3, pp. 194–195), which implies that all estimates of μ in $\mathcal{C}_u$ are unbiased. We also consider a subclass of $\mathcal{C}_u$ defined as

$$\mathcal{C}_0 = \{\hat{\mu}_{\phi_0} : \hat{\mu} = \bar{x}_1 + D\phi_0(s_1^2, s_2^2)\}.$$

Here we assume that both ϕ and ϕ_0 are smooth in the sense that they admit enough order derivatives with respect to their arguments.

Four popular estimates of μ in this context are given below:

$$\hat{\mu}_1 = \left(\frac{1}{s_1^2} + \frac{1}{s_2^2}\right)^{-1} \left(\frac{\bar{x}_1}{s_1^2} + \frac{\bar{x}_2}{s_2^2}\right),$$

$$\hat{\mu}_2 = \bar{x}_1 + D\frac{s_1^2 + D^2}{s_1^2 + s_2^2 + D^2} \quad \text{(Sinha and Mouqadem, 1982)},$$

$$\hat{\mu}_3 = \bar{x}_1 + D\min(0.5, \frac{s_1^2}{s_1^2 + s_2^2}) \quad \text{(Sinha, 1979)},$$

$$\hat{\mu}_4 = \bar{x}_1 + D\frac{s_1}{s_1 + s_2} \quad \text{(Sinha and Mouqadem, 1982)}.$$

Our comparison of the above estimates is essentially based on an expansion of their large-sample variances in n^{-1}. In order for an estimate to be first-order efficient (FOE), we expect the leading term of its variance (i.e., coefficient of n^{-1}) to be equal to the Rao-Cramer lower bound (Rao, 1973), which can be obtained by inverting the associated Fisher information matrix. The coefficient of n^{-2} in the large-sample variance of an unbiased estimate determines the nature of its second-order efficiency (SOE). The following result is established in Mitra and Sinha (2007).

Theorem 5.1. In the class $\mathcal{C}_0$, $\hat{\mu}_1$ is unique FOE. In the extended class $\mathcal{C}_u$, $\hat{\mu}_1$ is FOE (though not unique) and the condition of FOE determines second-order terms in the expansion of $\mathrm{Var}(\hat{\mu}_\phi)$.

As a byproduct of the proof of the above theorem, it is observed in Mitra and Sinha (2007) that the estimate $\hat{\mu}_4$ is not FOE. It is also proved there that the estimate $\hat{\mu}_3$ with $\phi = \min\{0.5, s_1^2/(s_1^2 + s_2^2)\}$, though lacks smoothness, is both FOE and SOE. Thus, its small-sample dominance over the Graybill-Deal estimate, which holds whenever $\sigma_1^2 \leq \sigma_2^2$, is not really true in large samples.

We now discuss the Bayes estimation of the common mean μ under Jeffrey's noninformative prior (Berger, 1980, p. 87), $\pi(\cdot)$, on the parameters $\boldsymbol{\theta} = (\mu, \sigma_1^2, \sigma_2^2)'$. Under this formulation, $\pi(\boldsymbol{\theta})$ is given by $\pi(\boldsymbol{\theta}) = \sqrt{\det I(\boldsymbol{\theta})}$, where $I(\boldsymbol{\theta})$ is the Fisher information matrix.

Note that for a bivariate normal distribution,

$$I(\mu, \sigma_1^2, \sigma_2^2) = \begin{pmatrix} \dfrac{n\,(\sigma_1^2 + \sigma_2^2)}{\sigma_1^2\,\sigma_2^2} & 0 & 0 \\ 0 & \dfrac{n}{2\,\sigma_1^4} & 0 \\ 0 & 0 & \dfrac{n}{2\,\sigma_2^4} \end{pmatrix}.$$

Hence, based on the Fisher information matrix, such a prior is given by

$$p(\mu, \sigma_1^2, \sigma_2^2) \propto \frac{(\sigma_1^2 + \sigma_2^2)^{1/2}}{(\sigma_1^2\,\sigma_2^2)^{3/2}}$$

where $-\infty < \mu < \infty$, σ_1^2, $\sigma_2^2 > 0$.

Combining this prior with the likelihood and writing

$$\mu_0 = \frac{\bar{x}_1/\sigma_1^2 + \bar{x}_2/\sigma_2^2}{1/\sigma_1^2 + 1/\sigma_2^2},$$

the posterior distribution of the parameters $(\mu, \sigma_1^2, \sigma_2^2)$ is given by

$$p(\mu, \sigma_1^2, \sigma_2^2 | \text{data})$$

$$\propto (\sigma_1^2\sigma_2^2)^{-\frac{n+3}{2}} \sqrt{\sigma_1^2 + \sigma_2^2}$$

$$\times \exp\left[-\frac{n(\bar{x}_1 - \mu)^2}{2\sigma_1^2} - \frac{n(\bar{x}_2 - \mu)^2}{2\sigma_2^2} - \frac{(n-1)s_1^2}{2\sigma_1^2} - \frac{(n-1)s_2^2}{2\sigma_2^2} \right]$$

$$= (\sigma_1^2)^{-(n+3)/2}\,(\sigma_2^2)^{-(n+3)/2} \sqrt{\sigma_1^2 + \sigma_2^2}\, \exp\left[-\frac{nD^2}{2(\sigma_1^2 + \sigma_2^2)} \right]$$

$$\times \exp\left[-\frac{n}{2}\Big(\frac{1}{\sigma_1^2} + \frac{1}{\sigma_2^2}\Big)(\mu - \mu_0)^2 \right] \exp\left[-\frac{(n-1)s_1^2}{2\sigma_1^2} - \frac{(n-1)s_2^2}{2\sigma_2^2} \right].$$

The joint posterior of $(\mu, \sigma_1^2, \sigma_2^2)$ can be viewed as:

(i) Conditionally given (σ_1^2, σ_2^2), the posterior of μ is $N\big(\mu_0, \sigma_1^2\sigma_2^2/[n(\sigma_1^2 + \sigma_2^2)]\big)$

(ii) Joint marginal posterior of σ_1^2, σ_2^2 is given by

$$p(\sigma_1^2, \sigma_2^2 | \text{data}) \propto (\sigma_1^2)^{-(n/2+1)}(\sigma_2^2)^{-(n/2+1)}$$

$$\times \exp\left[-\frac{nD^2}{2(\sigma_1^2 + \sigma_2^2)} - \frac{(n-1)s_1^2}{\sigma_1^2} - \frac{(n-1)s_2^2}{\sigma_2^2} \right].$$

As a Bayes estimate of μ, we choose the posterior mean, which is given by

$$
\begin{aligned}
\hat{\mu}_B &= \mathrm{E}(\mu|\,\mathrm{data}) \\
&= \mathrm{E}\left[\mathrm{E}(\mu|\sigma_1^2, \sigma_2^2, \mathrm{data})\right] \\
&= \bar{x}_1\,\mathrm{E}\left[\frac{\theta}{1+\theta}\,\Big|\,\mathrm{data}\right] + \bar{x}_2\,\mathrm{E}\left[\frac{1}{1+\theta}\,\Big|\,\mathrm{data}\right], \quad \text{where } \theta = \frac{\sigma_2^2}{\sigma_1^2}.
\end{aligned}
$$

Hence computation of $\hat{\mu}_B$ boils down to evaluating $\mathrm{E}[1/(1+\theta)|\,\mathrm{data}]$. To compute this term we need to find the posterior density of θ.

Upon making a transformation from $(\sigma_1^2, \sigma_2^2) \mapsto (\sigma_1^2, \theta)$ in (ii), we get the following:

$$
p(\sigma_1^2, \theta) \propto \theta^{-(n/2+1)}(\sigma_1^2)^{-(n+2)} \exp\left[-\frac{nD^2}{1+\theta} - (n-1)s_1^2 - \frac{(n-1)s_2^2}{\theta}\right].
$$

Now integrating the above expression with respect to σ_1^2, we get unnormalized posterior density of θ as

$$
p(\theta|\,\mathrm{data}) \propto \frac{\theta^{n/2}(\theta+1)^{n+1}}{(a\theta^2 + b\theta + c)^{n+1}}
$$

where $\theta > 0$ and $a = (n-1)s_1^2$, $b = (n-1)s_1^2 + (n-1)s_2^2 + nD^2$, $c = (n-1)s_2^2$. This leads to

$$
\mathrm{E}\left[\frac{1}{1+\theta}\,\Big|\,\mathrm{data}\right] = \frac{\displaystyle\int_0^\infty \frac{\theta^{n/2}(\theta+1)^n}{(a\theta^2+b\theta+c)^{n+1}}\,d\theta}{\displaystyle\int_0^\infty \frac{\theta^{n/2}(\theta+1)^{n+1}}{(a\theta^2+b\theta+c)^{n+1}}\,d\theta}
$$

The above integral is computed using the importance sampling method by choosing $g(\theta) = \exp(-\theta)$ (Gelman et al., 2004). It is obvious that the Bayes estimate of μ is unbiased. It is also proved in Mitra and Sinha (2007) that $\hat{\mu}_B$ is both FOE and SOE.

We end this section with a reference to Mitra and Sinha (2007), who reported the results of an extensive simulation study to compare the bias and variance of five unbiased estimates of μ: $\hat{\mu}_1, \hat{\mu}_2, \hat{\mu}_3, \hat{\mu}_4, \hat{\mu}_B$ for $n = 5, 10, 15$ and $\sigma_1^2 = 1$ and $\sigma_2^2 = 0.2(0.2)2$. Without any loss of generality, $\mu = 0$ is chosen for the simulation purpose. These simulation studies reveal that the Graybill-Deal estimate $\hat{\mu}_1$ and the Sinha-Mouqadem estimate $\hat{\mu}_2$ perform similarly and these two are better than the others. However, quite surprisingly, it turns out that the performance of the Bayes estimate is not satisfactory from the point of view of variance.

5.3 CONFIDENCE INTERVALS FOR THE COMMON MEAN

In this section we address the problem of constructing exact and approximate confidence intervals for μ. Our discussion is based on combinations of relevant component t or F statistics and also Fisher's P-values, as discussed in Chapter 3. We also provide a comparison of various methods based on their expected lengths of confidence intervals for μ. It should be noted that tests for μ are not separately discussed here because of the well-known connection between tests and confidence intervals.

The problem of constructing exact and approximate confidence intervals for the common mean μ of several normal populations with unequal and unknown variances arises in various contexts in statistical applications whenever two or more sources are involved with collecting data on the same basic characteristic of interest. We refer to Meier (1953), Eberhardt, Reeve, and Spiegelman (1989), and Skinner (1991) for some applications. However, although a lot of work has been done on point estimation of μ, as mentioned in Section 5.1, much less attention has been given to the problem of providing a meaningful confidence interval for μ. Several papers provide approximate confidence intervals for μ, centered at $\hat{\mu}_{GD}$, which are not quite useful because of the nature of underlying assumptions (see Meier, 1953; Eberhardt, Reeve, and Spiegelman, 1989). In one particular context of interblock analysis of a balanced incomplete block design, similar approximate confidence intervals centered at some combined estimator are known (see Brown and Cohen, 1974).

Our review of the literature given below includes an old work by Fairweather (1972) and a relatively recent work by Jordan and Krishnamoorthy (1996), which are based on inverting weighted linear combinations of Student's t statistics and F statistics, respectively, which are used to test hypotheses about μ. However, determination of the exact cut-off points of these test statistics can be done only numerically, and it seems to us that the full thrust of meta-analysis is not quite accomplished in these procedures. We mention below some exact confidence intervals for μ based on inverting exact tests for μ, which are constructed by combining the relevant P-values in a meaningful way (Yu, Sun, and Sinha, 2002). We also provide a comparison among them on the basis of their expected lengths. An approximate confidence interval for μ based on an unbiased estimator of $\text{Var}(\hat{\mu}_{GD})$ (see Sinha, 1985) is also given. For some related results, we refer to Rukhin (2007).

5.3.1 Approximate confidence intervals

Using the Graybill-Deal estimate and its estimated variance as given in Section 5.1, an approximate $100(1 - \alpha)\%$ confidence interval for μ can be constructed on the basis of a suitable normalization of $\hat{\mu}_{GD}$ and can be expressed as

$$\left[\hat{\mu}_{GD} - z_{\alpha/2} \sqrt{\widehat{\text{Var}}(\hat{\mu}_{GD})}, \ \hat{\mu}_{GD} + z_{\alpha/2} \sqrt{\widehat{\text{Var}}(\hat{\mu}_{GD})} \right],$$

where $z_{\alpha/2}$ is the standard normal upper $\alpha/2$ point. In practice, however, one can only use a first few terms from $\widehat{\text{Var}}(\hat{\mu}_{GD})$, depending on the sample sizes; see Eqs. (5.17) and (5.18). For better accuracy, one can use the fact that (Sinha, 1985) truncation of $\widehat{\text{Var}}(\hat{\mu}_{GD})$ at the $(m-1)$th term results in error not exceeding $n_{\min}^{-(m+1)}$ (see Proposition 5.6).

5.3.2 Exact confidence intervals

We now focus our attention on the construction of exact confidence intervals for μ. Since

$$t_i = \frac{\sqrt{n_i}(\bar{X}_i - \mu)}{S_i} \sim t_{n_i-1} \tag{5.28}$$

or, equivalently,

$$F_i = \frac{n_i(\bar{X}_i - \mu)^2}{S_i^2} \sim F_{1,n_i-1} \tag{5.29}$$

are standard test statistics for testing hypotheses about μ based on the ith sample, suitable linear combinations of $|t_i|$'s or F_i's or other functions thereof can be used as a pivot to construct exact confidence intervals for μ. This is precisely what is accomplished in Fairweather (1972), Cohen and Sackrowitz (1984), and Jordan and Krishnamoorthy (1996).

(a) Confidence interval for μ based on t_i's

Cohen and Sackrowitz (1984) suggested to use $M_t = \max_{1 \le i \le k}\{|t_i|\}$ as a test statistic for testing hypotheses about μ. We can use M_t to construct a confidence interval for μ once the cut-off point of the distribution of M_t is known, which is independent of any parameter. Thus, if $c_{\alpha/2}$ satisfies the condition

$$
\begin{aligned}
1 - \alpha &= \Pr[M_t \le c_{\alpha/2}] \\
&= \prod_{i=1}^{k} \Pr[|t_i| \le c_{\alpha/2}],
\end{aligned} \tag{5.30}
$$

an exact confidence interval for μ with confidence level $1 - \alpha$ is given by

$$\left[\max_{1 \le i \le k}\left\{ \bar{X}_i - \frac{c_{\alpha/2}S_i}{\sqrt{n_i}} \right\}, \min_{1 \le i \le k}\left\{ \bar{X}_i + \frac{c_{\alpha/2}S_i}{\sqrt{n_i}} \right\} \right]. \tag{5.31}$$

Determination of the cut-off point $c_{\alpha/2}$ is not easy in applications, and simulation may be necessary. An alternative approach is to use the confidence interval

$$\left[\max_{1 \le i \le k}\left\{ \bar{X}_i - \frac{c_{\alpha/2}^{(i)}S_i}{\sqrt{n_i}} \right\}, \min_{1 \le i \le k}\left\{ \bar{X}_i + \frac{c_{\alpha/2}^{(i)}S_i}{\sqrt{n_i}} \right\} \right], \tag{5.32}$$

where $c_{\alpha/2}^{(i)}$ satisfies $\Pr[|t_i| \le c_{\alpha/2}^{(i)}] = (1 - \alpha)^{1/k}$. This latter interval clearly also has an exact coverage probability $1 - \alpha$.

Fairweather (1972) suggested using a weighted linear combination of the t_i's, namely,

$$W_t = \sum_{i=1}^{k} u_i t_i, \quad u_i = \frac{[\text{Var}(t_i)]^{-1}}{\sum_{j=1}^{k}[\text{Var}(t_j)]^{-1}} \tag{5.33}$$

which is also a pivot. If $b_{\alpha/2}$ denotes the cut-off point of the distribution of W_t, satisfying the equation

$$1 - \alpha = \Pr[|W_t| \le b_{\alpha/2}], \tag{5.34}$$

then the confidence interval for μ is obtained as

$$\frac{\sum_{i=1}^{k} \sqrt{n_i} u_i \bar{X}_i / S_i}{\sum_{i=1}^{k} \sqrt{n_i} u_i / S_i} \pm \frac{b}{\sum_{i=1}^{k} \sqrt{n_i} u_i / S_i}. \tag{5.35}$$

It may be noted that

$$\mathrm{Var}(t_\nu) = \frac{\nu}{\nu - 2}, \quad \nu > 2. \tag{5.36}$$

(b) Confidence interval for μ based on F_i's

Jordan and Krishnamoorthy (1996) suggested using a linear combination of the F_i's such as $W_f = \sum_{i=1}^{k} w_i F_i$ for positive weights w_i's, which is again a pivot. Hence, if we can compute $a_{\alpha/2}$ such that

$$\Pr[W_f \le a_{\alpha/2}] = 1 - \alpha, \tag{5.37}$$

then, after simplification, an exact confidence interval for μ with confidence level $1 - \alpha$ is given by

$$\left[\sum_{i=1}^{k} p_i \bar{X}_i - \Delta, \ \sum_{i=1}^{k} p_i \bar{X}_i + \Delta \right] \tag{5.38}$$

where

$$p_i = \frac{w_i n_i / S_i^2}{\sum_{j=1}^{k} w_j n_j / S_j^2} \tag{5.39}$$

and

$$\Delta^2 = \frac{a_{\alpha/2}}{\sum_{i=1}^{k} w_i n_i / S_i^2} - \left[\sum_{i=1}^{k} p_i \bar{X}_i^2 - \left(\sum_{i=1}^{k} p_i \bar{X}_i \right)^2 \right]. \tag{5.40}$$

Jordan and Krishnamoorthy (1996) used w_i as inversely proportional to $\mathrm{Var}(F_i) = 2 m_i^2 (m_i - 1)/[(m_i - 2)^2 (m_i - 4)]$, where $m_i = n_i - 1$, resulting in w_i as

$$w_i = \frac{[(m_i - 2)^2 (m_i - 4)]/[m_i^2 (m_i - 1)]}{\sum_{j=1}^{k} [(m_j - 2)^2 (m_j - 4)]/[m_j^2 (m_j - 1)]}. \tag{5.41}$$

Of course, it is assumed that $n_i > 5$ for all the k studies.

(c) Confidence interval for μ based on P_i's

Since F_i, defined in (5.29), can be used for testing hypotheses about μ, we define the ith P-value, P_i, as

$$P_i = \int_{F_i}^{\infty} h_i(x) \, dx \tag{5.42}$$

where $h_i(x)$ denotes the pdf of the F distribution with 1 and $n_i - 1$ df. Recalling the fact that $P_1, \dots, P_k$ are iid uniformly distributed random variables, we can combine them using any of the methods described earlier in Chapter 3. In particular, we use below Tippett's method, Fisher's method, the inverse normal method, and the logit method.

1. Tippett's method (Tippett, 1931)

As already explained, if $P_{[1]}$ is the minimum of $P_1, P_2, \ldots, P_k$, then Tippett's method rejects the hypothesis about μ if $P_{[1]} < c_1 = 1 - (1 - \alpha)^{1/k}$. By inverting this rejection region, we have a confidence interval for μ with confidence coefficient $1 - \alpha$, given by

$$
\begin{aligned}
\text{CI} &= \{\mu : P_{[1]} \geq c_1\} \\
&= \{\mu : P_i \geq c_1, i = 1, \ldots, k\} \\
&= \left\{\mu : \int_{n_i(\bar{x}_i - \mu)^2 / s_i^2}^{\infty} f_i(x) \, dx \geq 1 - (1 - \alpha)^{1/k}, \ i = 1, \ldots, k\right\}.
\end{aligned}
\tag{5.43}
$$

2. Fisher's method (Fisher, 1932)

Since Fisher's method rejects hypotheses about μ when $-2\sum_{i=1}^{k} \ln P_i > \chi_{2k,\alpha}^2$, the confidence interval for μ obtained by inverting the acceptance region of this test is given by

$$
\begin{aligned}
\text{CI} &= \{\mu : -2 \sum_{i=1}^{k} \ln P_i \leq \chi_{2k,\alpha}^2\} \\
&= \{\mu : \prod_{i=1}^{k} P_i \geq e^{-2\chi_{2k,\alpha}^2}\} \\
&= \left\{\mu : \prod_{i=1}^{k} \int_{n_i(\bar{x}_i - \mu)^2 / s_i^2}^{\infty} f_i(x) \, dx \geq e^{-2\chi_{2k,\alpha}^2}\right\}
\end{aligned}
\tag{5.44}
$$

3. Inverse normal method (Stouffer et al., 1949)

Since this method rejects hypotheses about μ when $\left[\sum_{i=1}^{k} \Phi^{-1}(P_i)\right]/\sqrt{k} < -z_\alpha$ at level α, the $(1 - \alpha)$-level confidence interval for μ obtained by inverting this acceptance region is given by

$$
\text{CI} = \left\{\mu : \frac{\sum_{i=1}^{k} \Phi^{-1}(P_i)}{\sqrt{k}} \geq -z_\alpha\right\}.
\tag{5.45}
$$

4. Logit method (George, 1977)

This method rejects H_0 if $\sum_{i=1}^{k} \ln[P_i/(1 - P_i)] < c$, where c is a predetermined constant. It was mentioned earlier that the distribution of

$$
G^* = \left[-\sum_{i=1}^{k} \ln\left(\frac{P_i}{1 - P_i}\right)\right] \left[\frac{3}{k\pi^2}\right]^{1/2}
\tag{5.46}
$$

can be approximated by a standard normal distribution (see Chapter 3). Therefore a $(1 - \alpha)$-level confidence interval for μ can be obtained from

$$
\text{CI} = \{\mu : G^* < z_\alpha\}.
\tag{5.47}
$$

It is an interesting research problem to settle if the confidence regions for μ obtained from the above four methods are actually genuine intervals. The appendix at the end of this chapter makes an attempt to establish the same for Fisher's method on the basis of an expansion technique. See Yu, Sun, and Sinha (2002) for details.

5.4 APPLICATIONS

In this section we provide two examples to illustrate the methods described above.

Example 5.1. Here we examine the data reported in Meier (1953) and analyzed in Jordan and Krishnamoorthy (1996) about the percentage of albumin in plasma protein in human subjects. We would like to combine the results of four experiments in order to construct a confidence interval for the common mean μ. The data appear in Table 5.1.

Table 5.1 Percentage of albumin in plasma protein

Experiment	n_i	Mean	Variance
A	12	62.3	12.986
B	15	60.3	7.840
C	7	59.5	33.433
D	16	61.5	18.513

We have applied all the techniques described in this section and computed the two-sided confidence intervals with $\alpha = 0.05$. These are given in Table 5.2. The critical value for interval (5.31) is $c = 3.053$. For interval (5.32), the four critical values are determined as $2.9702, 2.8543, 3.5055$, and 2.8272. In interval (5.35), we have $b \doteq 1.102$ and, in interval (5.38), $a \doteq 3.191$. It is interesting to observe that most of the confidence intervals are centered at around the same value, and the one based on F turns out to be the best in the sense of having the smallest observed length.

Table 5.2 Interval estimates for μ in the albumin example

Method	95% CI on μ
Cohen and Sackrowitz (1984), interval (5.31)	60.82 ± 1.68
Cohen and Sackrowitz (1984), interval (5.32)	60.78 ± 1.58
Fairweather (1972), interval (5.35)	61.04 ± 1.15
Jordan and Krishnamoorthy (1996), interval (5.38)	61.00 ± 1.44
Fisher, interval (5.44)	61.00 ± 1.42
Inverse normal, interval (5.45)	61.00 ± 1.31
Logit, interval (5.47)	61.00 ± 1.35

Example 5.2. This is from Eberhardt, Reeve, and Spiegelman (1989) and deals with the problem of estimation of mean selenium in nonfat milk powder by combining the results of four methods. Data appear in the Table 5.3.

Table 5.3   Selenium in nonfat milk powder

Methods	n_i	Mean	Variance
Atomic absorption spectrometry	8	105.0	85.711
Neutron activation:			
1. Instrumental	12	109.75	20.748
2. Radiochemical	14	109.5	2.729
Isotope dilution mass spectrometry	8	113.25	33.640

Here again we have applied all the techniques described in this section and computed the two-sided confidence intervals for the common mean μ with $\alpha = 0.05$. These are given in Table 5.4. The critical value for interval (5.31) is here $c = 3.128$. For interval (5.32), the four critical values are determined as $3.321, 2.970, 2.886$, and 3.321. In interval (5.35), we have $b \doteq 1.118$ and, in interval (5.38), $a \doteq 3.341$. It is rather interesting to observe that most of the confidence intervals are centered at around the same value, namely, 109.6, and the one based on the normal method turns out to be the best in the sense of having the smallest observed length.

Table 5.4   Interval estimates for μ in the selenium example

Method	95% CI on μ
Cohen and Sackrowitz (1984), interval (5.31)	109.5 ± 1.38
Cohen and Sackrowitz (1984), interval (5.32)	109.5 ± 1.27
Fairweather (1972), interval (5.35)	109.7 ± 1.11
Jordan and Krishnamoorthy (1996), interval (5.38)	109.6 ± 1.08
Fisher, interval (5.44)	109.6 ± 1.09
Inverse normal, interval (5.45)	109.6 ± 0.93
Logit, interval (5.47)	109.6 ± 1.25

Appendix: Theory of Fisher's Method

Let $T_n(\mu) = -2\sum_{i=1}^{k} \ln P_i(\mu) \sim \chi_{2k}^2$ under H_0, where $P_i(\mu)$ is the P-value defined by

$$P_i(\mu) = \Pr[F_{1,n_i-1} > c_i(\mu)] \quad \text{with} \quad c_i(\mu) = \frac{n_i(\bar{x}_i - \mu)^2}{s_i^2}.$$

Hence, the $100(1 - \alpha)\%$ confidence interval for μ is

$$\{\mu : T_n(\mu) \leq \chi^2_{2k,\alpha}\}.$$

Now we approximate T_n by $\tilde{T}_n$, which is

$$\tilde{T}_n(\mu) = T_n(\hat{\mu}) + \sum_{i=1}^{k} b_i(c_i - \hat{c}_i),$$

where

$$\hat{\mu} = \frac{\sum_{i=1}^{k} n_i \bar{x}_i / s_i^2}{\sum_{i=1}^{k} n_i / s_i^2} \quad \text{the Graybill-Deal estimator}, \quad \hat{c}_i = c_i(\hat{\mu}),$$

and b_i is chosen such that $T_n(\mu) \approx \tilde{T}_n(\mu)$.

Suppose there exists μ_0 such that

$$c_i \equiv c_i^* = F_{\exp[-\chi^2_{2k,\alpha}/(2k)]}(1, n_i - 1)$$

and define $\varepsilon(\mu) = T_n(\mu) - \tilde{T}_n(\mu)$. Then, we have,

$$
\begin{aligned}
\varepsilon(\mu) &= T_n(\mu) - \tilde{T}_n(\mu) - \sum_{i=1}^{k} b_i(c_i - \hat{c}_i) \\
&\approx T_n(\mu)|_{c_i = c_i^*} - T_n(\hat{\mu}) - \sum_{i=1}^{k} b_i(c_i^* - \hat{c}_i) \\
&\quad + \sum_{i=1}^{k} \left(\frac{d\,T_n}{d\,c_i} - b_i\right)\Big|_{c_i = c_i^*}(c_i - c_i^*).
\end{aligned}
$$

If we put

$$b_i = \frac{d\,T_n}{d\,c_i}\Big|_{c_i = c_i^*} = -2\frac{P_i'(c_i)}{P_i(c_i)}\Big|_{c_i = c_i^*},$$

then

$$\varepsilon(\hat{\mu}) = 0 \quad \text{and} \quad \varepsilon(\mu|_{c_i - c_i^*}) \approx 0 \quad \text{(1st order)}.$$

Since

$$
\begin{aligned}
P_i'(c_i) &= \frac{d}{dc_i} \Pr(F_{1, n_i - 1} > c_i) \\
&= \frac{d}{dc_i} \int_{c_i}^{\infty} \frac{(\frac{1}{n_i - 1})^{1/2}}{B(\frac{1}{2}, \frac{n_i - 1}{2})} \frac{u^{-1/2}}{(1 + \frac{u}{n_i - 1})^{n_i/2}} \, d\,u \\
&= -\frac{\Gamma(n_i/2)}{\Gamma(1/2)\,\Gamma[(n - 1)/2]} \left(\frac{1}{n_i - 1}\right)^{1/2} c_i^{-1/2} \left(1 + \frac{c_i}{n_i - 1}\right)^{-n_i/2}
\end{aligned}
$$

and

$$P_i(c_i^*) = \Pr(F_{1,n_i-1} > c_i^*) = \exp\left(-\frac{\chi^2_{2k,\alpha}}{2k}\right).$$

Therefore,

$$\begin{aligned} b_i &= \frac{2\,\Gamma(n_i/2)}{\Gamma(1/2)\,\Gamma[(n_i-1)/2]} \left(\frac{1}{n_i-1}\right)^{1/2} c_i^{-1/2} \\ &\quad \times \left(1+\frac{c_i}{n_i-1}\right)^{-n_i/2} \exp\left(-\frac{\chi^2_{2k,\alpha}}{2k}\right). \end{aligned}$$

Hence,

$$\begin{aligned} T_n(\mu) &\le \chi^2_{2k,\alpha} \\ \implies \quad \tilde{T}_n(\mu) &\le \chi^2_{2k,\alpha} \\ \implies \quad \sum_{i=1}^{k} b_i\,c_i &\le \chi^2_{2k,\alpha} - T_n(\hat{\mu}) + \sum_{i=1}^{k} b_i\,\hat{c}_i \equiv a,\,\text{says}. \end{aligned}$$

As a result, the $100(1-\alpha)\%$ confidence interval for μ is

$$\mu \in \sum_{i=1}^{k} q_i\bar{x}_i \pm \left[\frac{a}{\sum_{i=1}^{k} b_i\,n_i/s_i^2} + \left(\sum_{i=1}^{k} q_i\,\bar{x}_i\right)^2 - \sum_{i=1}^{k} q_i\,\bar{x}_i^2\right]^{1/2},$$

where

$$q_i = \frac{b_i\,n_i/s_i^2}{\sum_{j=1}^{k} b_j\,n_j/s_j^2}.$$

CHAPTER 6

TESTS OF HOMOGENEITY IN META-ANALYSIS

As has been mentioned earlier, meta-analysis of results from different experiments or studies is quite common these days. However, as has been emphasized, it is equally important to make sure that the underlying effect sizes arising out of these experiments are indeed homogeneous before performing any meta-analysis or pooling of evidence or data so that an inference on a common effect makes sense.

In this chapter we discuss at length the problem of testing homogeneity of means in a one-way fixed effects model. We assume throughout that the observations are drawn from k independent univariate normal populations with means $\mu_1, \ldots, \mu_k$ and variances $\sigma_1^2, \sigma_2^2, \ldots, \sigma_k^2$, and the problem is to test the homogeneity hypothesis with respect to means, given by $H_0 : \mu_1 = \cdots = \mu_k$, against a general alternative. Once H_0 is accepted, we feel quite comfortable in pooling all the data sets in order to make suitable inference about the common unknown mean μ. The next chapter, Chapter 7, deals with the dual problem of testing homogeneity of means in a one-way random effects model, which indeed also has a long and rich history.

The problem of testing the homogeneity of means in a one-way analysis of variance (ANOVA) is one of the oldest problems in statistics with applications in many diverse fields (Cochran, 1937). Under the classical ANOVA assumption of normality, independence, and homogeneous error variances ($\sigma_1^2 = \sigma_2^2 = \cdots = \sigma_k^2$), one uses

Statistical Meta-Analysis with Applications. By Joachim Hartung, Guido Knapp, Bimal K. Sinha **63**
Copyright © 2008 John Wiley & Sons, Inc.

the standard likelihood ratio F test, which is also known to be the optimum from an invariance point of view. However, when one or more of these basic assumptions are violated, the F test ceases to be any good, let alone be optimum! This is especially true in the case of nonhomogeneous error variances, which is often the situation in meta-analysis. In the literature (Cochran, 1937; Welch, 1951), several tests of H_0 have been proposed and compared in the presence of heterogeneity of error variances. All these tests are approximate and work quite well in large samples.

The main goal of this chapter is to present a systematic development of these tests along with results of some simulation studies to compare them (Section 6.1). This chapter is based mostly on Hartung, Argac, and Makambi (2002). An exact solution based on a relatively new notion of generalized P-values is also presented in this chapter (Section 6.2). The chapter concludes with illustrations of four classic data sets. It should be noted that, for $k = 2$, the testing problem under consideration boils down to the famous Behrens-Fisher problem!

6.1 MODEL AND TEST STATISTICS

Let X_{ij} be the observation on the jth subject of the ith population/study, $i = 1, \ldots, k$ and $j = 1, \ldots, n_i$. Then the standard one-way ANOVA model is given by

$$X_{ij} = \mu_i + e_{ij} = \mu + \tau_i + e_{ij}, \quad i = 1, \ldots, k, \, j = 1, \ldots, n_i,$$

where μ is the common mean for all the k populations, τ_i is the effect of population i with $\sum_{i=1}^{k} \tau_i = 0$, and e_{ij} are error terms which are assumed to be mutually independent and normally distributed with

$$\mathrm{E}(e_{ij}) = 0, \quad \mathrm{Var}(e_{ij}) = \sigma_i^2, \quad i = 1, \ldots, k, \, j = 1, \ldots, n_i.$$

Under the above set-up, we are interested in testing the hypothesis

$$H_0 : \mu_1 = \cdots = \mu_k.$$

To test this hypothesis, we propose the following test statistics.

ANOVA F Test
The test statistics S_{an} is given by

$$S_{an} = \frac{N - k}{k - 1} \frac{\sum_{i=1}^{k} n_i \, (\bar{X}_{i.} - \bar{X}_{..})^2}{\sum_{i=1}^{k} (n_i - 1) \, S_i^2},$$

with $N = \sum_{i=1}^{k} n_i$, $\bar{X}_{i.} = \sum_{j=1}^{n_i} X_{ij}/n_i$, $\bar{X}_{..} = \sum_{i=1}^{k} n_i \bar{X}_{i.}/N$, and $S_i^2 = \sum_{j=1}^{n_i} (X_{ij} - \bar{X}_{i.})/(n_i - 1)$.

This test was originally meant to test for equality of population means under variance homogeneity and has an F distribution with $k - 1$ and $N - k$ df under the null hypothesis. The test rejects H_0 at level α if $S_{an} > F_{k-1,N-k;\alpha}$, where $F_{k-1,N-k;\alpha}$ is the upper $100\alpha\%$ point of the F distribution with $k - 1$ and $N - k$ df.

This ANOVA F test has the weakness of not being robust with respect to heterogeneity in the intrapopulation error variances (Brown and Forsythe, 1974).

Cochran's Test
This test suggested by Cochran in 1937 is based on

$$S_{\text{ch}} = \sum_{i=1}^{k} w_i \left(\bar{X}_{i.} - \sum_{j=1}^{k} h_j \bar{X}_{j.} \right)^2,$$

where $w_i = n_i/S_i^2, h_i = w_i / \sum_{i=1}^{k} w_i$. Under H_0, the Cochran statistic is distributed approximately as a χ^2 variable with $k - 1$ df. The test rejects H_0 at level α if $S_{\text{ch}} > \chi^2_{k-1;\alpha}$, where $\chi^2_{k-1;\alpha}$ is the upper $100\alpha\%$ point of the chi-square distribution with $k-1$ df. Cochran's test is often used as the standard test for testing homogeneity in meta-analysis. This test has been already introduced in Chapter 4 as the general large-sample test of homogeneity.

Welch Test
The Welch test is given by

$$S_{\text{we}} = \frac{\sum_{i=1}^{k} w_i \left(\bar{X}_{i.} - \sum_{j=1}^{k} h_j \bar{X}_{j.} \right)^2}{(k-1) + 2 \dfrac{k-2}{k+1} \sum_{i=1}^{k} \dfrac{1}{n_i - 1} (1 - h_i)^2},$$

where $w_i = n_i/S_i^2, h_i = w_i / \sum_{i=1}^{k} w_i$. This test is an extension of testing the equality of two means to more than two means (see Welch, 1951) in the presence of variance heterogeneity within populations. The Welch test is a modification of Cochran's test. Under H_0, the statistic S_{we} has an approximate F distribution with $k - 1$ and ν_g df, where

$$\nu_g = \frac{(k^2 - 1)/3}{\sum_{i=1}^{k} (1 - h_i)^2 / (n_i - 1)}.$$

This test rejects H_0 at level α if $S_{\text{we}} > F_{k-1,\nu_g;\alpha}$.

Brown-Forsythe (BF) Test
This test, also known as the modified F test, is based on

$$S_{\text{bf}} = \frac{\sum_{i=1}^{k} n_i (\bar{X}_{i.} - \bar{X}_{..})^2}{\sum_{i=1}^{k} (1 - n_i/N) S_i^2}.$$

When H_0 is true, S_{bf} is distributed approximately as an F variable with $k - 1$ and ν df, where

$$\nu = \frac{\left[\sum_{i=1}^{k} (1 - n_i/N) S_i^2 \right]^2}{\sum_{i=1}^{k} (1 - n_i/N)^2 S_i^4 / (n_i - 1)}.$$

The test rejects H_0 at level α if $S_{bf} > F_{k-1,\nu;\alpha}$. Using a simulation study, Brown and Forsythe (1974) demonstrated that their statistic is robust under heterogeneity of variances. If the population variances are close to being homogeneous, the BF test is closer to the ANOVA F test than to Welch's test.

Mehrotra (Modified Brown-Forsythe) Test

The test statistic

$$S_{bf(m)} = \frac{\sum_{i=1}^{k} n_i (\bar{X}_{i.} - \bar{X}_{..})^2}{\sum_{i=1}^{k} (1 - n_i/N) S_i^2}$$

was proposed by Mehrotra (1997) in an attempt to correct a "flaw" in the BF test. Under H_0, $S_{bf(m)}$ is distributed approximately as an F variable with ν_1 and ν df, where

$$\nu_1 = \frac{\left[\sum_{i=1}^{k} (1 - n_i/N) S_i^2 \right]^2}{\sum_{i=1}^{k} S_i^4 + \left(\sum_{i=1}^{k} n_i S_i^2 / N \right)^2 - 2 \sum_{i=1}^{k} n_i S_i^4 / N}$$

and ν is defined in the BF test. The test rejects H_0 at level α if $S_{bf(m)} > F_{\nu_1,\nu;\alpha}$.

Approximate ANOVA F Test

The test statistic

$$S_{aF} = \frac{N - k}{k - 1} \frac{\sum_{i=1}^{k} n_i (\bar{X}_{i.} - \bar{X}_{..})^2}{\sum_{i=1}^{k} (n_i - 1) S_i^2}$$

was proposed by Asiribo and Gurland (1990). Under H_0, the statistic S_{aF} is distributed approximately as an F variable with ν_1 and ν_2 df, where ν_1 is defined under Mehrotra test above and

$$\nu_2 = \frac{\left[\sum_{i=1}^{k} (n_i - 1) S_i^2 \right]^2}{\sum_{i=1}^{k} (n_i - 1) S_i^4}.$$

The test rejects H_0 at level α if $S_{aF} > \hat{c} \cdot F_{\nu_1,\nu_2;\alpha}$, where

$$\hat{c} = \frac{N - k}{N(k - 1)} \frac{\sum_{i=1}^{k} (N - n_i) S_i^2}{\sum_{i=1}^{k} (n_i - 1) S_i^2}.$$

We notice that the numerator df for S_{aF} and $S_{bf(m)}$ are equal. Further, for $n_i = n, i = 1, \ldots, k$, that is, for balanced data, the test statistic and the df for both the numerator and denominator of these two statistics are also equal.

Adjusted Welch Test

The Welch test uses weights $w_i = n_i/S_i^2$. We know that

$$E(w_i) = E\left(\frac{n_i}{S_i^2} \right) = c_i \cdot \frac{n_i}{\sigma_i^2},$$

where $c_i = (n_i - 1)/(n_i - 3)$. Therefore, an unbiased estimator of n_i/σ_i^2 is $n_i/(c_i S_i^2)$.

Defining $w_i^* = n_i/(c_i S_i^2)$, Hartung, Argac, and Makambi (2002) propose a test they called the adjusted Welch test, denoted by S_{aw}, which is given by

$$S_{\text{aw}} = \frac{\sum_{i=1}^{k} w_i^* \left(\bar{X}_{i.} - \sum_{j=1}^{k} h_j^* \bar{X}_{j.} \right)^2}{\left[(k-1) + 2 \frac{k-2}{k+1} \sum_{i=1}^{k} \frac{1}{n_i - 1} (1 - h_i^*) \right]^2},$$

where $h_i^* = w_i^* / \sum_{j=1}^{k} w_j^*, i = 1, \dots, k$. Under H_0, the adjusted Welch statistic, S_{aw}, is distributed approximately as an F variable with $k - 1$ and ν_g^* df, with

$$\nu_g^* = \frac{(k^2 - 1)/3}{\sum_{i=1}^{k} (1 - h_i^*)^2 / (n_i - 1)}.$$

The test rejects H_0 at level α if $S_{\text{aw}} > F_{k-1, \nu_g^*; \alpha}$. When the sample sizes are large, S_{aw} approaches the Welch test. With small sample sizes, this statistic will help to correct the overshooting of the Welch test with respect to α.

Extensive simulation studies by Hartung, Argac, and Makambi (2002) for both size and power under normal and nonnormal populations, under homogeneous and heterogeneous variances, and under balanced and unbalanced schemes reveal that the modified Brown-Forsythe test and the approximate F test are relatively least affected by changes from normal populations with homogeneous variances.

6.2   AN EXACT TEST OF HOMOGENEITY

We conclude this section with a brief discussion of the application of the generalized P-value for solving the underlying testing problem of homogeneity of means in the presence of heterogeneity variances. This procedure described below will produce an exact test. For details, we refer to Tsui and Weerahandi (1989), Thursby (1992), and Griffiths and Judge (1992).

We first discuss the case $k = 2$, that is, the Behrens-Fisher problem. Let $X = (\bar{X}_{1.} - \bar{X}_{2.}, S_1^2, S_2^2)$, $x = (\bar{x}_{1.} - \bar{x}_{2.}, s_1^2, s_2^2)$, $\theta = \mu_1 - \mu_2$, and $\eta = (\sigma_1^2, \sigma_2^2)$. Here S_1^2 and S_2^2 are the two sample variances which are unbiased estimates of σ_1^2 and σ_2^2, respectively. We then define $T(X; x, \theta, \eta)$ as

$$T(X; x, \theta, \eta) = (\bar{X}_{1.} - \bar{X}_{2.}) \left(\frac{\sigma_1^2}{n_1} + \frac{\sigma_2^2}{n_2} \right)^{-1/2} \left(\frac{s_1^2 \sigma_1^2}{S_1^2 n_1} + \frac{s_2^2 \sigma_2^2}{S_2^2 n_2} \right)^{1/2}.$$

Note that the *observed* value of T is $t = \bar{x}_{1.} - \bar{x}_{2.}$ and that E(T) increases with $\mu_1 - \mu_2$. Hence the generalized P-value can be defined as

$$
\begin{aligned}
\text{gen.}P &= \Pr\left[T \geq \bar{x}_{1.} - \bar{x}_{2.} \mid \mu_1 = \mu_2 \right] \\
&= \Pr\left[Z \left(\frac{s_1^2(n_1 - 1)}{U_1 n_1} + \frac{s_2^2(n_2 - 1)}{U_2 n_2} \right)^{1/2} \geq \bar{x}_{1.} - \bar{x}_{2.} \right]
\end{aligned}
$$

Table 6.4   Percentage of albumin in plasma protein

Experiment	n_i	Mean	Variance s_i^2
A	12	62.3	12.986
B	15	60.3	7.840
C	7	59.5	33.433
D	16	61.5	18.513

Table 6.5   Test statistics and P-values in the albumin example

Test	Value of test statistic	P-value
ANOVA F test	0.991	0.405
Cochran	3.186	0.364
Welch	0.993	0.417
Brown-Forsythe	0.833	0.491
Mehrotra	0.833	0.471
Approximate ANOVA F test	0.833	0.465
Adjusted Welch test	0.804	0.507
Generalized P-value		0.367

Example 6.3. Here we examine the data on selenium in nonfat milk powder from Eberhardt, Reeve, and Spiegelman (1989). The summary statistics are given in Table 6.6 and the values of the test statistics with corresponding P-values are reported in Table 6.7.

Table 6.6   Selenium in nonfat milk powder

Methods	n_i	Mean	Variance s_i^2
Atomic absorption spectrometry	8	105.0	85.711
Neutron activation:			
1. Instrumental	12	109.75	20.748
2. Radiochemical	14	109.5	2.729
Isotope dilution mass spectrometry	8	113.25	33.640

Here again all tests except the ANOVA F test lead to acceptance of the null hypothesis.

Table 6.7   Test statistics and P-values in the selenium example

Test	Value of test statistic	P-value
ANOVA F test	3.169	0.035
Cochran	5.208	0.157
Welch	1.589	0.235
Brown-Forsythe	2.428	0.104
Mehrotra	2.428	0.120
Approximate ANOVA F test	2.428	0.114
Adjusted Welch test	1.137	0.367
Generalized P-value		0.147

Example 6.4. Here we examine the data reported in Weerahandi (2004, p. 43). The individual data are reported in Table 6.8 and Table 6.9 contains the values of the test statistics as well as the corresponding P-values.

Table 6.8   Strength of four brands of reinforcing bars

Brand A	21.4, 13.5, 21.1, 13.3, 18.9, 19.2, 18.3
Brand B	27.3, 22.3, 16.9, 11.3, 26.3, 19.8, 16.2, 25.4
Brand C	18.7, 19.1, 16.4, 15.9, 18.7, 20.1, 17.8
Brand D	19.9, 19.3, 18.7, 20.3, 22.8, 20.8, 20.9, 23.6, 21.2

Table 6.9   Test statistics and P-values in the strength of reinforcing bars example

Test	Value of test statistic	P-value
ANOVA F test	1.608	0.211
Cochran	14.439	0.002
Welch	4.385	0.023
Brown-Forsythe	1.616	0.232
Mehrotra	1.616	0.234
Approximate ANOVA F test	1.616	0.236
Adjusted Welch test	3.086	0.063
Generalized P-value		0.021

It is interesting to observe that, as in Example 6.1, in this problem the Cochran test, Welch test, and generalized P-value test share the same conclusion of outright rejection of the null hypothesis while other tests strongly recommend its acceptance!

CHAPTER 7

ONE-WAY RANDOM EFFECTS MODEL

7.1 INTRODUCTION

As discussed in the previous chapter, tests for homogeneity of means or in general effect sizes are crucial before performing any meta-analysis or pooling of data. When tests for homogeneity lead to acceptance of the null hypothesis, thus supporting the evidence that the underlying population means or effect sizes can be believed to be the same, one feels quite comfortable in carrying out the meta-analysis in order to draw appropriate inference about the common mean or effect size. When, however, the tests lead to rejection of the null hypothesis of homogeneity of means, it is not proper to do meta-analysis of data unless we find reasons for heterogeneity and make an attempt to explain them. The lack of homogeneity could be due to several covariates which might behave differently for different studies or simply because the means themselves might arise from a so called superpopulation, thus leading to their variability and apparent differences. In this chapter we discuss at length the latter formulation, which is often known as the one-way random effects model.

There is a vast literature on the one-way random effects model with its root in meta-analysis. Under this model with normality assumption, the treatment means $\mu_1, \ldots, \mu_k$ corresponding to k different studies or experiments are modeled as arising

Statistical Meta-Analysis with Applications. By Joachim Hartung, Guido Knapp, Bimal K. Sinha
Copyright © 2008 John Wiley & Sons, Inc.

from a supernormal population with an overall mean μ and an overall variability σ_a^2. The parameters of interest are then the overall mean μ and the interstudy variability σ_a^2 in terms of their estimation, tests, and confidence intervals.

In the remainder of this chapter we discuss many results pertaining to the above problems. Most of the results presented here appear for the first time in a book on statistical meta-analysis! Recalling that in the context of meta-analysis ANOVA models existence of heterogeneous within-study variances (also known as error variances) is very much a possibility, we consider the two cases of homogeneous and heterogeneous error variances separately in Sections 7.2 and 7.3, respectively. It turns out that, as expected, statistical inference about the parameters of interest under the homogeneous error structure can be carried out much more easily compared to that under a heterogenous error structure. It is also true that the analysis of a balanced model is much easier than the analysis of an unbalanced model. Recall that a balanced model refers to the case when we have an equal number of observations or replications from all the populations.

As will be clear from what follows, this particular topic of research has drawn the attention of many statisticians from all over the world and has prompted the emergence of new statistical methods. Most notably among them is the method based on generalized P-values, which itself has a considerable amount of literature including a few textbooks. We will mention in the sequel some results based on the notion of generalized P-values. For details on generalized P-values, we refer to Weerahandi (1995) and Khuri, Mathew, and Sinha (1998).

We end this section with a simple description of the model to be analyzed. We consider the case of the one-way random effects model of ANOVA, that is,

$$Y_{ij} = \mu + a_i + e_{ij}, \qquad i = 1, \ldots, k, \;\; j = 1, \ldots, n_i \geq 1, \qquad (7.1)$$

where Y_{ij} denotes the observable variable, μ the fixed but unknown grand mean, a_i the unobservable random effect with mean 0 and variance σ_a^2, and e_{ij} the error term with mean 0 and variance σ_i^2. We assume that the random variables $a_1, \ldots, a_k, e_{11}, \ldots e_{kn_k}$ are normally distributed and mutually stochastically independent. Furthermore, we denote by $N = \sum_{i=1}^{k} n_i$, the total number of observations.

The basic statistics for the above model are the sample means $\bar{Y}_{i.}$ and sample sum of squares SS_i, defined by

$$\bar{Y}_{i.} = \sum_{j=1}^{n_i} \frac{Y_{ij}}{n_i}, \quad SS_i = \sum_{j=1}^{n_i}(Y_{ij} - \bar{Y}_{i.})^2, \quad i = 1, \ldots, k.$$

Then the overall or grand mean and the two well-known sums of squares, namely, between sum of squares (BSS) and within sum of squares (WSS), are defined as

$$\bar{Y}_{..} = \sum_{i=1}^{k} n_i \frac{\bar{Y}_{i.}}{N}, \quad BSS = \sum_{i=1}^{k} n_i(\bar{Y}_{i.} - \bar{Y}_{..})^2, \quad WSS = SS_1 + \cdots + SS_k.$$

Obviously, under the assumption of normality and independence, it holds that

$$\bar{Y}_{..} \sim N\left(\mu, \sum_{i=1}^{k} \frac{n_i^2(\sigma_a^2 + \sigma_i^2/n_i)}{N^2}\right).$$

When the homogeneity of error variances holds, that is, $\sigma_1^2 = \cdots = \sigma_k^2 = \sigma^2$, this reduces to

$$\bar{Y}_{..} \sim N\left(\mu, \sum_{i=1}^{k} \frac{n_i^2(\sigma_a^2 + \sigma^2/n_i)}{N^2}\right).$$

Furthermore, in case of balanced models, that is, $n_1 = \cdots = n_k = n$, and homogeneity of error variances, we get

$$\bar{Y}_{..} \sim N\left(\mu, \frac{\sigma_a^2 + \sigma^2/n}{k}\right).$$

For WSS, we readily have

$$\text{WSS} \sim \sum_{i=1}^{k} \sigma_i^2 \, \chi_{n_i-1}^2 \sim \sigma^2 \chi_{N-k}^2, \tag{7.2}$$

with the latter result holding in case of the homogeneity of error variances.

For BSS, the results are somewhat complicated except for the balanced case with homogeneous error variances. Quite generally, since BSS can be written as a quadratic form in the sample means (corrected for the mean μ, without any loss of generality), we can conclude that the general distribution of BSS can be written as a linear function of independent chi-square variables with coefficients depending on the variance components and the replications. Under homogeneous error variances and a balanced model, we get

$$\text{BSS} \sim (\sigma^2 + n\sigma_a^2) \, \chi_{k-1}^2. \tag{7.3}$$

Of course, under normality of errors and random effects, independence of BSS and WSS follows immediately even under the most general situation of unbalanced models and heterogeneous error variances. The between-group mean sum of squares $\text{BMS} = \text{BSS}/(k-1)$, denoted as MS_1, has the expected value given by (assuming homogeneity of variances)

$$E(\text{MS}_1) = \gamma \, \sigma_a^2 + \sigma^2, \qquad \gamma = \frac{1}{k-1} \frac{N^2 - \sum_{i=1}^{k} n_i^2}{N}. \tag{7.4}$$

For later reference, we note from Eq. (7.2) that, under the assumption of homogeneity of error variances, a $(1-\alpha)$-level confidence interval for σ^2 is given by

$$\text{CI}(\sigma^2): \left[\frac{(N-k)\text{MS}_2}{\chi_{N-k;\,\alpha/2}^2} \; ; \; \frac{(N-k)\text{MS}_2}{\chi_{N-k;\,1-\alpha/2}^2}\right], \tag{7.5}$$

where $MS_2 = WSS/(N - k)$ and $\chi^2_{N-k;\,\alpha/2}$ denotes the upper $100(\alpha/2)\%$ point of a chi-square distribution with $N - k$ df.

It should also be mentioned that the approximation of the distribution of MS_1 by a multiple of a χ^2 distribution in the general case is satisfactory only if the between-group variance σ_a^2 is close to 0. This explains why an easy extension of the confidence interval for σ_a^2 in the balanced case, independently proposed by Tukey (1951) and Williams (1962) and discussed later in this chapter, is not possible in the unbalanced case.

7.2   HOMOGENEOUS ERROR VARIANCES

Under the assumption of homogeneous error variances, that is, $\sigma_1^2 = \sigma_2^2 = \cdots = \sigma_k^2 = \sigma^2$, the above model clearly boils down to the familiar intraclass correlation model with just three parameters: overall mean μ, between-study variance σ_a^2, and within-study or error variance σ^2. For balanced models, that is, when the treatment replications $n_1, \ldots, n_k$ are the same, there are exactly three sufficient statistics, namely, the overall sample mean, the between sum of squares, and the within sum of squares, and it is easy to derive the UMVUEs of the three parameters. In case of unbalanced models, there are many sufficient statistics and an unbiased estimate of the between-study variance σ_a^2 is not unique! Moreover, applying a fundamental result of LaMotte (1973), it turns out that all unbiased estimates of σ_a^2 in both balanced and unbalanced models are bound to assume negative values, thus making them unacceptable in practice. A lot of research has been conducted in order to derive nonnegative estimates of σ_a^2 with good frequentist properties. Because our emphasis here is more on tests and confidence intervals than on estimation, we omit these details and refer to the excellent book by Searle, Casella, and McCulloch (1992).

7.2.1   Test for $\sigma_a^2 = 0$

Although the one-way random effects model postulates the presence of a random component, it is of interest to test if this random component a_i is indeed present in the model (7.1). Since the null hypothesis here corresponds to the equality of means in a standard ANOVA set-up, we can use the regular F test based on the ratio of between and within sums of squares, i.e.,

$$F = \frac{BSS/(k - 1)}{WSS/(N - k)}.$$

Although this F test is known to have some optimum properties in the balanced case, in the unbalanced case this F test, though valid, ceases to have optimum properties, and a locally best invariant test under a natural group of transformations was derived by Das and Sinha (1987). The test statistic F^*, whose sampling distribution does not follow any known tabulated distribution, is given by

$$F^* = \frac{\sum_{i=1}^{k} n_i^2 \left(\bar{Y}_{i.} - \bar{Y}_{..}\right)^2}{WSS}.$$

7.2.2 Approximate tests for $H_0 : \sigma_a^2 = \delta > 0$ and confidence intervals for σ_a^2

When the F test for the nullity of the between-study variability is rejected, it is of importance to test for other meaningful positive values of this parameter as well as to construct its appropriate confidence intervals. Quite surprisingly, this particular problem has been tackled by many researchers over the last 50 years. It is clear from Eq. (7.3) that even in the case of balanced models there is no obvious test for a positive value of σ_a^2, and also it is not clear how to construct an exact confidence interval for σ_a^2. This is the main reason for a lot of research on this topic. Fortunately, the relatively new notion of a generalized P-value can be used to solve these problems exactly even in the case of unbalanced models. We will discuss this solution in Section 7.2.3.

In this section, however, we provide a survey of some main results on the derivation of approximate confidence intervals for σ_a^2 mostly from a classical point of view. Once an appropriate confidence interval is derived, it can be used to test the significance of a suggested positive value of the parameter σ_a^2 in the usual way. It should be noted that most of the procedures discussed below provide approximate solutions to our problem, especially in unbalanced models. In the sequel, we discuss the two cases of balanced and unbalanced models separately.

Balanced models. In the case of a balanced design, one method for constructing a confidence interval for the between-group variance σ_a^2 was proposed by Tukey (1951) and also independently by Williams (1962). The Tukey-Williams method is based upon noting the distributional properties of BSS and WSS given in Eqs. (7.2) and (7.3). Since it is easy to construct confidence intervals for σ^2 and $\sigma^2 + n\sigma_a^2$, exact $1 - \alpha$ confidence intervals for these parameters can be easily calculated, and by solving the intersection of these two confidence intervals, a confidence interval of the between-group variance σ_a^2 can be obtained which has a confidence coefficient at least $1 - 2\alpha$ due to Bonferroni's inequality. The results of simulation studies conducted by Boardman (1974) indicated that the confidence coefficient of the Tukey-Williams interval is nearly $1 - \alpha$ (cf. also Graybill, 1976, p. 620), and Wang (1990) showed that the confidence coefficient of this interval is even at least $1 - \alpha$ for customary values of α. The explicit Tukey-Williams interval is given as

$$\text{CI}(\sigma_a^2) : \left[\frac{1}{n \, \chi_{k-1;\alpha/2}^2} \left(\text{BSS} - \frac{k-1}{N-k} \text{WSS} \, F_{k-1,N-k;\alpha/2} \right) , \right.$$
$$\left. \frac{1}{n \, \chi_{k-1;1-\alpha/2}^2} \left(\text{BSS} - \frac{k-1}{N-k} \text{WSS} \, F_{k-1,N-k;1-\alpha/2} \right) \right]$$

Unbalanced models. Following the Tukey-Williams approach, Thomas and Hultquist (1978) proposed a confidence interval for the between-group variance σ_a^2 in the unbalanced case. This is based on a suitable χ^2 approximation of the distribution of BSS. However, this approximation is not good if the design is extremely unbalanced or if the ratio of the between- and within-group variances is less than 0.25. To overcome this problem, Burdick, Maqsood, and Graybill (1986) considered a conservative confidence interval for the ratio of between- and within-group variance, which was used in Burdick and Eickman (1986) to construct a confidence interval for the between-group variance based on the ideas of the Tukey-Williams method. In Burdick and Eickman (1986), a comparison of the confidence coefficients of the Thomas-Hultquist interval and the Burdick-Eickman interval on the basis of some simulation studies is reported. The results of the simulation studies indicated that the confidence coefficient is near $1 - \alpha$ in most cases. If the approximation to a χ^2 distribution in the Thomas-Hultquist approach is not so good, the resulting confidence interval can be very liberal, while in these situations the Burdick-Eickman interval can be very conservative.

Hartung and Knapp (2000) proposed a confidence interval for the between-group variance in the unbalanced design which is constructed from an exact confidence interval for the ratio of between- and within-group variance derived from Wald (1940) and an exact confidence interval of the error variance. We also refer the reader to Searle, Casella, and McCulloch (1992, p. 78) and Burdick and Graybill (1992, p. 186f) in this connection.

We describe below all the three procedures mentioned above for constructing an approximate confidence interval for σ_a^2 based on the two familiar sums of squares, namely, between and within sums of squares.

Thomas-Hultquist confidence interval for σ_a^2. Instead of MS_1 from Eq. (7.4), Thomas and Hultquist (1978) considered the sample variance of the group means given by

$$MS_3 = \frac{1}{k-1} \sum_{i=1}^{k} \left(\bar{Y}_{i.} - \frac{1}{k} \sum_{i=1}^{k} \bar{Y}_{i.} \right)^2.$$

They showed that it holds approximately

$$\frac{(k-1)MS_3}{\sigma_a^2 + \sigma^2/\tilde{n}} \overset{\text{appr.}}{\sim} \chi_{k-1}^2, \tag{7.6}$$

where $\tilde{n}$ denotes the harmonic mean of the sample sizes of the k groups. Combining Eqs. (7.2) and (7.6), it is then easy to conclude that

$$\frac{\sigma^2}{\sigma_a^2 + \sigma^2/\tilde{n}} \frac{MS_3}{MS_2} \overset{\text{appr.}}{\sim} F_{k-1, N-k}. \tag{7.7}$$

From Eqs. (7.6) and (7.7), $(1-\alpha)$-level confidence intervals for $\sigma_a^2 + \sigma^2/\tilde{n}$ and σ_a^2/σ^2 can be constructed, and adopting the ideas of constructing a confidence interval by Tukey and Williams to the present situation leads to the following confidence interval for σ_a^2:

$$CI_{TH}(\sigma_a^2) : \left[\frac{k-1}{\chi_{k-1;\,\alpha/2}^2} \left(MS_3 - \frac{MS_2}{\tilde{n}} F_{k-1,\,N-k;\,\alpha/2} \right), \right.$$

$$\left. \frac{k-1}{\chi_{k-1;\,1-\alpha/2}^2} \left(MS_3 - \frac{MS_2}{\tilde{n}} F_{k-1,\,N-k;\,1-\alpha/2} \right) \right]. \tag{7.8}$$

Due to Bonferroni's inequality the confidence coefficient of the interval (7.8) is at least $1 - 2\alpha$, but one may hope that the actual confidence coefficient is nearly $1 - \alpha$. However, as mentioned earlier, Thomas and Hultquist (1978) reported that the χ^2 approximation in Eq. (7.6) is not good for extremely unbalanced designs where the ratio $\eta = \sigma_a^2/\sigma_e^2$ is less than 0.25. Thus, in such situations the confidence interval (7.8) can be a liberal one, that is, the confidence coefficient lies substantially below $1 - \alpha$.

Burdick-Eickman confidence interval for σ_a^2. Burdick, Maqsood, and Graybill (1986) suggested a confidence interval for the ratio $\eta = \sigma_a^2/\sigma^2$ which overcomes the problem with small ratios in the Thomas-Hultquist procedure and has a confidence coefficient of at least $1 - \alpha$. This interval is given by

$$\mathrm{CI}(\eta) : \left[\frac{\mathrm{MS}_3}{\mathrm{MS}_2} \frac{1}{F_{k-1,\,N-k;\,\alpha/2}} - \frac{1}{n_{\min}}, \frac{\mathrm{MS}_3}{\mathrm{MS}_2} \frac{1}{F_{k-1,\,N-k;\,\alpha/2}} - \frac{1}{n_{\max}} \right] \quad (7.9)$$

with $n_{\min} = \min\{n_1, \ldots, n_k\}$ and $n_{\max} = \max\{n_1, \ldots, n_k\}$.

Using interval (7.9) and the confidence interval for $\sigma_a^2 + \sigma^2/\tilde{n}$ from Eq. (7.6), Burdick and Eickman (1986) investigated the confidence interval for σ_a^2 constructed by the Tukey-Williams method. This interval is given by

$$\mathrm{CI}_{\mathrm{BE}}(\sigma_a^2) : \left[\left(\frac{\tilde{n}L}{1 + \tilde{n}L} \right) \frac{(k-1)\mathrm{MS}_3}{\chi_{k-1;\,\alpha/2}^2}, \left(\frac{\tilde{n}U}{1 + \tilde{n}U} \right) \frac{(k-1)\mathrm{MS}_3}{\chi_{k-1;\,\alpha/2}^2} \right], \quad (7.10)$$

with

$$L = \max \left\{ 0, \frac{\mathrm{MS}_3}{\mathrm{MS}_2} \frac{1}{F_{k-1,\,N-k;\,\alpha/2}} - \frac{1}{n_{\min}} \right\}$$

and

$$U = \max \left\{ 0, \frac{\mathrm{MS}_3}{\mathrm{MS}_2} \frac{1}{F_{k-1,\,N-k;\,1-\alpha/2}} - \frac{1}{n_{\max}} \right\}.$$

Hartung-Knapp confidence interval for σ_a^2. Instead of approximative confidence intervals for η as in the Thomas-Hultquist and Burdick-Eickman approaches, Hartung and Knapp (2000) considered the exact confidence interval for η given in Wald (1940) to construct a confidence interval for σ_a^2.

Following Wald (1940), we observe that

$$\mathrm{Var}(\bar{Y}_{i.}) = \sigma_a^2 + \frac{\sigma^2}{n_i} = \frac{\sigma^2}{w_i}$$

with $w_i = n_i/(1 + \eta\, n_i)$, $i = 1, \ldots, k$. Now, Wald considered the sum of squares

$$(k-1)\mathrm{MS}_4 = \sum_{i=1}^{k} w_i \left(\bar{Y}_{i.} - \frac{\sum_{i=1}^{k} w_i \bar{Y}_{i.}}{\sum_{i=1}^{k} w_i} \right)^2$$

and proved that

$$\frac{(k-1)\mathrm{MS}_4}{\sigma^2} \sim \chi^2_{k-1} \, .$$

Furthermore, MS_4 and MS_2 are stochastically independent so that

$$F_w(\eta) = \frac{\mathrm{MS}_4}{\mathrm{MS}_2} \sim F_{k-1,\, n-k} \, . \qquad (7.11)$$

Obviously, Eq. (7.11) can be used to construct an exact confidence interval for the ratio η.

Wald showed that $(k-1)\mathrm{MS}_4$ is a strictly monotonously decreasing function in η, and so the bounds of the exact confidence interval are given as the solutions of the following two equations:

$$\begin{aligned} \text{lower bound:} \quad & F_w(\eta) = F_{k-1,\, N-k,\, \alpha/2}, \\ \text{upper bound:} \quad & F_w(\eta) = F_{k-1,\, N-k,\, 1-\alpha/2}. \end{aligned} \qquad (7.12)$$

Since $F_w(\eta)$ is a strictly monotonously decreasing function in η, the solution of Eq. (7.12), if it exists, is unique. But due to the fact that η is nonnegative, $(k-1)\mathrm{MS}_4$ is bounded at $\eta = 0$, namely it holds that

$$(k-1)\mathrm{MS}_4 \leq \sum_{i=1}^{k} n_i \left(\bar{Y}_{i.} - \frac{\sum_{i=1}^{k} n_i \bar{Y}_{i.}}{\sum_{n=1}^{k} n_i} \right)^2 \, .$$

Thus, a nonnegative solution of Eq. (7.12) may not exist. If such a solution of one of the equations in (7.12) does not exist, the corresponding bound in the confidence interval is set equal to zero. Note that the existence of a nonnegative solution in Eq. (7.12) only depends on the chosen α.

Let us denote by η_L and η_U the solutions of the equations in Eq. (7.12). We then propose, using the confidence bounds from interval (7.5) for σ^2, the following confidence interval for σ_a^2:

$$\mathrm{CI}(\sigma_a^2) : \left[\frac{(N-k)\mathrm{MS}_2}{\chi^2_{N-k;\, \alpha}} \, \eta_L \, , \, \frac{(N-k)\mathrm{MS}_2}{\chi^2_{N-k;\, 1-\alpha}} \, \eta_U \right] , \qquad (7.13)$$

which has a confidence coefficient of at least $1 - 2\alpha$ according to Bonferroni's inequality. But due to the fact that the confidence coefficient of $[\sigma^2 \, \eta_L \, , \, \sigma^2 \, \eta_U]$ is exactly $1 - \alpha$, the resulting confidence interval (7.13) may be very conservative, that is, the confidence coefficient is larger than $1 - \alpha$. So, we also consider a confidence interval for σ_a^2 with the estimator MS_2 for σ^2 instead of the bounds of the confidence interval for σ^2, that is,

$$\widetilde{\mathrm{CI}}(\sigma_a^2) : [\mathrm{MS}_2 \, \eta_L \, , \, \mathrm{MS}_2 \, \eta_U] \, . \qquad (7.14)$$

Through extensive simulation studies conducted by Hartung and Knapp (2000), the observations of Burdick and Eickman (1986) are confirmed in the sense that the

Thomas-Hultquist interval may be very liberal for small σ_a^2, that is, the confidence coefficient lies considerably below $1 - \alpha$. In these situations, the Burdick-Eickman interval has a confidence coefficient which is always larger than $1 - \alpha$, but the interval can be very conservative. If σ_a^2 becomes larger, both intervals are very similar. The confidence interval deduced from Wald's confidence interval for the ratio η with the bounds of the confidence interval of the error variance as estimates for the error variance has always a confidence coefficient at least as great as $1 - \alpha$, but this interval can be very conservative for large σ_a^2. A good compromise for the whole range of σ_a^2 is the confidence interval (7.14), which has a confidence coefficient at least as great as $1 - \alpha$ for small σ_a^2, and for growing σ_a^2 the confidence interval only becomes moderately conservative.

7.2.3   Exact test and confidence interval for σ_a^2 based on a generalized P-value approach

In this section we describe the relatively new notion of a generalized P-value and its applications to our problem. The original ideas are due to Tsui and Weerahandi (1989) and Weerahandi (1993).

We start with a general description of the notion of a generalized P-value. If X is a random variable whose distribution depends on the scalar parameter θ of interest and a set of nuisance parameters η and the problem is to test

$$H_0 : \theta \leq \theta_0 \quad \text{versus} \quad H_1 : \theta > \theta_0,$$

a generalized P-value approach proceeds by judiciously specifying a test variable $T(X; x, \theta, \eta)$ which depends on the random variable X, its observed value x, and the parameters θ and η, satisfying the following three properties:

(i) The sampling distribution of $T(X; x, \theta, \eta)$ derived from that of X, for fixed x, is free of the nuisance parameter η.

(ii) The observed value of $T(X; x, \theta, \eta)$ when $X = x$, that is, $T(x; x, \theta, \eta)$, is free of the nuisance parameter η.

(iii) $\Pr[T(X; x, \theta, \eta) \geq t]$ is nondecreasing in θ for fixed x and η.

Under the above conditions, a generalized P-value is defined by

$$\text{gen}.P = \Pr[T(X; x, \theta_0, \eta) \geq t],$$

where $t = T(x; x, \theta_0, \eta)$.

In the same spirit as above, Weerahandi (1993) constructed a one-sided confidence bound for θ based on a test variable $T_1(X; x, \theta, \eta)$ satisfying the above three properties and also the added constraint that the observed value of T_1 is $T_1(x; x, \theta, \eta) = \theta$. Let $t_1(x)$ satisfy the condition

$$\Pr[T_1 \leq t_1(x)] = 1 - \alpha.$$

Then $t_1(x)$ can be regarded as a $(1 - \alpha)$-level upper confidence limit for θ.

We now turn our attention to the applications of this concept to our specific problem.

(a) **An exact test for $H_0 : \sigma_a^2 = \delta > 0$ in the balanced case.** This testing problem is commonly known in the literature as a nonstandard testing problem in the sense that there are no obvious pivots or exact tests for testing this null hypothesis based on the two sums of squares: BSS and WSS. Recall that, in the balanced case, this fact follows from the canonical form of the model based on two independent sums of squares, BSS $\sim (\sigma^2 + n\sigma_a^2)\chi_{(k-1)}^2$ and WSS $\sim \sigma^2 \chi_{k(n-1)}^2$. While it is obvious that an exact test for $\sigma_a^2 = 0$ or even for $\sigma_a^2/\sigma^2 = \delta$ can be easily constructed simply by taking the ratio of BSS and WSS, the same is not true for the null hypothesis $H_0 : \sigma_a^2 = \delta$ for some $\delta > 0$. We now describe a test for this hypothesis in the balanced case based on a generalized P-value.

In our context, taking $X = (\text{BSS}, \text{WSS})$, $x = (\text{bss}, \text{wss})$, the observed values of X, $\theta = \sigma_a^2$ and $\eta = \sigma^2$, we define

$$T(\text{BSS}, \text{WSS}; \text{bss}, \text{wss}, \sigma_a^2, \sigma^2) = \frac{n\,\sigma_a^2 + \text{wss}\,(\sigma^2/\text{WSS})}{\text{bss}\,[(n\,\sigma_a^2 + \sigma^2)/\text{BSS}]}$$

It is easy to verify that T defined above satisfies the conditions (i)–(iii), and hence the generalized P-value for testing $H_0 : \sigma_a^2 = \delta$ or $H_0 : \sigma_a^2 \leq \delta$ versus $H_1 : \sigma_a^2 > \delta$ is given by

$$\text{gen.}P = \Pr[T \geq 1] = \Pr\left[\frac{n\delta + \text{wss}/U_e}{\text{bss}/U_a} \geq 1\right]$$

where $U_a = \text{BSS}/(\sigma^2 + n\sigma_a^2) \sim \chi_{k-1}^2$ and $U_e = \text{WSS}/\sigma^2 \sim \chi_{k(n-1)}^2$. The test procedure rejects H_0 if the generalized P-value is small. We should point out that the computation of the generalized P-values in this and similar other problems can be easily done by simulation using standard statistical software.

(b) **One-sided confidence bound for σ_a^2 in the balanced case.** We define

$$T_1 = T(\text{BSS}, \text{WSS}; \text{bss}, \text{wss}, \sigma_a^2, \sigma^2)$$

$$= \frac{1}{n}\left[\frac{\text{bss}\,(n\sigma_a^2 + \sigma^2)}{\text{BSS}} - \frac{\text{wss}\,\sigma^2}{\text{WSS}}\right] = \frac{1}{n}\left[\frac{\text{bss}}{U_a} - \frac{\text{wss}}{U_e}\right]$$

It is then easy to verify that the sampling distribution of T_1, for fixed $x = (\text{bss}, \text{wss})$, does not depend on σ^2 and that the observed value of T_1 is indeed σ_a^2. Let $t_1(\text{bss}, \text{wss})$ satisfy the condition

$$\Pr[T_1 \leq t_1(\text{bss}, \text{wss})] = 1 - \alpha.$$

Then $t_1(\text{bss}, \text{wss})$ can be regarded as a $(1 - \alpha)$-level upper confidence limit for σ_a^2.

We now provide an example from Verbeke and Molenberghs (1997) to illustrate the application of this approach.

Example 7.1. This example demonstrating the application of a generalized P-value to find an upper confidence limit of σ_a^2 is taken from Verbeke and Molenberghs (1997). To measure the efficiency of an antibiotic after it has been stored for two years, eight batches of the drug are randomly selected from a population of available batches and a random sample of size 2 is taken from each selected batch (balanced design). Data representing the concentration of the active component are given in Table 7.1.

Table 7.1 Concentration of the active component

Batch:	1	2	3	4	5	6	7	8
Observations	40	33	46	55	63	35	56	34
	42	34	47	52	59	38	56	29

Employing the very natural one-way balanced random effects model here and doing some routine computations, the ANOVA in Table 7.2 is obtained. It is evident from the ANOVA table that a batch-to-batch variability is very much in existence in this problem, implying $\sigma_a^2 > 0$.

Table 7.2 ANOVA table for the active component example

	Sum of squares	df	Mean squares	Expected mean squares
Batches	BSS = 1708	7	BMS = 244.1	$2\sigma_a^2 + \sigma^2$
Error	WSS = 32.5	8	WMS = 4.062	σ^2

In order to derive a 95% upper confidence interval for the parameter σ_a^2, it is indeed possible to use the familiar Satterthwaite approximation which is as follows. The estimate of σ_a^2 is

$$\hat{\sigma}_a^2 = \frac{\text{BMS} - \text{WMS}}{2}.$$

Consider the approximation $\nu\,\hat{\sigma}_a^2/\sigma_a^2 \sim \chi_\nu^2$ and equating the second moments yields

$$\hat{\nu} = \frac{(\text{BMS}/2 - \text{WMS}/2)^2}{\text{BMS}^2/7 + \text{WMS}^2/8} = 1.69.$$

This leads to the interval

$$\sigma_a^2 \le \hat{\nu}\,\hat{\sigma}_a^2/\chi_{\hat{\nu};0.05}^2 = 3707.50,$$

which is just useless for this problem.

On the other hand, the application of a generalized confidence interval to this problem, as developed here, based on $T_1 = (1708/U_a - 32.5/U_e)/2$, yields $\sigma_a^2 \le 392.27$, which is much more informative than the previous bound.

(c) **An exact test for** $H_0 : \sigma_a^2 = \delta > 0$ **and a confidence bound for** σ_a^2 **in the unbalanced case**. For testing $H_0 : \sigma_a^2 = \delta > 0$ versus the alternative $H_1 : \sigma_a^2 > \delta$, a potential generalized test variable can be defined as follows.

Define

$$\rho = \frac{\sigma_a^2}{\sigma^2}, \quad w_i(\rho) = \frac{n_i}{1 + \rho\, n_i},$$

and

$$\bar{Y}_w(\rho) = \sum_{i=1}^{k} w_i(\rho)\, \bar{Y}_{i.} \Big/ \sum_{i=1}^{k} w_i(\rho) \sim N\left(\mu, \sigma^2 \Big/ \sum_{i=1}^{k} w_i(\rho)\right).$$

Let

$$S_{wB}(\rho) = \sum_{i=1}^{k} w_i(\rho)\left[\bar{Y}_{i.} - \bar{Y}_w(\rho)\right]^2 \sim \sigma^2 \chi_{k-1}^2.$$

Define $W_1 = \text{WSS}/\sigma^2 \sim \chi_{N-k}^2$ and $W_2 = S_{wB}(\rho)/\sigma^2 \sim \chi_{k-1}^2$, which are independent. Finally, let

$$T(S_{wB}(\rho), \text{WSS}; s_{wB}, \text{wss}, \sigma_a^2, \sigma^2)$$

$$= \frac{\text{wss}\, S_{wB}(\rho)}{\text{WSS}\, s_{wB}\left(\frac{\sigma_a^2}{\sigma^2}\frac{\text{WSS}}{\text{wss}}\right)} = \frac{W_2\, \text{wss}}{W_1\, s_{wB}\left(\frac{\sigma_a^2\, W_1}{\text{wss}}\right)}$$

It is easily seen from the second equality above that the distribution of the test variable $T(S_{wB}(\rho), \text{WSS}; s_{wB}, \text{wss}, \sigma_a^2, \sigma^2)$ depends only on the parameter of interest, namely, σ_a^2, and is independent of the nuisance parameter σ^2! It also follows from the first equality above that the observed value of $T(S_{wB}(\rho), \text{WSS}; s_{wB}, \text{wss}, \sigma_a^2, \sigma^2)$ is 1. Hence, the generalized P-value for testing $H_0 : \sigma_a^2 = \delta > 0$ versus the alternative $H_1 : \sigma_a^2 > \delta$ is given by

$$\begin{aligned}
\text{gen.}P &= \Pr[T(S_{wB}(\rho), \text{WSS}; s_{wB}, \text{wss}, \sigma_a^2, \sigma^2) \geq 1 \mid \sigma_a^2 = \delta] \\
&= \Pr\left[W_2 \geq \frac{W_1}{\text{wss}}\, s_{wB}\, \frac{W_2 \delta}{\text{wss}}\right]
\end{aligned}$$

The generalized confidence bounds for σ_a^2 can be obtained by solving the equations

$$\Pr\left[W_2 \geq \frac{W_1}{\text{wss}}\, s_{wB}\, \frac{W_2\, \delta_1}{\text{wss}}\right] = \frac{\alpha}{2}$$

$$\Pr\left[W_2 \geq \frac{W_1}{\text{wss}}\, s_{wB}\, \frac{W_2\, \delta_2}{\text{wss}}\right] = 1 - \frac{\alpha}{2}$$

in which case $[\delta_2, \delta_1]$ is the $100(1 - \alpha)\%$ generalized confidence interval for σ_a^2.

7.2.4   Tests and confidence intervals for μ

In this section we discuss some tests and confidence intervals for the overall mean parameter μ. Clearly, an unbiased estimate of μ is given by the overall sample mean $\bar{y} = \sum \bar{y}_i/k$ whose distribution is normal with mean μ and variance $\eta^2 = \sum(\sigma_a^2 + \sigma^2/n_i)/k^2$. In the balanced case when $n_1 = \cdots = n_k = n$, $\bar{Y}_i$'s are iid with a common mean μ and a common variance $\sigma_a^2 + \sigma^2/n$ so that a t test can be carried out to test hypotheses about μ and also the usual t statistic can be used to derive confidence limits for μ. In the unbalanced case, however, only some approximate tests and confidence intervals for μ can be developed. We can easily estimate the common within-study variance σ^2 by just combining the within-sample variances MS_2 with a combined df $N - k$. As for the other variance component, namely, the between-study variance σ_a^2, since the usual ANOVA estimate can assume negative values, many modifications of it are available in the literature. A normal approximation is then used for the distribution of the so-called studentized variable $t = (\bar{Y} - \mu)/\hat{\sigma}(\bar{Y})$ to obtain approximate tests and confidence intervals for μ. Details can be found in Rukhin and Vangel (1998) and Rukhin, Biggerstaff, and Vangel (2000).

An exact test for μ in the unbalanced case is described in Iyer, Wang, and Mathew (2004) using the notion of the generalized P-value. However, the solution is rather complicated and we omit the details.

7.3   HETEROGENEOUS ERROR VARIANCES

In this section we discuss the problem of drawing appropriate inferences about the overall mean μ and the between-study variability σ_a^2 under the more realistic scenario of heterogeneous error or within-study variances. It is obvious that one can estimate a within-study variance σ_i^2 from replicated observations from the ith study. However, the associated inference problems for μ and σ_a^2 here are quite hard and some satisfactory solutions have been offered only recently.

7.3.1   Tests for $H_0 : \sigma_a^2 = 0$

It is of course clear that testing the nullity of the between-study variance $H_0 : \sigma_a^2 = 0$ is easy to carry out because, under the null hypothesis, one has the usual fixed effects model with heterogeneous error or within-study variances. Thus, all the test procedures described in Chapter 6 are applicable here. Argac, Makambi, and Hartung (2001) performed some simulation in the context of this problem in an attempt to compare the proposed tests in terms of power and recommended the use of an adjusted Welch test (see Chapter 6) in most cases.

7.3.2   Tests for $H_0 : \sigma_a^2 = \delta > 0$

In many situations it is known a priori that some positive level of between-study variability may be present and it is desired to prescribe a test for a designated positive value for this parameter. Due to the heterogeneous error variances, it is clear that the testing problem here is quite difficult. We provide below two solutions to this problem.

Solution 1. Hartung, Makambi, and Argac (2001) proposed a test statistic for this problem which they called an extended ANOVA test statistic, and this is given by

$$F_A^* = \frac{\sum_{i=1}^k h_i \left(\bar{Y}_{i.} - \sum_{j=1}^k h_j \, \bar{Y}_{j.} \right)^2 / (k-1)}{\delta \sum_{i=1}^k h_i^2 + \sum_{i=1}^k h_i^2 \, S_i^2 / n_i}$$

with $h_i = w_i / \sum_{j=1}^k w_j$, $w_i = 1/\tilde{\tau}_i^2$, and $\tilde{\tau}_i^2 = \delta + S_i^2 / n_i$. Under the null hypothesis $H_0 : \sigma_a^2 = \delta$, the test statistic F_A^* is approximately F distributed with $k - 1$ and $\hat{\nu}_A$ degrees of freedom, where

$$\hat{\nu}_A = \frac{\left(\sum_{i=1}^k h_i^2 \, \tilde{\tau}_i^2 \right)^2}{\sum_{i=1}^k h_i^4 \, S_i^4 \, / \, [n_i^2 \, (n_i + 1)]} - 2.$$

So, we reject $H_0 : \sigma_a^2 = \delta$ at level α if $F^* > F_{m-1, \hat{\nu}_R; \alpha}$.

Solution 2. Hartung and Argac (2002) derived an extension of the Welch test statistic given by

$$F_W^* = \frac{\sum_{i=1}^k w_i \left(\bar{y}_{i.} - \sum_{j=1}^k h_j \bar{y}_{j.} \right)^2}{(k-1) + 2(k-2)(k-1)^{-1} \sum_{i=1}^k (1 - h_i)^2 / \hat{\nu}_i}$$

with $h_i = w_i / \sum_{j=1}^k w_j$, $w_i = 1/(\delta + S_i^2 / n_i)$, and

$$\hat{\nu}_i = \frac{2(\delta + S_i^2 / n_i)^2}{2 S_i^2 / [n_i^2 \, (n_i + 1)]}.$$

The test statistic F_W^* is approximately F distributed under the null hypothesis with $k - 1$ and $\hat{\nu}_W$ degrees of freedom, where

$$\hat{\nu}_W = \frac{k^2 - 1}{3 \sum_{i=1}^k (1 - h_i)^2 / \hat{\nu}_i}.$$

The null hypothesis is rejected at level α if $F_W^* > F_{k-1, \hat{\nu}_W; \alpha}$.

In the next section, appropriate confidence intervals of σ_a^2 will be presented, which in turn can also be used to test the significance of a designated positive value of this parameter.

7.3.3   Nonnegative estimation of σ_a^2 and confidence intervals

In this section we discuss various procedures to derive nonnegative estimates of the central parameter of interest, namely, σ_a^2, and also procedures to derive its confidence interval. We point out that the estimators are based either on quadratic forms of y or on likelihood methods.

Rao, Kaplan, and Cochran (1981) discussed extensively the parameter estimation in the one-way random effects models. We present here three estimators of σ_a^2 from this paper that are generally eligible for use in meta-analysis. With the between- and within-class sum of squares, the unbiased ANOVA-type estimator of σ_a^2 has the form

$$\hat{\sigma}_a^2 = \left(\frac{N}{N^2 - \sum_{i=1}^k n_i^2} \right) \left(\sum_{i=1}^k n_i (\bar{Y}_{i.} - \bar{Y}_{..})^2 - \sum_{i=1}^k \left(1 - \frac{n_i}{n} \right) S_i^2 \right). \quad (7.15)$$

Based on the unweighted sum of squares, the unbiased ANOVA-type estimator of the between-group variance is given by

$$\hat{\sigma}_a^2 = \frac{1}{k-1} \sum_{i=1}^k \left(\bar{Y}_i - \bar{Y}^* \right)^2 - \frac{1}{k} \sum_{i=1}^k \frac{S_i^2}{n_i} \quad (7.16)$$

with $\bar{Y}^* = \sum_{i=1}^k \bar{Y}_i / k$ as the mean of the group means. Both estimators (7.15) and (7.16) are unbiased estimators of σ_a^2. However, both estimators can yield negative values. Based on Rao's (1972) MINQUE principle without the condition of unbiasedness, Rao, Kaplan, and Cochran (1981) also provided an always nonnegative estimator of σ_a^2 as

$$\hat{\sigma}_a^2 = \frac{1}{k} \sum_{i=1}^k \ell_i^2 \left(\bar{Y}_{i.} - \bar{\bar{Y}}_{..} \right)^2, \quad (7.17)$$

where $\ell_i = n_i / (n_i + 1)$ and $\bar{\bar{Y}}_{..} = (\sum_{i=1}^k \ell_i \bar{Y}_{i.}) / (\sum_{i=1}^k \ell_i)$.

In the biomedical literature, an estimator proposed by DerSimonian and Laird (1986) is widely used. Based on Cochran's homogeneity statistic (see Chapters 4 and 6) and using the method-of-moment approach in the one-way random effects model assuming known within-group variances σ_i^2, they derived the estimator

$$\hat{\sigma}_a^2 = \frac{\sum_{i=1}^k w_i (\bar{Y}_{i.} - \tilde{Y}_{..})^2 - (k-1)}{\sum_{i=1}^k w_i - \sum_{i=1}^k w_i^2 / \sum_{i=1}^k w_i}, \quad (7.18)$$

where $\tilde{Y}_{..} = \sum_{i=1}^k w_i \bar{Y}_{i.} / \sum_{i=1}^k w_i$ and in the present model $w_i = n_i / \sigma_i^2$. The estimator (7.18) is an unbiased estimator of σ_a^2 given known σ_i^2. In practice, estimates of the within-group variances have to be plugged in and then, naturally, the resultant estimator of σ_a^2 is no longer unbiased. Moreover, like the unbiased ANOVA-type estimators (7.15) and (7.16), the DerSimonian-Laird estimator can yield negative estimates with positive probability.

Using the general approach of nonnegative minimum-biased invariant quadratic estimation of variance components proposed by Hartung (1981), Heine (1993) derived the nonnegative minimum-biased estimator of σ_a^2 in the present model. If $N - 2n_i \geq 0$, $i = 1, \ldots, k$, this estimator reads

$$\hat{\sigma}_a^2 = \frac{n^2 \sum_{i=1}^k n_i^2 \prod_{\ell' \neq \ell}(N - 2n_{\ell'})(\bar{Y}_{i.} - \bar{Y}_{..})^2}{\left(\sum_{\ell=1}^k n_\ell^2 + 1\right) \sum_{\ell=1}^k n_\ell(N - n_\ell)\prod_{\ell' \neq \ell}(N - 2n_{\ell'})}.$$

Hartung and Makambi (2002) proposed two further nonnegative estimators of σ_a^2. We present their ideas here in more detail. Let $b = (b_1, \ldots, b_k)'$ be weights such that $\sum_{i=1}^k b_i = 1$. Then, $\hat{\mu}(b) = \sum_{i=1}^k b_i \bar{Y}_{i.}$ is an unbiased estimator of μ. Define the quadratic form

$$Q(b) = \sum_{i=1}^k \gamma_i \left[\bar{Y}_{i.} - \hat{\mu}(b)\right]^2,$$

where $\gamma_i = b_i^2/\{(1 - 2\, b_i)\sum_{j=1}^k b_j(1 - b_j)/(1 - 2\, b_j)\}$. Note that none of the weights is allowed to be equal to 0.5. Hartung and Makambi (2002) then show that

$$\hat{\sigma}_a^2 = \frac{1}{\sum_{j=1}^k b_j^2}\left(Q(b) - \sum_{i=1}^k b_i^2 \frac{S_i^2}{n_i}\right) \tag{7.19}$$

is an unbiased estimator for σ_a^2 given that the weights b_i are known. In case the weights b_i depend on unknown parameters which have to be estimated, then, by plugging in the estimated weights in (7.19), the resulting estimator is no longer unbiased for σ_a^2. Like the unbiased ANOVA-type estimators and the DerSimonian-Laird estimator, the estimator (7.19) also can yield negative estimates. Thus, Hartung and Makambi are led to derive a nonnegative estimator of σ_a^2. Starting with the quadratic form $Q_1(b) = Q(b)/\sum_{i=1}^k b_i^2$ as a possible nonnegative estimator of σ_a^2 and bias adjusting this estimator according to the uniformly minimum-bias principle by Hartung (1981), they obtain the estimator

$$\hat{\sigma}_a^2 = \frac{Q_1(b)}{Q_1(b) + 2\sum_{i=1}^k r_i\hat{\sigma}_i^2/n_i}\, Q_1(b)$$

where $r_i = b_i^2/\sum_{j=1}^k b_j^2$.

Using the same principle as above, Hartung and Makambi (2002) also derive a nonnegative estimator based on Cochran's homogeneity statistic

$$Q_C = \sum_{i=1}^k w_i(\bar{Y}_{i.} - \tilde{Y}_{..})^2,$$

which is the basic quadratic form in the DerSimonian-Laird estimator (7.18). Their second nonnegative estimator is given by

$$\hat{\sigma}_a^2 = \frac{\lambda}{\sum_{i=1}^k w_i - \sum_{i=1}^k w_i^2/\sum_{i=1}^k w_i}\, Q_C, \tag{7.20}$$

where

$$\lambda = \frac{Q_C}{2(k-1) + Q_C}.$$

Maximum likelihood estimation in the present model has already been discussed by Cochran (1954). Rukhin, Biggerstaff, and Vangel (2000) provide the estimation equations of the maximum likelihood (ML) and the restricted maximum likelihood estimator (REML) estimator of σ_a^2. Moreover, Rukhin, Biggerstaff, and Vangel (2000) show that the REML estimator of σ_a^2 is closed to the Mandel-Paule (1970) estimator.

The Mandel-Paule estimator is based on the quadratic form

$$Q = \sum_{i=1}^{k} \omega_i \left(\bar{Y}_{i.} - \bar{Y}_\omega \right)^2$$

with $\bar{Y}_\omega = \sum_{i=1}^{k} \omega_i \bar{Y}_{i.} / \sum_{i=1}^{k} \omega_i$ and $\omega_i = (\sigma_a^2 + \sigma_i^2/n_i)^{-1}$. For known variance components, Q is a chi-square distributed random variable with $k-1$ df. By plugging in estimates of σ_i^2 in Q, we obtain

$$\tilde{Q}(\sigma_a^2) = \sum_{i=1}^{k} \tilde{\omega}_i \left(\bar{Y}_{i.} - \bar{Y}_{\tilde{\omega}} \right)^2 \tag{7.21}$$

with $\bar{Y}_{\tilde{\omega}} = \sum_{i=1}^{k} \tilde{\omega}_i \bar{Y}_{i.} / \sum_{i=1}^{k} \tilde{\omega}_i$ and $\tilde{\omega}_i = (\sigma_a^2 + S_i^2/n_i)^{-1}$. The quadratic form $\tilde{Q}(\sigma_a^2)$ is a strictly monotone decreasing function in σ_a^2, so that $\tilde{Q}(0) > \tilde{Q}(\sigma_a^2)$ for $\sigma_a^2 > 0$. Furthermore, $\tilde{Q}(\sigma_a^2)$ can be well approximated by a chi square random variable with $k-1$ df. The Mandel-Paule estimator for σ_a^2 is then given as the solution of the equation

$$\tilde{Q}(\sigma_a^2) = k - 1. \tag{7.22}$$

In case, $Q(0) < k - 1$, the estimate is set to zero.

In the one-way random effects model, usually all the data are available. Sometimes, only summary statistics are available and then we obtain the following model, which can be seen as a special case of the one-way random effects model. Let $(\bar{Y}_{1.}, S_1^2), (\bar{Y}_{2.}, S_2^2), \ldots, (\bar{Y}_{k.}, S_k^2)$ be independent observations representing summary estimates $\bar{Y}_{i.}$ of some parameter μ of interest from k independent sources, together with estimates S_i^2/n_i of the variances of $\bar{Y}_{i.}$, and n_i denotes the corresponding sample size. Then we consider the model

$$\bar{Y}_{i.} = \mu + a_i + e_i, \quad i = 1, \ldots, k, \tag{7.23}$$

where a_i are normally distributed random variables with mean zero and variance σ_a^2, representing the between-group variance, and e_i are normally distributed random variables with mean zero and variance σ_i^2/n_i. In model (7.23), we assume that the variances σ_i^2 are reasonably well estimated by the S_i^2 within the independent groups. So, we assume the σ_i^2 are known and simply replace them by their estimates s_i^2.

Taking the σ_i^2 as known, the estimating equations of the maximum likelihood estimators of μ and σ_a^2 are given by

$$\mu = \frac{\sum_{i=1}^{k} w_i(\sigma_a^2)\, \bar{Y}_{i.}}{\sum_{i=1}^{k} w_i(\sigma_a^2)}, \tag{7.24}$$

$$\sum_{i=1}^{k} w_i^2(\sigma_a^2)\,(\bar{Y}_{i.} - \mu)^2 = \sum_{i=1}^{k} w_i(\sigma_a^2), \tag{7.25}$$

where $w_i(\sigma_a^2) = (\sigma_a^2 + s_i^2/n_i)^{-1}$. A convenient form of Eq. (7.25) for iterative solution is given by

$$\sigma_a^2 = \frac{\sum_{i=1}^{k} w_i^2(\sigma_a^2)[(\bar{Y}_{i.} - \mu)^2 - s_i^2/n_i]}{\sum_{i=1}^{k} w_i^2(\sigma_a^2)}. \tag{7.26}$$

The restricted likelihood estimate of σ_a^2 is found numerically by iterating

$$\sigma_a^2 = \frac{\sum_{i=1}^{k} w_i^2(\sigma_a^2)[(\bar{Y}_{i.} - \hat{\mu}(\sigma_a^2))^2 - s_i^2/n_i]}{\sum_{i=1}^{k} w_i^2(\sigma_a^2)} + \frac{1}{\sum_{i=1}^{k} w_i(\sigma_a^2)}. \tag{7.27}$$

We conclude the discussion on point estimation with a classical example quoted from Snedecor and Cochran (1967, p. 290). The observed sample means and variances of the means are given in Table 7.3.

Table 7.3   Summary data on artificial insemination of cows

Bull number	Sample size n_i	Mean $\bar{Y}_i$	Variance S_i^2/n_i
1	5	41.2	35.14
2	2	64.5	30.25
3	7	56.3	18.99
4	5	39.6	101.06
5	7	67.1	38.64
6	9	53.2	27.72

Applying most of the estimators presented in this section to the data set, we obtain the estimates given in Table 7.4. There is substantial variation between the point estimates. The maximum likelihood estimate (7.26) yields the smallest value with 51.35 and the ANOVA-type estimate (7.16) the largest one with 89.68.

Recently, Hartung and Knapp (2005a) as well as Viechtbauer (2007) proposed a confidence interval using the quadratic form (7.21) which Mandel and Paule (1970) have used for their estimate of σ_a^2 in Eq. (7.22). Hartung and Knapp (2005a) derived the first two moments of $\tilde{Q}(\sigma_a^2)$ and discussed the accuracy of the approximation to the χ^2 distribution with $k - 1$ df.

Table 7.4 Estimates for the variation between the bulls

Formula	Estimate	Formula	Estimate
Eq. (7.15)	76.42	Eq. (7.20)	58.44
Eq. (7.16)	89.68	Eq. (7.22)	81.40
Eq. (7.17)	73.43	Eq. (7.26)	51.35
Eq. (7.18)	64.80	Eq. (7.27)	72.83

Hartung and Knapp (2005a) showed that $\tilde{Q}(\sigma_a^2)$ is a monotone decreasing function in σ_a^2 and thus proposed a $1 - \alpha$ confidence region for the among-group variance defined by

$$\text{CI}(\sigma_a^2) = \left\{ \sigma_a^2 \geq 0 \mid \chi_{k-1;1-\alpha/2}^2 \leq \tilde{Q}(\sigma_a^2) \leq \chi_{k-1;\alpha/2}^2 \right\}. \qquad (7.28)$$

Since $\tilde{Q}(\sigma_a^2)$ is a monotone decreasing function in $\sigma_a^2 \geq 0$, the function $\tilde{Q}(\sigma_a^2)$ has its maximal value at $\tilde{Q}(0)$. For $\tilde{Q}(0) < \chi_{k-1;\alpha/2}^2$, we define $C_1(\sigma_a^2) = \{0\}$; otherwise the confidence region $C_1(\sigma_a^2)$ is a genuine interval. Note that the validity of the inequality $\tilde{Q}(0) < \chi_{k-1;\alpha/2}^2$ only depends on the choice of α. To determine the bounds of the confidence interval one has to solve the two equations for σ_a^2, namely

$$\begin{array}{ll} \text{lower bound:} & \tilde{Q}(\sigma_a^2) = \chi_{k-1;\alpha/2}^2, \\ \text{upper bound:} & \tilde{Q}(\sigma_a^2) = \chi_{k-1;1-\alpha/2}^2. \end{array} \qquad (7.29)$$

Likelihood-based confidence intervals have been proposed by Hardy and Thompson (1996), Biggerstaff and Tweedie (1997), and Viechtbauer (2007). Recall that

$$\bar{Y}_i \sim N\left(\mu, \sigma_a^2 + \frac{\sigma_i^2}{n_i} \right), \quad i = 1, \ldots, k;$$

then it holds for the log-likelihood function of μ and σ_a^2,

$$l(\mu, \tau^2) \propto -\frac{1}{2} \sum_{i=1}^{k} \ln\left(\tau^2 + \frac{\sigma_i^2}{n_i} \right) - \frac{1}{2} \sum_{i=1}^{k} \frac{(\bar{Y}_i - \mu)^2}{\sigma_a^2 + \sigma_i^2}.$$

The two estimating equations for μ and σ_a^2 are

$$\hat{\mu} = \frac{\sum_{i=1}^{k} w_i \bar{Y}_i}{\sum_{i=1}^{k} w_i} \qquad (7.30)$$

and

$$\hat{\sigma}_a^2 = \frac{w_i^2 \left[(\bar{Y}_i - \hat{\mu})^2 - \sigma_i^2/n_i \right]}{\sum_{i=1}^{k} w_i^2} \qquad (7.31)$$

with $w_i = 1/(\sigma_a^2 + \sigma_i^2/n_i)$, $i = 1, \ldots, k$. Let $\hat{\mu}_{\text{ML}}$ and $\hat{\sigma}_{a,\text{ML}}^2$ denote the ML estimators. A confidence interval for σ_a^2 can then be obtained by profiling the likelihood ratio statistic; see Hardy and Thompson (1996). Denote $\tilde{\mu}$ as that value of (7.30) with $w_i = 1/(\tilde{\sigma}_a^2 + \sigma_i^2/n_i)$. Then, a $100(1-\alpha)\%$ confidence interval for σ_a^2 is given by

$$\mathrm{CI}(\sigma_a^2) : \left\{\tilde{\sigma}_a^2 \mid -2\left[l(\tilde{\mu}, \tilde{\sigma}_a^2) - l(\hat{\mu}_{\mathrm{ML}}, \hat{\sigma}_{a,\mathrm{ML}}^2)\right] < \chi_{1;\alpha}^2\right\}$$
$$= \left\{\tilde{\sigma}_a^2 \mid l(\tilde{\mu}, \tilde{\sigma}_a^2) > l(\hat{\mu}_{\mathrm{ML}}, \hat{\sigma}_{a,\mathrm{ML}}^2) - \chi_{1;\alpha}^2/2\right\}. \tag{7.32}$$

Alternatively, one can base the confidence interval on the restricted log-likelihood. Following Viechtbauer (2007), it holds for the restricted log-likelihood for σ_a^2,

$$l_R(\sigma_a^2) \propto -\frac{1}{2}\sum_{i=1}^{k} \ln\left(\sigma_a^2 + \frac{\sigma_i^2}{n_i}\right) - \frac{1}{2}\sum_{i=1}^{k}\frac{1}{\sigma_a^2 + \sigma_i^2/n_i} - \frac{1}{2}\sum_{i=1}^{k}\frac{(\bar{Y}_i - \hat{\mu})^2}{\sigma_a^2 + \sigma_i^2/n_i}.$$

The estimating equation for σ_a^2 is given by

$$\hat{\sigma}_a^2 = \frac{\sum_{i=1}^{k} w_i^2\left[(\bar{Y}_i - \hat{\mu})^2 - \sigma_i^2/n_i\right]}{\sum_{i=1}^{k} w_i^2} + \frac{1}{\sum_{i=1}^{k} w_i}.$$

Let $\hat{\sigma}_{a,\mathrm{REML}}^2$ denote the REML estimate. Then, a $100(1-\alpha)\%$ confidence interval for σ_a^2 is given by

$$\mathrm{CI}(\sigma_a^2) : \left\{\tilde{\sigma}_a^2 \mid -2\left[l_R(\tilde{\sigma}_a^2) - l_R(\hat{\sigma}_{a,\mathrm{REML}}^2)\right] < \chi_{1;\alpha}^2\right\}$$
$$= \left\{\tilde{\sigma}_a^2 \mid l_R(\tilde{\sigma}_a^2) > l_R(\hat{\sigma}_{a,\mathrm{REML}}^2) - \chi_{1;\alpha}^2/2\right\} \tag{7.33}$$

The asymptotic sampling variances of the ML and REML estimates of σ_a^2 can be obtained by taking the inverse of the Fisher information. Following Viechtbauer (2007), these variances are, respectively, equal to

$$\mathrm{Var}\left(\hat{\sigma}_{a,\mathrm{ML}}^2\right) = 2\left(\sum_{i=1}^{k} w_i\right)^{-1} \tag{7.34}$$

and

$$\mathrm{Var}\left(\hat{\sigma}_{a,\mathrm{REML}}^2\right) = 2\left(\sum_{i=1}^{k} w_i^2 - 2\frac{\sum_{i=1}^{k} w_i^3}{\sum_{i=1}^{k} w_i} + \frac{\left(\sum_{i=1}^{k} w_i^2\right)^2}{\left(\sum_{i=1}^{k} w_i\right)^2}\right)^{-1}. \tag{7.35}$$

Estimates of the sampling variances are obtained by setting $w_i = 1/(\hat{\sigma}_{a,\mathrm{ML}}^2 + \sigma_i^2/n_i)$ and $w_i = 1/(\hat{\sigma}_{a,\mathrm{REML}}^2 + \sigma_i^2/n_i)$ in Eqs. (7.34) and (7.35), respectively.

Based on the asymptotic normality assumption of ML and REML estimates, $100(1-\alpha)\%$ Wald-type confidence intervals for σ_a^2 are given by

$$\mathrm{CI}(\sigma_a^2) : \hat{\sigma}_{a,\mathrm{ML}}^2 \pm \sqrt{\widehat{\mathrm{Var}}\left(\hat{\sigma}_{a,\mathrm{ML}}^2\right)}\, z_{\alpha/2} \tag{7.36}$$

Table 7.5   95% confidence intervals for σ_a^2 in the artificial insemination example

Method	95% CI
Confidence interval (7.29)	$[5.739, 737.953]$
Confidence interval (7.32)	$[< 0.001, 346.477]$
Confidence interval (7.33)	$[< 0.001, 523.007]$
Confidence interval (7.36)	$[0, 148.593]$
Confidence interval (7.37)	$[0, 208.206]$

and

$$\text{CI}(\sigma_a^2) : \hat{\sigma}_{\text{REML}}^2 \pm \sqrt{\widehat{\text{Var}}\left(\hat{\sigma}_{\text{REML}}^2\right)}\, z_{\alpha/2}. \tag{7.37}$$

Applying the five confidence intervals to the data set from Table 7.3, we obtain the approximate 95% confidence intervals for σ_a^2 given in Table 7.5.

The Q-profiling confidence interval (7.29) is the widest one and clearly excludes the value zero, and the profile REML confidence interval (7.33) is the second widest in this example. The two Wald-type confidence intervals include the value zero; the lower bounds of the profile-type confidence intervals are tight to zero but positive.

Extensive simulation studies by Hartung and Knapp (2005a) and Viechtbauer (2007) have shown that the confidence interval (7.29) has, in general, the best actual confidence coefficient compared to the nominal one, so that this interval can generally be recommended.

7.3.4   Inference about μ

In the last section of this chapter, we present some results on estimation, tests, and confidence intervals of the overall mean μ.

Let us recall $\bar{Y}_i \sim N(\mu, \sigma_a^2 + \sigma_i^2/n_i)$. Then, when the within-study variances are known, the uniformly minimum variance unbiased estimator of μ is given by

$$\hat{\mu} = \frac{\sum_{i=1}^k w_i\, \bar{Y}_i}{\sum_{i=1}^k w_i},$$

where $w_i = (\sigma_a^2 + \sigma_i^2/n_i)^{-1}, i = 1, \ldots, k$. Then it holds for the standardized variable

$$Z = \frac{\hat{\mu}}{\left(\sum_{i=1}^k w_i\right)^{-1/2}} \sim N(\mu, 1).$$

However, in practice, we have to estimate the usually unknown variances. The within-population variances σ_i^2 are estimated by their sample counterparts, and the between-population variance σ_a^2 can be estimated using an estimator from the previous section. Finally, we obtain an approximate $100(1 - \alpha)\%$ confidence interval for μ as

$$\hat{\mu} = \frac{\sum_{i=1}^k \hat{w}_i\, \bar{Y}_i}{\sum_{i=1}^k \hat{w}_i} \pm \left(\sum_{i=1}^k \hat{w}_i\right)^{-1/2} z_{\alpha/2} \tag{7.38}$$

with $\hat{w}_i = (\hat{\sigma}_a^2 + \hat{\sigma}_i^2/n_i)^{-1}$.

As is well known, in small to moderate samples, which is mostly the case in applications, this confidence interval suffers from the same weaknesses as its fixed effects counterpart. Namely, the actual confidence coefficient is below the nominal one. Consequently, the corresponding test on the overall mean yields too many unjustified significant results.

Several modifications of the above normal test and confidence interval have been suggested in the literature (Hartung, 1999b; Hartung and Knapp; 2001a,b; Sidik and Jonkman, 2002; Hartung, Böckenhoff, and Knapp, 2003). We should mention that most of the modifications are very similar. We present below some results from Hartung and Knapp (2001a,b).

The basic results for the improved test are that the quadratic form

$$\sum_{i=1}^{k} w_i \, (\bar{Y}_{i.} - \hat{\mu})^2$$

is a chi-square random variable with $k - 1$ df, stochastically independent of $\hat{\mu}$, and that

$$q := \widehat{\text{Var}}(\hat{\mu}) = \frac{1}{k-1} \frac{\sum_{i=1}^{k} w_i \, (\bar{Y}_{i.} - \hat{\mu})^2}{\sum_{i=1}^{k} w_i} \tag{7.39}$$

is an unbiased estimator of the variance of $\hat{\mu}$. Consequently, under $H_0 : \mu = 0$,

$$T = \frac{\hat{\mu}}{\widehat{\text{Var}}(\hat{\mu})} \tag{7.40}$$

is a t-distributed random variable with $k - 1$ degrees of freedom. The test statistic T depends on the unknown variance components which have to be replaced by appropriate estimates in practice. By substituting the variance components by their estimates, the resulting test statistic is then approximately t distributed with $k - 1$ df. So, the alternative approximate $100(1 - \alpha)\%$ confidence interval for μ reads

$$\hat{\hat{\mu}} = \frac{\sum_{i=1}^{k} \hat{w}_i \, \bar{Y}_i}{\sum_{i=1}^{k} \hat{w}_i} \pm \sqrt{\hat{q}} \, t_{k-1,\alpha/2} \tag{7.41}$$

with $\hat{q}$ the estimate according (7.39) with w_i replaced by $\hat{w}_i$.

Hartung and Knapp (2001a,b) conducted an extensive simulation study to compare the attained type I error rates for the commonly used confidence interval (7.38) and the proposed modified confidence interval (7.41). It turns out that the interval (7.41) greatly improves the attained confidence coefficient. Moreover, the good performance of the interval (7.41) does not heavily depend on the choice of the between-group variance estimator.

An exact test for μ in the present model is described in Iyer, Wang, and Mathew (2004) using the notion of the generalized P-value. However, the solution is rather complicated and we omit the details.

To conclude this chapter, let us analyze the data set from Table 7.3 and compute the approximate 95% confidence intervals for μ. The results are given in Table 7.6, where we have used three different estimates of the between-group variance from Table 7.4.

Table 7.6 Confidence intervals for μ in the artificial insemination example

Method for estimating σ_a^2	Estimate for μ	95% CI for μ based on (7.38)	95% CI for μ based on (7.41)
DSL from Eq. (7.18)	54.70	$[46.62, 62.77]$	$[43.34, 66.05]$
MLE from Eq. (7.26)	54.80	$[47.30, 62.29]$	$[43.54, 66.05]$
REML from Eq. (7.27)	54.64	$[46.25, 63.04]$	$[43.25, 66.04]$

Recall from Table 7.4 that the estimate for σ_a^2 from Eq. (7.18) is 64.80, from Eq. (7.26) is 51.35, and from Eq. (7.27) is 72.83. The overall estimate for μ is not so much affected by the choice of the between-group variance estimate. However, the confidence interval (7.38) is more affected by the estimate of σ_a^2. The larger the estimate of σ_a^2, the wider the interval. In contrast, the length of the interval (7.41) is relatively stable with respect to the estimate of σ_a^2.

response ratios is indicated which is of independent interest, for instance, in the field of ecology.

8.1   DIFFERENCE OF MEANS

Let us assume that in general there are k independent trials comparing a treatment (T) versus a control (C). Let X_{Tij}, $j = 1, \ldots, n_{Ti}$, $i = 1, \ldots, k$, be iid observations in the treatment group from a normal distribution with mean μ_{Ti} and variance σ_{Ti}^2 and X_{Cij}, $j = 1, \ldots, n_{Ci}$, $i = 1, \ldots, k$, be iid observations in the control group from a normal distribution with mean μ_{Ci} and variance σ_{Ci}^2. Define $\bar{X}_{Ti}$ and S_{Ti}^2 as well as $\bar{X}_{Ci}$ and S_{Ci}^2 as

$$
\bar{X}_{Ti} = \frac{1}{n_{Ti}} \sum_{j=1}^{n_{Ti}} X_{Tij}, \quad S_{Ti}^2 = \frac{1}{n_{Ti} - 1} \sum_{j=1}^{n_{Ti}} \left(X_{Tij} - \bar{X}_{Ti} \right)^2,
$$

and

$$
\bar{X}_{Ci} = \frac{1}{n_{Ci}} \sum_{j=1}^{n_{Ci}} X_{Cij}, \quad S_{Ci}^2 = \frac{1}{n_{Ci} - 1} \sum_{j=1}^{n_{Ci}} \left(X_{Cij} - \bar{X}_{Ci} \right)^2.
$$

Then it follows that

$$
\bar{X}_{Ti} \sim N\left(\mu_{Ti}, \frac{\sigma_{Ti}^2}{n_{Ti}} \right), \quad (n_{Ti} - 1)S_{Ti}^2 \sim \sigma_{Ti}^2 \, \chi_{n_{Ti}-1}^2, \tag{8.1}
$$

and

$$
\bar{X}_{Ci} \sim N\left(\mu_{Ci}, \frac{\sigma_{Ci}^2}{n_{Ci}} \right), \quad (n_{Ci} - 1)S_{Ci}^2 \sim \sigma_{Ci}^2 \, \chi_{n_{Ci}-1}^2. \tag{8.2}
$$

Note that the statistics (8.1) and (8.2) are all mutually independent. Assuming that in each trial the population variances are identical, that is, $\sigma_i^2 = \sigma_{Ti}^2 = \sigma_{Ci}^2$, $i = 1, \ldots, k$, then the pooled sample variance is given by

$$
S_i^{*2} = \frac{1}{n_{Ti} + n_{Ci} - 2} \left[(n_{Ti} - 1)S_{Ti}^2 + (n_{Ci} - 1)S_{Ci}^2 \right] \tag{8.3}
$$

and it follows that

$$
(n_{Ti} + n_{Ci} - 2)S_i^{*2} \sim \sigma_i^2 \chi_{n_{Ti}+n_{Ci}-2}^2. \tag{8.4}
$$

Let $\mu_{Di} = \mu_{Ti} - \mu_{Ci}$, $i = 1, \ldots, k$, be the parameter of interest in each study; then

$$
D_i = \bar{X}_{Ti} - \bar{X}_{Ci}
$$

is an unbiased estimator of μ_{Di} with

$$
D_i \sim N\left(\mu_{Di}, \frac{\sigma_{Ti}^2}{n_{Ti}} + \frac{\sigma_{Ci}^2}{n_{Ci}} \right)
$$

in general or

$$D_i \sim N\left(\mu_{Di}, \frac{n_{Ti} + n_{Ci}}{n_{Ti} \, n_{Ci}} \, \sigma_i^2\right)$$

for identical population variances in each trial.

The variance of D_i can be unbiasedly estimated either by

$$\widehat{\mathrm{Var}}(D_i) = \frac{S_{Ti}^2}{n_{Ti}} + \frac{S_{Ci}^2}{n_{Ci}}$$

or by

$$\widehat{\mathrm{Var}}(D_i) = \frac{n_{Ti} + n_{Ci}}{n_{Ti} \, n_{Ci}} \, S_i^{*2}.$$

Note that the latter variance estimator is an exactly scaled chi-square distributed random variable [see Eq. (8.4)], whereas the distribution of $S_{Ti}^2/n_{Ti} + S_{Ci}^2/n_{Ci}$, which is a linear combination of two independent chi-square variables, can only be approximated, for instance, by Satterthwaite's (1946) approximation if the population variances are different. In this case, the Satterthwaite approximation yields

$$\frac{S_{Ti}^2}{n_{Ti}} + \frac{S_{Ci}^2}{n_{Ci}} \overset{\mathrm{approx.}}{\sim} \left(\frac{\sigma_{Ti}^2}{n_{Ti}} + \frac{\sigma_{Ci}^2}{n_{Ci}}\right) \chi_{\nu_i}^2$$

with

$$\nu_i - \frac{\sigma_{Ti}^2}{n_{Ti} - 1} + \frac{\sigma_{Ci}^2}{n_{Ci} - 1}.$$

Since the degrees of freedom depend on the unknown variances, they must be estimated in practice, say by $\hat{\nu}_i = S_{Ti}^2/(n_{Ti} - 1) + S_{Ci}^2/(n_{Ci} - 1)$.

In the rest of this section, for ease of presentation, we consider the case that the variances of the two populations are identical in each trial and we always use the pooled variance estimator (8.4). If the assumption of equal variances is not fulfilled in a trial, the estimator (8.4) has to be replaced by $S_{Ti}^2/n_{Ti} + S_{Ci}^2/n_{Ci}$. Note that exact statements using Eq. (8.4) only approximately hold if $S_{Ti}^2/n_{Ti} + S_{Ci}^2/n_{Ci}$ must be used.

Under the assumption of equality of difference of means in all the trials, that is, it holds that

$$\mu_{D1} = \mu_{D2} = \cdots = \mu_{Dk} = \mu_D, \tag{8.5}$$

we have the common mean problem from Chapter 5. Based on (D_i, S_i^{*2}), $i = 1, \ldots, k$, the analogous estimator to the Graybill-Deal estimator (see Chapter 5) has the form

$$\hat{\mu}_D = \sum_{i=1}^{k} \frac{n_{Ti} \, n_{Ci}}{n_{Ti} + n_{Ci}} \frac{D_i}{S_i^{*2}} \Bigg/ \sum_{i=1}^{k} \frac{n_{Ti} \, n_{Ci}}{n_{Ti} + n_{Ci}} \frac{1}{S_i^{*2}}.$$

Using the mutual independence of D_i and S_i^*, it is readily verified that $\hat{\mu}_D$ is an unbiased estimator of μ_D.

8.1.1 Approximate confidence intervals for the common mean difference

If we can find an unbiased estimator, say $\widehat{\mathrm{Var}}(\hat{\mu}_D)$, of $\mathrm{Var}(\hat{\mu})$, then the studentized version $(\hat{\mu}_D - \mu_D)/\sqrt{\widehat{\mathrm{Var}}(\hat{\mu}_D)}$ follows $N(0,1)$ asymptotically. This can be used for testing as well as for interval estimation of μ_D at least in large samples.

Following the lines of Proposition 5.6 (see Chapter 5) and writing $\widehat{\mathrm{Var}}(D_i) = S_i^{*2}/f_i$ with $f_i = n_{Ti}\, n_{ci}/(n_{Ti} + n_{Ci})$, $i = 1, \ldots, k$, a first order approximation of $\widehat{\mathrm{Var}}(\hat{\mu}_D)$, say $\widehat{\mathrm{Var}}_{(1)}(\hat{\mu}_D)$, is obtained as

$$\widehat{\mathrm{Var}}_{(1)}(\hat{\mu}_D) =$$
$$\left(\sum_{i=1}^{k} \frac{f_i}{S_i^{*2}} \right)^{-1} \left[1 + \sum_{i=1}^{k} \frac{4}{n_{Ti} + n_{Ci}} \left(\frac{f_i/S_i^{*2}}{\sum_{j=1}^{k} f_j/S_j^{*2}} - \frac{f_i^2/S_i^{*4}}{\left(\sum_{j=1}^{k} f_j/S_j^{*2} \right)^2} \right) \right].$$
$$(8.6)$$

This approximation is comparable to the approximation when Meier's (1953) general result is applied in the present model. Meier's approximation yields

$$\widehat{\mathrm{Var}}_{(2)}(\hat{\mu}_D) =$$
$$\left(\sum_{i=1}^{k} \frac{f_i}{S_i^{*2}} \right)^{-1} \left[1 + \sum_{i=1}^{k} \frac{4}{n_{Ti} + n_{Ci} - 2} \left(\frac{f_i/S_i^{*2}}{\sum_{j=1}^{k} f_j/S_j^{*2}} - \frac{f_i^2/S_i^{*4}}{\left(\sum_{j=1}^{k} f_j/S_j^{*2} \right)^2} \right) \right].$$
$$(8.7)$$

Note that the general estimated (asymptotic) variance (see Chapter 4) is

$$\widehat{\mathrm{Var}}_{(3)}(\hat{\mu}_D) = \left(\sum_{i=1}^{k} \frac{f_i}{S_i^{*2}} \right)^{-1}. \qquad (8.8)$$

Using the above variance estimators, an approximate $100(1 - \alpha)\%$ confidence interval for μ_D can be constructed as

$$\left[\hat{\mu}_D - z_{\alpha/2} \sqrt{\widehat{\mathrm{Var}}(\hat{\mu}_D)} \,,\; \hat{\mu}_D + z_{\alpha/2} \sqrt{\widehat{\mathrm{Var}}(\hat{\mu}_D)} \right]. \qquad (8.9)$$

8.1.2 Exact confidence intervals for the common mean difference

All the exact confidence intervals for the common mean (see Section 5.3.2) can also be applied in the present situation. Recall that

$$t_i = \frac{\sqrt{f_i}\,(D_i - \mu_D)}{S_i^*} \sim t_{n_{Ti} + n_{Ci} - 2}$$

and, equivalently,

$$F_i = \frac{f_i(D_i - \mu_D)^2}{S_i^{*2}} \sim F_{1, n_{Ti} + n_{Ci} - 2} \tag{8.10}$$

are standard test statistics for testing hypotheses about μ_D in the ith trial. Consequently, suitable linear combinations of $|t_i|$'s or F_i's can be used as a pivot to construct exact confidence intervals for μ_D.

By replacing throughout $\bar{X}_i$ by D_i, S_i^2 by S_i^{*2}, and n_i by f_i, we obtain exact confidence intervals in analogy to the intervals (5.31), (5.32), and (5.35) as

$$\left[\max_{1 \le i \le k} \left\{ D_i - \frac{c_{\alpha/2} \, S_i^*}{\sqrt{f_i}} \right\} \;,\; \min_{1 \le i \le k} \left\{ D_i + \frac{c_{\alpha/2} \, S_i^*}{\sqrt{f_i}} \right\} \right], \tag{8.11}$$

where $c_{\alpha/2}$ satisfies

$$1 - \alpha = \prod_{i=1}^{k} \Pr\left(|t_i| \le c_{\alpha/2} \right) \;,$$

$$\left[\max_{1 \le i \le k} \left\{ D_i - \frac{c_{\alpha/2}^{(i)} \, S_i^*}{\sqrt{f_i}} \right\} \;,\; \min_{1 \le i \le k} \left\{ D_i + \frac{c_{\alpha/2}^{(i)} \, S_i^*}{\sqrt{f_i}} \right\} \right], \tag{8.12}$$

where $c_{\alpha/2}^{(i)}$ satisfies

$$\Pr\left(|t_i| \le c_{\alpha/2} \right) = (1 - \alpha)^{1/k} \;,$$

and

$$\frac{\sum_{i=1}^{k} \sqrt{f_i} \, u_i \, D_i / S_i^*}{\sum_{i=1}^{k} \sqrt{f_i} \, u_i / S_i^*} \pm \frac{b_{\alpha/2}}{\sum_{i=1}^{k} \sqrt{f_i} \, u_i / S_i^*}, \tag{8.13}$$

where $u_i = \text{Var}(t_i)^{-1} / \sum_{j=1}^{k} \text{Var}(t_j)^{-1}$, $i = 1, \ldots, k$, and $b_{\alpha/2}$ satisfies

$$1 - \alpha = \Pr\left(\sum_{i=1}^{k} u_i \, |t_i| \le b_{\alpha/2} \right).$$

Similarly, the exact confidence interval (5.38) for the common mean can be applied by additionally setting $m_i = n_{Ti} + n_{Ci} - 2$ in the present context. We omit the detailed presentation here.

Using F_i defined in (8.10), one can construct the exact confidence intervals (5.43), (5.44), (5.45), and (5.47) based on the P-values after calculating the P-values as

$$P_i = \int_{F_i}^{\infty} h_i(x) \, dx$$

where here $h_i(x)$ denote the pdf of the F distribution with 1 and $(n_{Ti} + n_{Ci} - 2)$ df.

Example 8.1. Let us reanalyze the dentifrice data from Example 4.4. Recall that the homogeneity test does not reject the homogeneity assumption. The estimate of the common difference of means is $\hat{\mu}_D = 0.2833$ with large-sample 95% confidence interval of $[0.1022, 0.4644]$. Using the estimates (8.6) or (8.7) instead of (8.8), the resulting bounds of the interval (8.9) only slightly change. Applying the exact confidence intervals to this data set, we obtain the results in Table 8.1.

Table 8.1   Interval estimates for μ_D in the dentifrice example

Method	95% CI on μ
Cohen and Sackrowitz (1984), in analogy to interval (5.31)	$[-0.1815, 0.5615]$
Cohen and Sackrowitz (1984), in analogy to interval (5.32)	$[-0.1800, 0.5600]$
Fairweather (1972), in analogy to interval (5.35)	$[0.1193, 0.5365]$
Jordan and Krishnamoorthy (1996), in analogy to interval (5.38)	$[-0.2495, 1.1377]$
Fisher, in analogy to interval (5.44)	$[-0.0186, 0.6141]$
Inverse normal, in analogy to interval (5.45)	$[0.0024, 0.6777]$
Logit, in analogy to interval (5.47)	$[-0.0036, 0.6396]$

It is interesting to observe that the exact interval based on Fairweather (1972) is the shortest one and clearly excludes the value zero like the approximate confidence intervals. The lower bounds of the exact intervals based on P-values are around the value zero, whereas the other three intervals clearly include this value.

8.1.3   Testing homogeneity

The crucial assumption of the underlying meta-analysis in the Sections 8.1.1 and 8.1.2 is the assumption (8.5) of identical mean differences in all the trials. Formally, we can test this homogeneity hypothesis

$$H_0 : \mu_{D1} = \mu_{D2} = \cdots = \mu_{Dk} \tag{8.14}$$

using test statistics from Section 6.1. However, note that we cannot extend all test statistics from this section but can extend only those which depend on the sample means and not on the overall mean. This restriction leads to the use of Cochran's test, Welch's test, and the adjusted Welch test in the present situation. These are described below.

Define $w_i = f_i / S_i^{*2}$, $i = 1, \ldots, k$, and $h_i = w_i / \sum_{j=1}^{k} w_j$; then Cochran's statistic for testing H_0 is given as

$$S_{ch} = \sum_{i=1}^{k} w_i \left(D_i - \sum_{j=1}^{k} h_j D_j \right)^2, \tag{8.15}$$

which is approximately chi-square distributed with $k - 1$ degrees of freedom under H_0.

The Welch test is given as

$$S_{\text{we}} = \frac{\sum_{i=1}^{k} w_i \left(D_i - \sum_{j=1}^{k} h_j D_j \right)^2}{(k-1) + 2[(k-2)/(k+1)] \sum_{i=1}^{k} (1-h_i)^2 / (n_{Ti} + n_{Ci} - 2)}$$

Under H_0, the statistic S_{we} has an approximate F distribution with $k - 1$ and ν_g degrees of freedom, where

$$\nu_g = \frac{(k^2 - 1)/3}{\sum_{i=1}^{k} (1 - h_i)^2 / (n_{Ti} + n_{Ci} - 2)}.$$

Following the lines of Hartung, Argac, and Makambi (2002), we know that

$$E\left(\frac{f_i}{S_i^{*2}}\right) = \frac{c_i f_i}{S_i^{*2}}$$

with $c_i = (n_{Ti} + n_{Ci} - 2)/(n_{Ti} + n_{Ci} - 4)$. Defining $w_i^* = f_i/(c_i S_i^{*2})$ and $h_i* = w_i^*/\sum_{j=1}^{k} w_j*$, $i = 1, \ldots, k$, leads to the adjusted Welch test statistic

$$S_{\text{aw}} = \frac{\sum_{i=1}^{k} w_i^* \left(D_i - \sum_{j=1}^{k} h_j^* D_j \right)^2}{(k-1) + 2[(k-2)/(k+1)] \sum_{i=1}^{k} (1-h_i^*)^2 / (n_{Ti} + n_{Ci} - 2)}.$$

Under H_0, the statistic S_{aw} is approximately distributed as an F variate with $k - 1$ and ν_g^* degrees of freedom, where

$$\nu_g^* = \frac{(k^2 - 1)/3}{\sum_{i=1}^{k} (1 - h_i^*)^2 / (n_{Ti} + n_{Ci} - 2)}.$$

8.1.4 Analysis in the random effects model

In case the homogeneity assumption (8.5) is not fulfilled, the meta-analysis using the random effects model is appropriate and methods from Chapter 7 may be appealing to extend to the present model. Since the heteroscedastic error case is the usual scenario in practice, we restrict the presentation here to the model

$$D_i \sim N\left(\mu_D, \ \sigma_a^2 + \frac{\sigma_i^2}{f_i}\right),$$

where σ_a^2 is the parameter for the variability between the studies. Recall that the pooled within-study variance estimator of σ_i^2 is given as

$$S_i^{*2} = \frac{1}{n_{Ti} + n_{Ci} - 2} \left[(n_{Ti} - 1)S_{Ti}^2 + (n_{Ci} - 1)S_{Ci}^2 \right]$$

with

$$(n_{Ti} + n_{Ci} - 2)S_i^{*2} \sim \sigma_i^2 \, \chi_{n_{Ti}+n_{Ci}-2}^2.$$

Estimates of σ_a^2 are available from the methods of Chapter 7 and we restrict the discussion of estimating σ_a^2 in the present model to four methods which are often used in practice.

In analogy to the estimator (7.16), an unbiased ANOVA-type estimator of σ_a^2 is given as

$$\hat{\sigma}_a^2 = \frac{1}{k-1} \sum_{i=1}^{k} (D_i - \bar{D})^2 - \frac{1}{k} \sum_{i=1}^{k} \frac{S_i^{*2}}{f_i} \tag{8.16}$$

with $\bar{D} = \sum_{i=1}^{k} D_i/k$ as the overall mean of the group mean differences. Recall that although estimator (8.16) is an unbiased one, it can yield negative values which are usually truncated to zero in practice. The truncated estimator, of course, is no longer an unbiased estimator.

Following the DerSimonian-Laird (1986) approach [see Eq. (7.18] we obtain the estimator

$$\hat{\sigma}_a^2 = \frac{\sum_{i=1}^{k} w_i (D_i - \tilde{D})^2 - (k-1)}{\sum_{i=1}^{k} w_i - \sum_{i=1}^{k} w_i^2 / \sum_{i=1}^{k} w_i}, \tag{8.17}$$

where $\tilde{D} = \sum_{i=1}^{k} w_i D_i / \sum_{i=1}^{k} w_i$, and in the present model, $w_i = f_i/\sigma_i^2$. Again, the estimator (8.17) is an unbiased estimator of σ_a^2 given known σ_i^2. In practice, estimates of the within-group variances have to be plugged in and then, naturally, the resultant estimator of σ_a^2 is no longer unbiased. Moreover, like the unbiased ANOVA-type estimator (8.16), the DerSimonian-Laird estimator can yield negative estimates with positive probability.

The Mandel-Paule (1970) estimator for σ_a^2 [see Eqs. (7.21) and (7.22)] is based on the quadratic form

$$\tilde{Q}(\sigma_a^2) = \sum_{i=1}^{k} \tilde{\omega}_i \left(D_i - \bar{D}_{\tilde{\omega}} \right)^2 \tag{8.18}$$

with $\bar{D}_{\tilde{\omega}} = \sum_{i=1}^{k} \tilde{\omega}_i D_i / \sum_{i=1}^{k} \tilde{\omega}_i$ and $\tilde{\omega}_i = (\sigma_a^2 + S_i^{*2}/f_i)^{-1}$. Since $\tilde{Q}(\sigma_a^2)$ can be well approximated by a chi-square random variable with $k-1$ degrees of freedom, the Mandel-Paule estimator for σ_a^2 is then given as the solution of the following equation:

$$\tilde{Q}(\sigma_a^2) = k - 1.$$

In case $Q(0) < k - 1$, the estimate is set to zero.

Taking the σ_i^2's as known, the estimating equations of the maximum likelihood estimators of μ and σ_a^2 are given by

$$\mu = \frac{\sum_{i=1}^{k} w_i(\sigma_a^2) \, D_i}{\sum_{i=1}^{k} w_i(\sigma_a^2)}, \tag{8.19}$$

$$\sum_{i=1}^{k} w_i^2(\sigma_a^2) \, (D_i - \mu_D)^2 = \sum_{i=1}^{k} w_i(\sigma_a^2), \tag{8.20}$$

where $w_i(\sigma_a^2) = (\sigma_a^2 + s_i^{*2}/f_i)^{-1}$. A convenient form of Eq. (8.20) for iterative solution is given by

$$\sigma_a^2 = \frac{\sum_{i=1}^{k} w_i^2(\sigma_a^2)[(D_i - \mu_D)^2 - s_i^{*2}/f_i]}{\sum_{i=1}^{k} w_i^2(\sigma_a^2)}. \tag{8.21}$$

The restricted maximum likelihood estimate of σ_a^2 is found numerically by iterating

$$\sigma_a^2 = \frac{\sum_{i=1}^{k} w_i^2(\sigma_a^2)[(D_i - \hat{\mu}_D(\sigma_a^2))^2 - s_i^{*2}/f_i]}{\sum_{i=1}^{k} w_i^2(\sigma_a^2)} + \frac{1}{\sum_{i=1}^{k} w_i(\sigma_a^2)}. \tag{8.22}$$

By profiling the restricted log-likelihood for σ_a^2, we can construct a $100(1 - \alpha)\%$ confidence interval for σ_a^2. Recall that the restricted log-likelihood function can be written as

$$l_R(\sigma_a^2) \propto -\frac{1}{2} \sum_{i=1}^{k} \ln\left(\sigma_a^2 + \frac{s_i^{*2}}{f_i}\right) - \frac{1}{2} \sum_{i=1}^{k} \frac{1}{\sigma_a^2 + s_i^{*2}/f_i} - \frac{1}{2} \sum_{i=1}^{k} \frac{(D_i - \hat{\mu}_D)^2}{\sigma_a^2 + s_i^{*2}/f_i}$$

Let $\hat{\sigma}_{a,\mathrm{REML}}^2$ denote the REML estimate according to Eq. (8.22). Then, a $100(1-\alpha)\%$ confidence interval for σ_a^2 is given by

$$\mathrm{CI}(\sigma_a^2) : \left\{ \tilde{\sigma}_a^2 \mid -2\left[l_R(\tilde{\sigma}_a^2) - l_R(\hat{\sigma}_{a,\mathrm{REML}}^2)\right] < \chi_{1;\alpha}^2 \right\}$$

$$= \left\{ \tilde{\sigma}_a^2 \mid l_R(\tilde{\sigma}_a^2) > l_R(\hat{\sigma}_{a,\mathrm{REML}}^2) - \chi_{1;\alpha}^2/2 \right\}.$$

Using the quadratic form (8.18) and following Hartung and Knapp (2005a) or Viechtbauer (2007), a further approximate $100(1 - \alpha)\%$ confidence interval can be obtained as

$$\mathrm{CI}(\sigma_a^2) = \left\{ \sigma_a^2 \geq 0 \mid \chi_{k-1;1-\alpha/2}^2 \leq \tilde{Q}(\sigma_a^2) \leq \chi_{k-1;\alpha/2}^2 \right\}.$$

To determine the bounds of the confidence interval explicitly one has to solve the two equations for σ_a^2, namely:

$$\text{lower bound:} \qquad \tilde{Q}(\sigma_a^2) = \chi_{k-1;\alpha/2}^2,$$

$$\text{upper bound:} \qquad \tilde{Q}(\sigma_a^2) = \chi_{k-1;1-\alpha/2}^2.$$

Finally, we can consider the statistical inference for μ_D, the primary parameter of interest. Let us recall $D_i \sim N(\mu_D, \sigma_a^2 + \sigma_i^2/f_i)$. Then, when the between-study variance and the within-study variances are known, the uniformly minimum variance unbiased estimator of μ_D is given by

$$\hat{\mu}_D = \frac{\sum_{i=1}^{k} w_i D_i}{\sum_{i=1}^{k} w_i},$$

where $w_i = (\sigma_a^2 + \sigma_i^2/f_i)^{-1}$, $i = 1, \ldots, k$. Then it holds for the standardized variable

$$Z = \frac{\hat{\mu}_D}{(\sum_{i=1}^{k} w_i)^{-1/2}} \sim N(\mu_D, 1),$$

Since we have to plug in estimates of all the unknown variances in practice, we obtain an approximate $100(1 - \alpha)\%$ confidence interval for μ_D as

$$\hat{\mu}_D = \frac{\sum_{i=1}^{k} \hat{w}_i \, D_i}{\sum_{i=1}^{k} \hat{w}_i} \pm \left(\sum_{i=1}^{k} \hat{w}_i \right)^{-1/2} z_{\alpha/2} \tag{8.23}$$

with $\hat{w}_i = (\hat{\sigma}_a^2 + \hat{\sigma}_i^2/f_i)^{-1}$.

As is well known, in small to moderate samples, this confidence interval suffers from the same weaknesses as its fixed effects counterpart. Namely, the actual confidence coefficient is below the nominal one. Consequently, the corresponding test on the overall mean yields too many unjustified significant results.

Using the modification proposed by Hartung and Knapp (2001a,b), an unbiased estimator of the variance of $\hat{\mu}_D$ is given as

$$q := \widehat{\text{Var}}(\hat{\mu}_D) = \frac{1}{k-1} \frac{\sum_{i=1}^{k} w_i \, (D_i - \hat{\mu}_D)^2}{\sum_{i=1}^{k} w_i}. \tag{8.24}$$

By replacing the unknown variances by their appropriate estimates, we finally obtain the improved approximate $100(1 - \alpha)\%$ confidence interval for μ_D,

$$\hat{\mu}_D = \frac{\sum_{i=1}^{k} \hat{w}_i \, D_i}{\sum_{i=1}^{k} \hat{w}_i} \pm \sqrt{\hat{q}} \, t_{k-1,\alpha/2}, \tag{8.25}$$

with $\hat{q}$ being the estimate (8.24) where w_i is replaced by $\hat{w}_i$.

Example 8.2. As an example let us consider the amlodipine data set from Section 18.4. Using a pooled variance estimate in each trial, the observed mean differences with corresponding standard errors are given in Table 8.2.

The meta-analysis results are summarized in Table 8.3. In the random effects model, we have used the DerSimonian-Laird (DSL) estimate (8.17) and the REML estimate solving Eq. (8.22) for estimating the between-study variance. Since the estimate of the heterogeneity parameter is close to zero, the results in the fixed effects and random effects model are nearly same. Note that the interval (8.25) is always wider than the interval (8.23). But in all the intervals the value zero is not included so we can reject the null hypothesis of no treatment difference.

Table 8.2 Mean differences and standard errors (s.e.)
in the amlodipine example

Study	Mean difference	s.e.
1	0.2343	0.0686
2	0.2541	0.0967
3	0.1451	0.0968
4	−0.1347	0.1251
5	0.1566	0.0762
6	0.0894	0.0980
7	0.6669	0.2506
8	0.1423	0.0734

Table 8.3 Meta-analysis results in the amlodipine example

Model	Method	$\hat{\tau}^2$	$\hat{\mu}_D$	95% CI for μ_D based on (8.23)	95% CI for μ_D based on (8.25)
Fixed effects		0	0.1624	$[0.0994, 0.2254]$	$[0.0613, 0.2634]$
Random effects	DSL	0.0066	0.1590	$[0.0713, 0.2467]$	$[0.0390, 0.2790]$
	REML	0.0003	0.1620	$[0.0978, 0.2262]$	$[0.0600, 0.2641]$

8.2 STANDARDIZED DIFFERENCE OF MEANS

The standardized mean difference as an effect size based on means has already been
introduced in Section 2.1. Several estimators of this effect size have also been discussed there. In this section, we will discuss the combination of estimates of this
effect size in the random effects model of meta-analysis, where the results can be
easily applied to the fixed effects model of meta-analysis by setting the value of the
between-study variability equal to zero. For $i = 1, \ldots, k$ independent experiments
or studies, let $\bar{X}_{Ti}$, S_{Ti}^2, and n_{Ti} denote sample mean, sample variance, and sample
size in the ith experimental (treatment) group, respectively, and likewise $\bar{X}_{Ci}$, S_{Ci}^2,
and n_{Ci} the sample mean, sample variance, and sample size in the ith control group,
respectively, as defined in (8.1) and (8.2).

Recall from Section 2.1 that the standardized mean difference in the ith study is
defined as

$$\theta_i = \frac{\mu_{Ti} - \mu_{Ci}}{\sigma},$$

where σ denotes either the standard deviation σ_{Ci} of the population control group or
an average population standard deviation (namely, an average of σ_{Ti} and σ_{Ci}).

In the remainder of this section we will exclusively consider Hedges's g from
Section 2.1 as the estimate of θ_i, $i = 1, \ldots, k$. Using the notation in the present

chapter, this estimator is given by

$$g_i = \frac{\bar{X}_{Ti} - \bar{X}_{Ci}}{S_i^*}$$

with S_i^{*2} being the pooled sample variance from Eq. (8.3). Since g_i is biased for θ_i, an approximately unbiased estimate of θ_i (see Section 2.1) is given as

$$g_i^* = \left(1 - \frac{3}{4n_i - 9}\right) g_i$$

with $n_i = n_{Ti} + n_{Ci}$, $i = 1, \ldots, k$, the total sample size in the ith study.

The variance of g_i in large samples is given as

$$\mathrm{Var}(g_i) \approx \frac{n_{Ti} + n_{Ci}}{n_{Ti}\, n_{Ci}} + \frac{\theta_i^2}{2\,(n_{Ti} + n_{Ci} - 2)},$$

which can be estimated by

$$\widehat{\mathrm{Var}}(g_i) = \frac{n_{Ti} + n_{Ci}}{n_{Ti}\, n_{Ci}} + \frac{g_i^2}{2\,(n_{Ti} + n_{Ci} - 2)}.$$

The homogeneity hypothesis

$$H_0 : \theta_1 = \theta_2 = \cdots = \theta_k,$$

that is, all standardized mean differences are identical, can be tested using Cochran's homogeneity statistic. In analogy to (8.15), defining now $w_i = 1/\widehat{\mathrm{Var}}(g_i)$ and $h_i = w_i/\sum_{j=1}^{k} w_j$, $i = 1, \ldots, k$, the test statistic can be obtained as

$$Q = \sum_{i=1}^{k} w_i \left(g_i - \sum_{j=1}^{k} h_j\, g_i\right)^2. \tag{8.26}$$

Under H_0, Q is approximately chi-square distributed with $k - 1$ degrees of freedom. If the homogeneity assumption holds, the fixed effects meta-analysis model is quite appropriate; otherwise, the combination of the results should be carried out in a random effects model.

Recall that the random effects model is given here as

$$g_i \sim N\left[\theta, \sigma_a^2 + \left(\frac{n_{Ti} + n_{Ci}}{n_{Ti}\, n_{Ci}} + \frac{\theta_i^2}{2\,(n_{Ti} + n_{Ci} - 2)}\right)\right], \tag{8.27}$$

where θ denotes the overall effect size and σ_a^2 stands for the between-study variability.

Following the DerSimonian-Laird (1986) approach [see also (8.17)] an estimate of σ_a^2 can be obtained as

$$\hat{\sigma}_a^2 = \frac{Q - (k-1)}{\sum w_i - \sum w_i^2 / \sum w_i} \tag{8.28}$$

with Q from Eq. (8.26), where negative estimates are set to zero.

Let $w_i^* = 1/[\hat{\sigma}_a^2 + \widehat{Var}(g_i)]$, $i = 1, \ldots, k$, denote the estimate of the inverse of the variance in model (8.27); then the estimate of the overall effect θ is given by

$$\hat{\theta} = \frac{\sum_{i=1}^{k} w_i^* g_i}{\sum_{i=1}^{k} w_i}.$$

The large-sample variance of $\hat{\theta}$ is given as

$$\widehat{Var}_{(1)}(\hat{\theta}) = \left(\sum_{i=1}^{k} w_i^* \right)^{-1}.$$

Following Hartung (1999b), another estimator of the variance of $\hat{\theta}$ is given as

$$\widehat{Var}_{(2)}(\hat{\theta}) = \frac{1}{k-1} \frac{\sum_{i=1}^{k} w_i^* (g_i - \hat{\theta})^2}{\sum_{i=1}^{k} w_i^*}.$$

Consequently, a large-sample $100(1 - \alpha)\%$ confidence interval for θ is given as

$$\hat{\theta} \pm \sqrt{\widehat{Var}_{(1)}(\hat{\theta})} \, z_{\alpha/2}, \tag{8.29}$$

which can be improved with respect to the actual coverage probability for a small number of studies through

$$\hat{\theta} \pm \sqrt{\widehat{Var}_{(2)}(\hat{\theta})} \, t_{k-1;\alpha/2}. \tag{8.30}$$

See Hartung and Knapp (2001a) for details.

Example 8.3. Let us again consider the amlodipine data set from Section 18.4. Now assume that the standardized mean difference is the parameter of interest. The observed standardized mean differences with corresponding standard errors are given in Table 8.4.

The meta-analysis results are summarized in Table 8.5. Again we have used the DSL estimate (8.28) and the REML estimate solving Eq. (8.22) for estimating the between-study variance in the random effects model. Since the estimates of the heterogeneity parameter is close to zero, the results in the fixed effects and random effects models are rather close together. The interval (8.29) is again always wider than the interval (8.30), but in all the intervals the value zero is not included so we can reject the null hypothesis of no treatment difference.

Table 8.4   Standardized mean differences and standard errors (s.e.) in the amlodipine example

Study	Mean difference	s.e.
1	0.6987	0.2125
2	0.6946	0.2759
3	0.2459	0.1656
4	−0.4245	0.4128
5	0.5000	0.2501
6	0.2287	0.2548
7	0.7139	0.2807
8	0.3989	0.2095

Table 8.5   Meta-analysis results in the amlodipine example

Model	Method	$\hat{\tau}^2$	$\hat{\theta}$	95% CI for θ based on (8.29)	95% CI for θ based on (8.30)
Fixed effects		0	0.4204	[0.2574, 0.5835]	[0.1880, 0.6529]
Random effects	DSL	0.0227	0.4238	[0.2259, 0.6218]	[0.1757, 0.6720]
	REML	0.0076	0.4229	[0.2469, 0.5987]	[0.1841, 0.6614]

8.3   RATIO OF MEANS

The response ratio, that is, the ratio of mean outcome in the experimental group to that in the control group, and closely related measures of proportionate change are often used as measures of effect sizes in ecology; see Hedges, Gurevitch, and Curtis (1999).

For $i = 1, \ldots, k$ independent experiments, let $\bar{X}_{Ti}$, S_{Ti}^2, and n_{Ti} denote sample mean, sample variance, and sample size (number of replicates) in the ith experimental (treatment) group, respectively, and likewise $\bar{X}_{Ci}$, S_{Ci}^2, and n_{Ci} the sample mean, sample variance, and sample size in the ith control group, respectively, as defined in Eqs. (8.1) and (8.2). The parameter of interest is the ratio of the population means, that is, $\rho_i = \mu_{Ti}/\mu_{Ci}$. The sample response ratio $R_i = \bar{X}_{Ti}/\bar{X}_{Ci}$ is an estimate of ρ_i in the ith experiment. Usually, the combination of the response ratios R_i is carried out on the metric of the natural logarithm for two reasons. First, the natural logarithm linearizes the metric, that is, deviations in the numerator are treated the same as deviations in the denominator. Second, the sampling distribution of R_i is skewed and the sampling distribution of $\ln(R_i)$ is much more normal in small sample sizes than that of R_i. For further discussion on this topic, we refer to Hedges, Gurevitch, and Curtis (1999).

Let $\zeta_i = \ln(\mu_{Ti}) - \ln(\mu_{Ci})$ be the natural logarithm of the ratio of population means in the ith experiment. Then, ζ_i can be estimated by

$$\hat{\zeta}_i = \ln(\bar{X}_{Ti}) - \ln(\bar{X}_{Ci})$$

with

$$\mathrm{Var}(\hat{\zeta}_i) \approx \frac{\sigma_{Ti}^2}{n_{Ti}\,\mu_{Ti}^2} + \frac{\sigma_{Ci}^2}{n_{Ci}\,\mu_{Ci}^2}$$

or

$$\mathrm{Var}(\hat{\zeta}_i) \approx \sigma_i^2 \left(\frac{1}{n_{Ti}\,\mu_{Ti}^2} + \frac{1}{n_{Ci}\,\mu_{Ci}^2} \right),$$

where the latter holds for $\sigma_i^2 = \sigma_{Ti}^2 = \sigma_{Ci}^2$.

Let us assume in the rest of this section that $\sigma_i^2 = \sigma_{Ti}^2 = \sigma_{Ci}^2$ holds. Then, the variance of $\hat{\zeta}_i$ can be estimated as

$$\widehat{\mathrm{Var}}(\hat{\zeta}_i) = S_i^{*\,2} \left(\frac{1}{n_{Ti}\,\bar{X}_{Ti}^2} + \frac{1}{n_{Ci}\,\bar{X}_{Ci}^2} \right),$$

where $S_i^{*\,2}$ is the pooled sample variance (8.3).

The homogeneity hypothesis that all the ratios of population means are equal, that is,

$$H_0 : \rho_1 = \rho_2 = \cdots = \rho_k \quad \text{or equivalently} \quad H_0^* : \zeta_1 = \zeta_2 = \cdots = \zeta_k,$$

can be tested using Cochran's homogeneity statistic. In analogy to the test statistic (8.15), defining now $w_i = 1/\widehat{\mathrm{Var}}(\hat{\zeta}_i)$ and $h_i = w_i / \sum_{j=1}^{k} w_j$, $i = 1, \ldots, k$, the test statistic can be obtained as

$$Q = \sum_{i=1}^{k} w_i \left(\hat{\zeta}_i - \sum_{j=1}^{k} h_j\,\hat{\zeta}_j \right)^2. \tag{8.31}$$

Under H_0 and H_0^*, respectively, Q is approximately chi-square distributed with $k - 1$ degrees of freedom. If the homogeneity assumption holds, the fixed effects meta-analysis model is quite appropriate; otherwise, the combination of the results should be carried out in a random effects model.

Recall that the random effects model is given here as

$$\hat{\zeta}_i \sim N \left[\zeta, \sigma_a^2 + \sigma_i^2 \left(\frac{1}{n_{Ti}\,\mu_{Ti}^2} + \frac{1}{n_{Ci}\,\mu_{Ci}^2} \right) \right], \tag{8.32}$$

where ζ denotes the overall effect size on the logarithmic scale and σ_a^2 stands for the between-study variability.

Following the DerSimonian-Laird (1986) approach, an estimate of σ_a^2 can be obtained as

$$\hat{\sigma}_a^2 = \frac{Q - (k - 1)}{\sum w_i - \sum w_i^2 / \sum w_i}$$

with Q obtained from Eq. (8.31). This estimator may yield negative values which are set to zero in practice.

Let $w_i^* = 1/[\hat{\sigma}_a^2 + \widehat{\mathrm{Var}}(\hat{\zeta}_i)]$, $i = 1, \ldots, k$, denote the estimate of the inverse of the variance in model (8.32); then the estimate of the overall effect ζ is given by

$$\hat{\zeta} = \frac{\sum_{i=1}^k w_i^* \hat{\zeta}_i}{\sum_{i=1}^k w_i}.$$

The large-sample variance of $\hat{\zeta}$ is given as

$$\widehat{\mathrm{Var}}_{(1)}(\hat{\zeta}) = \left(\sum_{i=1}^k w_i^*\right)^{-1}.$$

For a small number of studies, Hedges, Gurevitch, and Curtis (1999) recommend the use of the variance estimator

$$\widehat{\mathrm{Var}}_{(2)}(\hat{\zeta}) =$$
$$\left(\sum_{i=1}^k w_i^*\right)^{-1} \left(1 + 4 \sum_{i=1}^k \frac{1}{n_{Ti} + n_{Ci} - 2} \left(\frac{w_i^*}{w_i}\right)^2 \frac{w_i^*[\sum_{j=1}^k w_j^* - w_i^*]}{(\sum_{j=1}^k w_j^*)^2}\right).$$

Following Hartung (1999b), another estimator of the variance of $\hat{\zeta}$ is given as

$$\widehat{\mathrm{Var}}_{(3)}(\hat{\zeta}) = \frac{1}{k-1} \frac{\sum_{i=1}^k w_i^*(\hat{\zeta}_i - \hat{\zeta})^2}{\sum_{i=1}^k w_i^*}.$$

A large-sample $100(1 - \alpha)\%$ confidence interval for ζ is given as

$$\hat{\zeta} \pm \sqrt{\widehat{\mathrm{Var}}_{(1)}(\hat{\zeta})}\, z_{\alpha/2},$$

which can be improved with respect to the actual coverage probability for a small number of studies through

$$\hat{\zeta} \pm \sqrt{\widehat{\mathrm{Var}}_{(2)}(\hat{\zeta})}\, z_{\alpha/2}.$$

Following Hartung and Knapp (2001a), an alternative $100(1 - \alpha)\%$ confidence interval for ζ can be obtained as

$$\hat{\zeta} \pm \sqrt{\widehat{\mathrm{Var}}_{(3)}(\hat{\zeta})}\, t_{k-1,\alpha/2}.$$

After combining the results on the log scale, the results will naturally be transformed to the original scale using antilogs. Backtransforming the mean of logs introduces a bias into the estimate of the mean response ratio due to the convexity of the log transform. This bias also arises, for example, in the averaging of correlation coefficients by backtransforming the average of several Fisher's z transforms, or in the averaging of odds ratios by backtransforming the average of several log-odds ratios. However, since the magnitude of the bias depends upon the variance of the weighted mean, this bias is usually expected to be slight.

CHAPTER 9

COMBINING CONTROLLED TRIALS WITH DISCRETE OUTCOMES

An important application of meta-analysis, especially in biometry and epidemiology, is the combination of results from comparative trials with binary outcomes. Often in clinical trials or observational studies, the outcome can be generally characterized as success and failure or as positive and negative. The effect size measures for binary outcomes have already been introduced in Chapter 2. The meta-analytical methods described in Chapter 4 as well as the methods of the one-way random effects model presented in Chapter 7 can be generally applied to the case of binary data. In the first section of this chapter, we discuss some additional features of meta-analysis of binary data. In the second section, we consider a natural extension, namely, the meta-analysis of outcomes with more than two classification categories or, in other words, the meta-analysis of ordinal data.

First, we briefly summarize the crucial results from Chapters 4 and 7 which can be directly used for combining results from controlled trials with binary or ordinal outcome.

Let θ_i be the parameter of interest in the ith trial and let us assume that each independent trial provides an estimate of θ_i, say $\hat{\theta}_i$, $i = 1, \ldots, k$, as well as an estimate of $\text{Var}(\hat{\theta}_i) = \sigma_i^2(\theta_i)$, say $\hat{\sigma}_i^2(\theta_i)$. Note that quite often the variance $\sigma_i^2(\theta_i)$ may functionally depend on the parameter of interest. In the random effects model

Statistical Meta-Analysis with Applications. By Joachim Hartung, Guido Knapp, Bimal K. Sinha
Copyright © 2008 John Wiley & Sons, Inc.

of meta-analysis, we have, at least approximatively,

$$\hat{\theta}_i \sim N\left[\theta, \tau^2 + \sigma_i^2(\theta_i)\right], \ i = 1, \ldots, k. \tag{9.1}$$

Here θ stands for the overall effect size and τ^2 denotes the parameter for the between-study variance, also called the heterogeneity parameter. If $\tau^2 = 0$, we have the fixed effects model of meta-analysis and θ is then the common effect size in all the studies; see Chapter 4.

For testing the homogeneity hypothesis, $H_0 : \tau^2 = 0$, we can use Cochran's homogeneity test (see Chapters 4 and 6), which is given here as

$$Q = \sum_{i=1}^{k} \hat{v}_i \left(\hat{\theta}_i - \tilde{\theta}\right)^2 \tag{9.2}$$

with $\hat{v}_i = 1/\hat{\sigma}_i^2(\theta_i)$, $i = 1, \ldots, k$, and $\tilde{\theta} = \sum_{i=1}^{k} \hat{v}_i \hat{\theta}_i / \sum_{i=1}^{k} \hat{v}_i$. Under H_0, the statistic Q is approximately chi-square distributed with $k - 1$ degrees of freedom and H_0 is rejected at level α if $Q > \chi_{k-1;\alpha}^2$ with $\chi_{k-1;\alpha}^2$ being the upper α percentage point of the chi-square distribution with $k - 1$ degrees of freedom.

For estimating the heterogeneity parameter τ^2, the DSL estimator or the REML estimator (see Chapter 7) are commonly used in the present setting. The DSL estimator of τ^2 is given here as

$$\hat{\tau}_{\text{DSL}}^2 = \frac{Q - (k-1)}{\sum_{i=1}^{k} \hat{v}_i - \sum_{i=1}^{k} \hat{v}_i^2 / \sum_{i=1}^{k} \hat{v}_i} \tag{9.3}$$

with Q from Eq. (9.2).

Let $w_i(\tau^2) = 1/[\tau^2 + \hat{\sigma}_i^2(\theta_i)]$, $i = 1, \ldots, k$, and

$$\hat{\theta}(\tau^2) = \frac{\sum_{i=1}^{k} w_i(\tau^2) \hat{\theta}_i}{\sum_{i=1}^{k} w_i(\tau^2)}.$$

Then, the REML estimate of τ^2 can be found numerically by iterating

$$\tau^2 = \frac{\sum_{i=1}^{k} w_i^2(\tau^2) \left\{[\hat{\theta} - \hat{\theta}(\tau^2)]^2 - \hat{\sigma}_i^2(\theta_i)\right\}}{\sum_{i=1}^{k} w_i^2(\tau^2)} + \frac{1}{\sum_{i=1}^{k} w_i(\tau^2)} \tag{9.4}$$

starting with an initial guess of τ^2, say τ_0^2, on the right-hand side of the above equation.

By profiling the restricted log-likelihood for τ^2, we can construct a $100(1 - \alpha)\%$ confidence interval for τ^2 as follows. Recall that the restricted log-likelihood function can be written as

$$l_R(\tau^2) \propto -\frac{1}{2} \sum_{i=1}^{k} \ln[\tau^2 + \hat{\sigma}_i^2(\theta_i)] - \frac{1}{2} \sum_{i=1}^{k} \frac{1}{\tau^2 + \hat{\sigma}_i^2(\theta_i)} - \frac{1}{2} \sum_{i=1}^{k} \frac{[\hat{\theta}_i - \hat{\theta}(\tau^2)]^2}{\tau^2 + \hat{\sigma}_i^2(\theta_i)}.$$

Let $\hat{\tau}^2_{\text{REML}}$ denote the REML estimate; see Eq. (9.4). Then, a $100(1-\alpha)\%$ confidence interval for τ^2 is given by

$$\text{CI}(\tau^2) : \left\{ \tilde{\tau}^2 \mid -2\left[l_R(\tilde{\tau}^2) - l_R(\hat{\tau}^2_{\text{REML}})\right] < \chi^2_{1;\alpha} \right\}$$
$$= \left\{ \tilde{\tau}^2 \mid l_R(\tilde{\tau}^2) > l_R(\hat{\tau}^2_{\text{REML}}) - \chi^2_{1;\alpha}/2 \right\}$$

with $\chi^2_{1;\alpha}$ being the upper α percentage point of the chi-square distribution with 1 df.
Using the quadratic form

$$\tilde{Q}(\tau^2) = \sum_{i=1}^{k} \tilde{w}_i \left(\hat{\theta}_i - \hat{\theta}_{\tilde{w}} \right)^2$$

with $\hat{\theta}_{\tilde{w}} = \sum_{i=1}^{k} \tilde{w}_i \hat{\theta}_i / \sum_{i=1}^{k} \tilde{w}_i$ and $\tilde{w}_i = [\tau^2 + \hat{\sigma}_i^2(\theta_i)]^{-1}$ and following Hartung and Knapp (2005a) or Viechtbauer (2007), a further approximate $100(1-\alpha)\%$ confidence interval for τ^2 can be obtained as

$$\text{CI}(\tau^2) = \left\{ \tau^2 \geq 0 \mid \chi^2_{k-1;1-\alpha/2} \leq \tilde{Q}(\tau^2) \leq \chi^2_{k-1;\alpha/2} \right\}.$$

To determine the bounds of the confidence interval explicitly one has to solve the two equations for τ^2, namely:

$$\text{lower bound:} \qquad \tilde{Q}(\tau^2) = \chi^2_{k-1;\alpha/2},$$
$$\text{upper bound:} \qquad \tilde{Q}(\tau^2) = \chi^2_{k-1;1-\alpha/2}.$$

Let $\hat{w}_i = 1/[\hat{\tau}^2 + \hat{\sigma}_i^2(\hat{\theta}_i)]$ be the inverse of the estimated variance in model (9.1), with $\hat{\tau}^2$ being a suitable estimate of τ^2. Then the estimate of the overall effect size is given as

$$\hat{\theta} = \frac{\sum_{i=1}^{k} \hat{w}_i \hat{\theta}_i}{\sum_{i=1}^{k} \hat{w}_i}.$$

The standard approximate $100(1-\alpha)\%$ confidence interval of θ is then given as

$$\hat{\theta} \pm \left(\sum_{i=1}^{k} \hat{w}_i \right)^{-1/2} z_{\alpha/2} \qquad (9.5)$$

whereas the modified approximate $100(1-\alpha)\%$ confidence interval according to Hartung and Knapp (2001b) is obtained as

$$\hat{\theta} = \pm\sqrt{\hat{q}} \, t_{k-1,\alpha/2} \quad \text{with} \quad \hat{q} = \frac{1}{k-1} \frac{\sum_{i=1}^{k} \hat{w}_i \left(\hat{\theta}_i - \hat{\theta} \right)^2}{\sum_{i=1}^{k} \hat{w}_i} \qquad (9.6)$$

and $t_{k-1,\alpha/2}$ the upper $\alpha/2$ percentage point of the t distribution with $k-1$ df.

9.1   BINARY DATA

Recalling from Chapter 2, let π_T and π_C denote the population proportions of two groups, say treatment and control groups. The observed frequencies on the two binary characteristics can then be arranged in a 2×2-table; see Table 9.1. Hereby, m_T and m_C are the number of successes in the treatment and control group, respectively, and n_T and n_C are the corresponding samples sizes.

Table 9.1   Observed frequencies on two binary characteristics

	Success	Failure	Total
Treatment	m_T	$n_T - m_T$	n_T
Control	m_C	$n_C - m_C$	n_C

9.1.1   Effect size estimates

Three prominent parameters of the difference of two groups with binary outcome, namely, probability difference, relative risk, and odds ratio, and their estimates have already been introduced in Chapter 2. Standard large-sample meta-analysis results are summarized in Chapter 4. In this section, we discuss some properties of the estimates with emphasis on sparse data situations. Given zero cells in Table 9.1, some estimates and their variances cannot be computed.

Probability difference. The probability difference is defined as $\theta_1 = \pi_T - \pi_C$ and can be unbiasedly estimated by the difference of the observed success probabilities

$$\hat{\theta}_1 = \frac{m_T}{n_T} - \frac{m_C}{n_C}. \tag{9.7}$$

The unbiased estimate of the variance of (9.7) is

$$\widehat{\mathrm{Var}}(\hat{\theta}_1) = \frac{m_T\,(n_T - m_T)}{n_T^2\,(n_T - 1)} + \frac{m_C\,(n_C - m_C)}{n_C^2\,(n_C - 1)}. \tag{9.8}$$

Critical data situations occur only in extreme cases, namely, when $m_T = m_C = 0$ or $m_T = n_T$ and $m_C = 0$ or $m_T = 0$ and $m_C = n_C$. In the first case, the estimated difference is zero, in the second case the estimate is $+1$, and in the last case it is -1. But in all the three cases, the variance estimate is zero! Hence, the inverse of the variance is infinity and a trial with such an extreme data situation cannot be incorporated in the usual way in the meta-analysis. The two extreme cases with estimates $+1$ and -1 may be only of theoretical interest. But the case of $m_T = m_C = 0$ may be of practical interest. Consider a controlled clinical trial and suppose the number of adverse events is of interest. Especially for small sample sizes, the situation might occur that no adverse events were observed in both treatment groups.

Relative risk. Setting $\theta_2 = \ln(\pi_T/\pi_C)$, the logarithm of the relative risk, an estimate of θ_2 may be defined as

$$\hat{\theta}_2 = \ln \left(\frac{m_T \, / \, n_T}{m_C \, / \, n_C} \right). \tag{9.9}$$

However, estimate (9.9) cannot be computed when $m_T = 0$ or $m_C = 0$. Moreover, there does not exist an unbiased estimate of the log relative risk. So, different proposals exist in the literature for estimating this parameter. Pettigrew, Gart, and Thomas (1986) discuss the proposed estimators with respect to bias and variance, and there is no optimal solution. The "optimal" solution always depends on the true, but unknown, success probabilities. One widely used estimate in this context is

$$\hat{\theta}_2 = \ln \left[\frac{(m_T + 0.5) \, / \, (n_T + 0.5)}{(m_C + 0.5) \, / \, (n_C + 0.5)} \right]. \tag{9.10}$$

The variance of estimate (9.10) is estimated without bias except for terms of order $O(n^{-3})$ by

$$\widehat{\mathrm{Var}}(\hat{\theta}_2) = \frac{1}{m_T + 0.5} - \frac{1}{n_T + 0.5} + \frac{1}{m_C + 0.5} - \frac{1}{n_C + 0.5}.$$

This variance estimate is always positive if $m_T \neq n_T$ or $m_C \neq n_C$. If $m_T = n_T$ or $m_C = n_C$, then the value 0.5 will not be added to n_T and n_C to ensure the positiveness of the variance estimate.

Odds ratio. Setting $\theta_3 = \ln\{[\pi_T/(1 - \pi_T)]/[\pi_C/(1 - \pi_C)]\}$, the logarithm of the odds ratio, an estimate of θ_3 is obtained as

$$\hat{\theta}_3 = \ln \left[\frac{m_T \, / \, (n_T - m_T)}{m_C \, / \, (n_C - m_C)} \right] = \ln \left[\frac{m_T \, (n_C - m_C)}{(n_T - m_T) \, m_C} \right]. \tag{9.11}$$

As in the case of the log relative risk, the estimate (9.11) cannot be computed when there are no successes or only successes in at least one group. Again, no unbiased estimate of the log odds ratio exists and Gart and Zweifel (1967) investigate several estimates of this parameter with respect to bias and variance. One estimate, originally proposed by Haldane (1955), is widely used, namely,

$$\begin{aligned} \hat{\theta}_3 &= \ln \left[\frac{(m_T + 0.5) \, / \, (n_T - m_T + 0.5)}{(m_C + 0.5) \, / \, (n_C - m_C + 0.5)} \right] \\ &= \ln \left[\frac{(m_T + 0.5) \, (n_C - m_C + 0.5)}{(n_T - m_T + 0.5) \, (m_C + 0.5)} \right]. \end{aligned} \tag{9.12}$$

The variance of estimate (9.12) is unbiasedly estimated, except terms of order $O(n^{-3})$, by

$$\widehat{\mathrm{Var}}(\hat{\theta}_3) = \frac{1}{m_T + 0.5} + \frac{1}{n_T - m_T + 0.5} + \frac{1}{m_C + 0.5} + \frac{1}{n_C - m_C + 0.5}.$$

9.1.2 Homogeneity tests

Before combining the results from the available experiments, a test of homogeneity of treatment effects should be carried out. In experiments with binary outcome, however, the choice of the measure of treatment difference may introduce a variability between the study results. For instance, homogeneity on the risk difference scale does not in general imply homogeneity on the log odds scale and vice versa.

The test of homogeneity is usually carried out in the framework of the fixed effects model for testing the equality of the means, but the hypothesis of homogeneity can be equivalently formulated in the random effects model for testing the hypothesis that no between-study variance is present; see Chapters 6 and 7.

The commonly used test of homogeneity in meta-analysis is Cochran's (1954) test; see Chapter 4 and Eq. (9.2). The test is based on a weighted least-squares statistic and compares the study-specific estimates of the effect measure with an estimate of the common homogeneous effect measure. For the effect measure log odds ratio, Cochran's test can be very conservative. Consequently, this test does not have sufficient power to detect heterogeneity. However, for the effect measure probability difference, Cochran's test can be very liberal so that the null hypothesis of homogeneity is falsely rejected too often. Based on the random effects meta-analysis approach, Hartung and Knapp (2004) suggest another test of homogeneity which is derived from an unbiased estimator of the variance of the common effect measure in the random effects model, proposed by Hartung (1999b); see Chapter 7. Hartung and Knapp (2004) discuss tests of homogeneity for both the outcome measures probability difference and log odds ratio and work out some improvements with respect to level and power of their new test.

In different areas of application there exist further tests of homogeneity for binary outcome measures. For instance, Lipsitz et al. (1998) consider homogeneity tests for the risk difference and Liang and Self (1985) for the (logarithmic) odds ratio. We omit the details here.

9.1.3 Binomial-normal hierarchical models in meta-analysis

A critical assumption in the fixed effects or random effects model is perhaps the assumption that the estimator of the treatment difference is normally distributed, especially for small sample sizes. When the number of successes in the treatment groups are known, that is, the observed 2×2 table is given, one can make direct use of the binomially distributed number of successes. In the random effects approach this can be done in a binomial-normal hierarchical model that can be analyzed within the Bayesian framework using Markov chain Monte Carlo (MCMC) methods. Here we will only present the basic ideas of the model formulations.

Smith, Spiegelhalter, and Thomas (1995) first present the formulation for the log odds ratio that is straightforward. Then Warn, Thompson, and Spiegelhalter (2002) also consider the binomial-normal hierarchical model for the risk difference. All three models have one common feature, namely, that the number of successes m_{Ti} and m_{Ci} are both binomially distributed with parameters n_{Ti} and π_{Ti} and n_{Ci}

and π_{Ci}, respectively in each study i, $i = 1, \ldots, k$. Then let $\mu_i = \text{logit}(\pi_{Ci}) = \ln[\pi_{Ci}/(1 - \pi_{Ci})]$ be the logarithmic odds in the control group and assume that the logarithmic odds in the treatment group is $\mu_i + \theta_i$. Consequently, θ_i is the study-specific treatment difference on the log odds ratio scale. Finally, assume that θ_i comes from a normal distribution with mean θ, the overall effect of treatment difference, and variance τ^2, the heterogeneity parameter.

In summary, we may write the binomial-normal hierarchical model for the log odds ratio as

$$
\begin{aligned}
m_{Ci} &\sim \text{Bin}\left(n_{Ci}, \pi_{Ci}\right), \\
m_{Ti} &\sim \text{Bin}\left(n_{Ti}, \pi_{Ti}\right), \\
\mu_i &= \text{logit}(\pi_{Ci}), \\
\text{logit}(\pi_{Ti}) &= \mu_i + \theta_i, \\
\theta_i &\sim N(\theta, \tau^2).
\end{aligned}
\tag{9.13}
$$

Note that each value of θ_i from the normal distribution yields admissible values of the success probabilities π_{Ti} and π_{Ci}.

For the log relative risk, we set $\mu_i = \ln(\pi_{Ci})$, that is, the logarithm of the success probability in the control group. Then the logarithm of the success probability in the treatment group is parameterized as $\ln(\pi_{Ti}) = \mu_i + \theta_i$ and θ_i is the log relative risk. Again, assume that θ_i comes from a normal distribution with mean θ, the overall effect of treatment difference, and variance τ^2, the heterogeneity parameter. But now, the value θ_i needs to be constrained so that $\pi_{Ti} \in [0, 1]$. Following Warn, Thompson, and Spiegelhalter (2002) this is equivalent to constraining $\ln(\pi_{Ti})$ to the interval $(-\infty, 0]$, which is achieved by confining θ_i to be less than $-\ln(\pi_{Ci})$. Let θ_i^U be the minimum of θ_i and $-\ln(\pi_{Ci})$; then θ_i^U can take any value in the range $(-\infty, -\ln(\pi_{Ci}))$. The full model can then be summarized as

$$
\begin{aligned}
m_{Ci} &\sim \text{Bin}\left(n_{Ci}, \pi_{Ci}\right), \\
m_{Ti} &\sim \text{Bin}\left(n_{Ti}, \pi_{Ti}\right), \\
\mu_i &= \ln(\pi_{Ci}), \\
\ln(\pi_{Ti}) &= \mu_i + \min\left\{\theta_i, -\ln(\pi_{Ci})\right\}, \\
\theta_i &\sim N(\theta, \tau^2).
\end{aligned}
\tag{9.14}
$$

Finally, we consider the third effect measure probability difference. Let $\mu_i = \pi_{Ci}$ be the success probability in the control group. Then the success probability in the treatment group is parameterized as $\pi_{Ti} = \mu_i + \theta_i$, and as before assume that θ_i arises from a normal distribution with mean θ, the overall effect of treatment difference, and variance τ^2, the heterogeneity parameter. As in the previous case, the value θ_i needs to be constrained so that $\pi_{Ti} \in [0, 1]$, that is, $\theta_i \in [-\pi_{Ci}, 1 - \pi_{Ci}]$. Define two new parameters θ_i^U and θ_i^L, corresponding to upper and lower bounds for θ_i. Let θ_i^L be the maximum of θ_i and $-\pi_{Ci}$; then θ_i^L can take any value in the range $[-\pi_{Ci}, \infty)$. Similarly, let θ_i^U be the minimum of θ_i^L and $1 - \pi_{Ci}$; then θ_i is confined to the required range $[-\pi_{Ci}, 1 - \pi_{Ci}]$. The full model is then given by

$$
\begin{aligned}
m_{Ci} &\sim \mathrm{Bin}\,(n_{Ci}, \pi_{Ci})\,, \\
m_{Ti} &\sim \mathrm{Bin}\,(n_{Ti}, \pi_{Ti})\,, \\
\mu_i &= \pi_{Ci}, \\
\pi_{Ti} &= \mu_i + \min\{\max\{\theta_i, -\pi_{Ci}\}, 1 - \pi_{Ci}\}\,, \\
\theta_i &\sim N(\theta, \tau^2).
\end{aligned}
\tag{9.15}
$$

For a full Bayesian analysis in the models (9.13), (9.14), and (9.15), appropriate prior distributions have to be determined for the hyperparameters θ and τ^2 as well as for the success probabilities p_{Ci} in the control groups, which may also be called baseline risk. A Bayesian meta-analysis can be conducted using the software WinBUGS.

9.1.4   An example for combining results from controlled clinical trials

Hartung and Knapp (2001b) put together the results of 13 controlled trials of a drug named cisapride compared to placebo for the treatment of nonulcer dyspepsia. The data are given in Section 18.5 with further information of the research problem. The originally conducted meta-analysis was done with the probability difference as the effect size; see Allescher et al. (2001). Besides the probability difference, we also consider here the log odds ratio as effect size for demonstration purposes. Table 9.2 contains the estimates of the probability difference (PD) and the log odds ratio [ln(OR)] with corresponding standard errors.

Table 9.2   Estimates of probability difference and log odds ratio with corresponding standard errors for the 13 cisapride studies

Study	PD	s.e.(PD)	ln(OR)	s.e.[ln(OR)]
1	0.3750	0.1425	2.4567	1.1492
2	0.6875	0.1281	3.8067	1.1832
3	0.3235	0.1065	1.6401	0.5937
4	0.1964	0.0889	0.8835	0.4093
5	0.3636	0.1431	1.5404	0.6524
6	0.5057	0.0825	2.2860	0.4559
7	0.3569	0.1639	1.6740	0.8201
8	0.1034	0.0927	0.4200	0.3755
9	0.5143	0.1647	2.3026	0.8756
10	0.4316	0.1253	1.8888	0.6199
11	0.5970	0.0848	2.8574	0.5537
12	-0.0782	0.1217	-0.3697	0.5684
13	0.0526	0.1159	0.2113	0.4601

Let us first combine the results for the probability difference. Cochran's homogeneity statistic [see Eq. (9.2)] yields $Q = 49.44$ and, compared to 21.03, the 5%

cut-off point of the chi-square distribution with 12 degrees of freedom, leads to a rejection of the homogeneity hypothesis. This indicates that the use of the random effects meta-analysis model is appropriate. The DerSimonian-Laird estimate of the heterogeneity parameter is $\hat{\tau}^2_{\text{DSL}} = 0.0391$ and the REML estimate of τ^2 is $\hat{\tau}^2_{\text{REML}} = 0.0376$. Both estimates are rather close, so we will use the value of $\hat{\tau}^2_{\text{DSL}}$ for further analysis. The overall estimate for the probability difference is 0.3375 with 95% confidence interval $[0.2119, 0.4632]$ using interval (9.5) and 95% confidence interval $[0.2021, 0.4730]$ using interval (9.6). For applying the binomial-hierarchical model for the probability difference [see model (9.15)], we use as prior distributions for θ the uniform distribution on the interval $[-1, 1]$ and for τ, the standard deviation between the studies, the uniform distribution on the interval $[0, 2]$. Finally, we have to specify priors for p_{Ci}, the underlying or baseline risk. We use two different approaches. First, we use the noninformative prior $U[0, 1]$, the uniform distribution on the interval $[0, 1]$ (method A) and, second, we use as prior for p_{Ci} the beta distribution with parameters α and β and as priors for both parameters of the beta distribution the uniform distribution on the intervals $[1, 100]$ (method B). Method A produces an estimate of τ^2 as 0.034. Then, the estimate of the overall probability difference is 0.300 with 95% credible interval $[0.174, 0.425]$. With method B, the estimate of τ^2 is 0.014, and the estimate of the overall probability difference is 0.310 with 95% credible interval $[0.221, 0.405]$.

On the log odds ratio scale, Cochran's homogeneity statistic is $Q = 41.67$ and again the homogeneity hypothesis is rejected. The DerSimonian-Laird estimate is $\hat{\tau}^2_{\text{DSL}} = 0.8086$ and the REML estimate $\hat{\tau}^2_{\text{REML}} = 0.8155$. Again using $\hat{\tau}^2_{\text{DSL}}$ for further analysis leads to an overall estimate of the log odds ratio of 1.4911 with 95% confidence interval $[0.8881, 2.0941]$ using interval (9.5) and 95% confidence interval $[0.8206, 2.1617]$ using interval (9.6). To apply the binomial-hierarchical model (9.13), we use the same priors as above except that we now take $N(0, 10)$ as the prior for θ. Method A produces an estimate of τ^2 as 1.122, and the estimate of the overall log odds ratio is 1.445 with 95% credible interval $[0.782, 2.206]$. With method B, the estimate of τ^2 is 0.494, and the estimate of the overall log odds ratio difference is 1.491 with 95% credible interval $[1.039, 1.963]$.

9.1.5 An example for combining results from observational studies

As an example for combining results of observational studies we use the studies on second-hand smoking from Section 18.6. Since only estimates of relative risk with corresponding 95% confidence intervals are provided, we have to extract the standard error of the estimates using the general method described in Section 17.1. Usually the effects are estimated on the log scale and then the estimates are transformed to the original scale. Consequently, we first use the logarithms of the bounds of the confidence limits and then extract the standard error of the logarithm of the estimate. The results are summarized in Table 9.3.

For testing homogeneity on the logarithmic relative risk scale, Cochran's homogeneity test yields a value of 17.204 corresponding to a P-value of 0.509. Thus, the homogeneity assumption cannot be rejected and we feel quite confident to apply the

Table 9.3   Nineteen studies on second-hand smoking

Study	Relative risk	95% CI on RR	$\ln(RR)$	$\text{s.e.}(\ln(RR))$
1	1.52	$[0.88 - 2.63]$	0.419	0.279
2	1.52	$[0.39 - 5.99]$	0.419	0.697
3	0.81	$[0.34 - 1.90]$	-0.211	0.439
4	0.75	$[0.43 - 1.30]$	-0.288	0.282
5	2.07	$[0.82 - 5.25]$	0.728	0.477
6	1.19	$[0.82 - 1.73]$	0.174	0.190
7	1.31	$[0.87 - 1.98]$	0.270	0.210
8	2.16	$[1.08 - 4.29]$	0.770	0.352
9	2.34	$[0.81 - 6.75]$	0.850	0.541
10	2.55	$[0.74 - 8.78]$	0.936	0.631
11	0.79	$[0.25 - 2.45]$	-0.236	0.582
12	1.55	$[0.90 - 2.67]$	0.438	0.277
13	1.65	$[1.16 - 2.35]$	0.501	0.180
14	2.01	$[1.09 - 3.71]$	0.698	0.312
15	1.03	$[0.41 - 2.55]$	0.030	0.466
16	1.28	$[0.76 - 2.15]$	0.247	0.265
17	1.26	$[0.57 - 2.82]$	0.231	0.408
18	2.13	$[1.19 - 3.83]$	0.756	0.298
19	1.41	$[0.54 - 3.67]$	0.344	0.489

results in the fixed effects model from Chapter 4. The overall estimate of the log relative risk is 0.351 with 95% confidence interval $[0.212, 0.490]$ using interval (9.5), which yields an estimate of $\exp(0.351) = 1.421$ on the relative risk scale with 95% confidence interval $[\exp(0.212), \exp(0.490)] = [1.236, 1.633]$. The DerSimonian-Laird estimator for the between-study variance is equal to zero, as expected from the result of the homogeneity test, but the restricted maximum likelihood estimator of the between-study variance is slightly positive, namely, $\tau^2_{REML} = 0.00089$, but this does not essentially change the overall meta-analysis result. Moreover, applying interval (9.6) to the present data situation results in a slightly wider 95% confidence interval for the relative risk, namely, $[1.228, 1.643]$, but this does not change the overall conclusion from this meta-analysis.

9.2   ORDINAL DATA

The data from a controlled trial with ordinal outcome can be arranged in a $2 \times r$ contingency table as in Table 9.4, where r denotes the number of categories of the response variable. In Table 9.4, n_{Tj} denotes the number of subjects in the first group with response in the jth category and n_{Cj} the corresponding number of subject in the control group. The sample sizes in the two groups are $n_{T.} = \sum_{j=1}^{r} n_{Tj}$ and $n_{C.} = \sum_{j=1}^{r} n_{Cj}$, respectively.

Table 9.4 Data from a controlled trial with ordinal outcome

	Category				
	1	2	$\cdots$	r	Total
Treatment	n_{T1}	n_{T2}	$\cdots$	n_{Tr}	$n_{T.}$
Control	n_{C1}	n_{C2}	$\cdots$	n_{Cr}	$n_{C.}$

Let $\pi_{1j} > 0$, $j = 1, \ldots, r$, be the probability of observing a response in the jth category in the first group and $\pi_{2j} > 0$ be the corresponding probability in the second group. Note that $\sum_{j=1}^{r} \pi_{1j} = \sum_{j=1}^{r} \pi_{2j} = 1$. We assume that the categories are ordered in terms of desirability: category 1 is the best and category r is the worst.

Let Y_T denote the response variable in the first sample and Y_C the one in the second sample. Then, in view of the ordering of the categories, the treatment is superior to the control when Y_C is stochastically larger than Y_T. If Y_C is stochastically larger than Y_T, then it holds that $\Pr(Y_C > Y_T) \geq \Pr(Y_C < Y_T)$. However, if the inequality is true, then it does not necessarily follow that Y_C is stochastically larger than Y_T. In the following two sections, we consider two effect measures that may be used to describe the difference of the response variables in a controlled trial with ordinal outcome.

9.2.1 Proportional odds model

The proportional odds model was introduced by McCullagh (1980). Consider the cumulative probabilities $q_{1j} = \sum_{i=1}^{j} \pi_{1i}$ and $q_{2j} = \sum_{i=1}^{j} \pi_{2i}$, respectively, up to category j, $j = 1, \ldots, r - 1$; then the odds ratio given cut-off point category j is

$$\theta_j = \frac{q_{1j}(1 - q_{2j})}{(1 - q_{1j})q_{2j}}, \qquad j = 1, \ldots, r - 1. \tag{9.16}$$

The proportional odds assumption reads

$$\theta_1 = \theta_2 = \cdots = \theta_{r-1} =: \theta. \tag{9.17}$$

If $\theta > 1$, then the treatment is superior to the control in view of the above ordering of the categories. This implies that Y_C is stochastically larger than Y_T. But, through the model assumption of proportional odds, the nature of how Y_C is stochastically larger than Y_T is restricted. The proportional odds model can be analyzed using standard statistical software packages for linear logistic regression like SAS or R. These software packages usually yield the maximum likelihood estimate of the log odds ratio and the corresponding standard error. Additional remarks for the analysis in the proportional odds model can be found in Whitehead and Jones (1994). Note that the proportional odds model can be considered as arising from a latent continuous variable, where this latent variable has a logistic distribution; see Whitehead et al. (2001) for further details.

9.2.2 Agresti's α

Agresti (1980) proposed a measure of association, here briefly named Agresti's α, which, in case of a $2 \times r$ contingency table, can be seen as a generalized odds ratio. Agresti's α is the ratio of $\Pr(Y_C > Y_T)$ and $\Pr(Y_C < Y_T)$, that is, in the present context, the probability to observe a worse response in the control group than in the treatment group divided by the probability to observe a better response in the control group than in the treatment group. In symbols, Agresti's α can be written as

$$\alpha = \frac{\sum_{j>i} \pi_{Ti}\, \pi_{Cj}}{\sum_{j<i} \pi_{Ti}\, \pi_{Cj}}. \tag{9.18}$$

Note that, if Y_C is stochastically larger than Y_t, then $\alpha > 1$. However, $\alpha > 1$ does not necessarily mean that Y_C is stochastically larger than Y_T. In case Y_C is stochastically larger than Y_T, Agresti's α is a meaningful measure of the difference of all possible distributions of Y_T and Y_C. If the distributions of Y_T and Y_C are identical, then $\alpha = 1$ and $\theta = 1$. However, $\alpha = 1$ again does not necessarily mean that the two distributions are identical. It only means that the two probabilities, $\Pr(Y_C > Y_T)$ and $\Pr(Y_C < Y_T)$, are identical. Of course, for 2×2 tables, Agresti's α is the odds ratio.

Agresti's α is easily estimated by plugging in the observed proportions $\hat{p}_{Ti} = n_{Ti}/n_T$ and $\hat{p}_{Ci} = n_{Ci}/n_C$, $i = 1, \ldots, r$, in Eq. (9.18) and we denote this estimator by $\hat{\alpha}$. Note that $\hat{\alpha}$ does not exist when "zeros occur".

Agresti (1980) provided a large-sample estimator of the variance of the estimator of α. This variance estimator reads

$$\hat{\sigma}(\hat{\alpha}) = \left(\sum_{i>j} \hat{p}_{Ti}\hat{p}_{Ci}\right)^{-2} \left[\frac{1}{n_T} \sum_j \hat{p}_{Tj}\left(\hat{\alpha} \sum_{i<j} \hat{p}_{Ci} - \sum_{i>j} \hat{p}_{Ci}\right)^2 \right.$$
$$\left. + \frac{1}{n_C} \sum_j \hat{p}_{Cj}\left(\hat{\alpha} \sum_{i>j} \hat{p}_{Ti} - \sum_{i<j} \hat{p}_{Ti}\right)^2.\right] \tag{9.19}$$

For constructing confidence intervals for Agresti's α, it is convenient to make the inference first on $\ln(\alpha)$ since the distribution of $\ln(\hat{\alpha})$ tends to be more symmetric and is likely to converge to normality faster than the distribution of $\hat{\alpha}$. According to Agresti (1980), the large-sample $1 - \kappa$ confidence interval for α is then given as $\exp\left(\ln(\hat{\alpha}) \pm z_{\kappa/2}\, \hat{\sigma}(\hat{\alpha}) \,/\, \hat{\alpha}\right)$ with z_γ being the γ cut-off point of the standard normal distribution.

9.2.3 An example of combining results from controlled clinical trials

For illustration purposes, we take an example from Whitehead and Jones (1994). The data as well as a more detailed description of the research problem are given in Section 18.7. Briefly, the extent of gastrointestinal damage was assessed for patients suffering from arthritis using a drug named misoprostol compared to patients not using this drug. In the different studies, the number of classification categories were different ranging from two to five. Score tests on proportional odds assumptions do not reveal any violation of this assumption in all the trials; see Whitehead and Jones (1994). Besides the meta-analysis on the log odds ratio scale, we describe the meta-analysis using Agresti's α as the measure of effect size. Table 9.5 contains the study-specific estimates along with standard errors as well as the corresponding 95% confidence intervals for both effect size measures considered here.

Table 9.5 Study-specific estimates, their standard errors, and 95% confidence intervals in the misoprostol example

	Proportional odds			Agresti's α		
Study	$\ln(\hat{\theta})$	s.e.$[\ln(\hat{\theta})]$	95% CI	$\ln(\hat{\alpha})$	s.e.$[\ln(\hat{\alpha})]$	95% CI
1	3.55	0.66	[2.25, 4.84]	3.04	0.56	[1.95, 4.14]
2	4.05	0.72	[2.64, 5.46]	3.58	0.62	[2.36, 4.79]
3	1.91	0.53	[0.87, 2.95]	1.69	0.46	[0.78, 2.60]
4	3.75	0.69	[2.40, 5.10]	3.04	0.59	[1.88, 4.19]
5	6.51	2.28	[2.04, 10.98]	4.02	1.96	[0.19, 7.86]
6	1.18	0.40	[0.40, 1.95]	1.12	0.38	[0.38, 1.86]
7	1.19	0.39	[0.43, 1.96]	1.19	0.39	[0.43, 1.94]
8	1.84	1.07	[−0.26, 3.94]	1.84	1.07	[−0.25, 3.92]
9	2.96	1.04	[0.93, 5.00]	2.96	1.04	[0.93, 5.00]
10	2.49	0.75	[1.01, 3.96]	2.49	0.75	[1.01, 3.96]
11	2.57	0.80	[1.00, 4.13]	2.37	0.78	[0.83, 3.91]
12	0.65	0.34	[−0.02, 1.31]	0.60	0.31	[−0.01, 1.21]
13	1.11	0.71	[−0.28, 2.50]	1.04	0.65	[−0.24, 2.31]

For both effect measures, the meta-analysis in a random effects model is appropriate. The values of Cochran's homogeneity statistic are 49.49 (log odds ratio) and 42.30 (log α), leading to P-values less than 0.0001. The DerSimonian-Laird estimate for the heterogeneity parameter is 1.1074 on the log odds ratio scale and 0.7672 on the log Agresti's α scale. The combined estimate is 2.2614 (95% CI: $[1.4665, 3.0561]$) for the log odds ratio and 2.0160 (95% CI: $[1.3906, 2.6413]$) for log Agresti's α, where the confidence intervals have been computed using interval (9.6).

CHAPTER 10

META-REGRESSION

As mentioned in the introduction, in case of substantial heterogeneity between the studies, possible causes of the heterogeneity should be explored. In the context of meta-analysis this can be done by either covariates on the study level that could explain the differences between the studies or covariates on the subject level. However, the latter approach is only possible when individual data are available. Since often only information on the study level is available, explaining and investigating heterogeneity by covariates on the study level have drawn much attention in applied sciences. The term meta-regression used to describe such analysis goes back to papers by Bashore, Osman, and Heffley (1989), Jones (1992), Greenland (1994), and Berlin and Antman (1994).

Since the number of studies in a meta-analysis is usually quite small, there is a great danger of overfitting. So, there is only room for a few explanatory variables in a meta-regression, whereas a lot of characteristics of the studies may be identified as potential causes of heterogeneity. Higgins and Thompson (2004) remark that explorations of heterogeneity are noted to be potentially misleading. Investigations of differences between the studies and their results are observational associations and are subject to biases (such as aggregation bias) and confounding (resulting from correlation between study characteristics). Consequently, there is a clear danger

Statistical Meta-Analysis with Applications. By Joachim Hartung, Guido Knapp, Bimal K. Sinha **127**
Copyright © 2008 John Wiley & Sons, Inc.

of misleading conclusions if P-values from multiple meta-regression analyses are interpreted naïvely.

This chapter is organized as follows. In Section 10.1 we describe in detail the analysis of the fixed and random effects meta-regression with one covariate. Section 10.2 contains the general analysis of meta-regression with more than one covariate. At the end of Section 10.2, an example with three covariates is worked out in detail. Finally, in Section 10.3, several meta-regression-type models will be presented which deal with other aspects of meta-analysis than explaining heterogeneity. However, the general analysis methods from Section 10.2 can be used to fit these models.

10.1   MODEL WITH ONE COVARIATE

In the fixed effects meta-regression we write

$$Y_i \sim N\left(\theta_i,\, \sigma_i^2\right), \quad i = 1, \ldots, k,$$

where Y_i is the statistic in the ith study. The study-specific mean θ_i is parameterized as

$$\theta_i = \theta + \beta x_i,$$

where x_i denotes a quantitative covariate or an indicator variable for a factor with only two levels, that is, $x_i = 0$ or $x_i = 1$. In case of a factor with two levels, θ represents the treatment effect given $x_i = 0$ and β is the difference of the treatment effect given $x_i = 1$ compared to $x_i = 0$. For a quantitative covariate, β stands for the change in the treatment effect given a unit change in the covariate. When the quantitative covariate is centered around its mean, θ represents the treatment effect given the mean of the quantitative covariate.

Additionally to the parameterization of the mean of the study-specific treatment effect, we can allow for a parameter of the still unexplained variation between the trials. That is, we can consider, in analogy to the random effects model of meta-analysis (see Chapter 7) the following two-stage model:

$$\begin{aligned} Y_i &\sim N\left(\theta_i,\, \sigma_i^2\right), \\ \theta_i &\sim N\left(\theta + \beta x_i,\, \sigma_a^2\right). \end{aligned}$$

The random effects meta-regression with one covariate is given as the marginal two-stage model, that is,

$$Y_i \sim N\left(\theta + \beta x_i,\, \sigma_a^2 + \sigma_i^2\right). \tag{10.1}$$

In the following, we will present the analysis in the random effects meta-regression. The corresponding analysis in the fixed effects meta-regression can be performed by setting $\sigma_a^2 = 0$.

Let $w_i = 1/\left(\sigma_a^2 + \sigma_i^2\right)$, $i = 1, \ldots, k$, be the true inverse of the variance of Y_i, $w = \sum_{i=1}^{k} w_i$, and $\lambda_i = w_i/w$, $i = 1, \ldots, k$, the normed weights; then the weighted least-squares estimators of θ and β are given by

$$\tilde{\beta} = \frac{\sum_{i=1}^{k} \lambda_i \, x_i \, Y_i - \sum_{i=1}^{k} \lambda_i \, x_i \, \sum_{i=1}^{k} \lambda_i \, Y_i}{\sum_{i=1}^{k} \lambda_i \, x_i^2 - \left(\sum_{i=1}^{k} \lambda_i x_i \right)^2} \tag{10.2}$$

and

$$\tilde{\theta} = \sum_{i=1}^{k} \lambda_i \, Y_i - \tilde{\beta} \sum_{i=1}^{k} \lambda_i \, x_i. \tag{10.3}$$

The variances and the covariance of the estimators $\tilde{\theta}$ and $\tilde{\beta}$ are

$$\text{Var}(\tilde{\theta}) = \left[\sum_{i=1}^{k} w_i - \left(\sum_{i=1}^{k} w_i \, x_i \right)^2 \Big/ \sum_{i=1}^{k} w_i \, x_i^2 \right]^{-1}, \tag{10.4}$$

$$\text{Var}(\tilde{\beta}) = \left[\sum_{i=1}^{k} w_i \, x_i^2 - \left(\sum_{i=1}^{k} w_i \, x_i \right)^2 \Big/ \sum_{i=1}^{k} w_i \right]^{-1}, \tag{10.5}$$

and

$$\text{Cov}(\tilde{\theta}, \tilde{\beta}) = \frac{- \sum_{i=1}^{k} w_i \, x_i}{\sum_{i=1}^{k} w_i \, \sum_{i=1}^{k} w_i \, x_i^2 - \left(\sum_{i=1}^{k} w_i \, x_i \right)^2}. \tag{10.6}$$

Usually, every study provides an estimate of the within-study variance σ_i^2. The between-study variance σ_a^2 can be estimated using the different estimation procedures discussed in Chapter 7 adapted for the meta-regression model with one covariate. In the following we will confine ourselves to the extension of the DerSimonian-Laird estimator and to the restricted maximum likelihood estimator; see Chapter 7.

Let $\hat{w}_i = 1/(\hat{\sigma}_a^2 + \hat{\sigma}_i^2)$, $i = 1, \ldots, k$, denote the consistent estimators of w_i, and by plugging in these estimators in Eqs. (10.2) and (10.3), we obtain the weighted least-squares estimators, denoted by $\hat{\theta}$ and $\hat{\beta}$.

The method of moments (MM) estimator of the between-study variance σ_a^2 can be derived from the statistic $Q_1 = \sum_{i=1}^{k} w_i^* (Y_i - \hat{\theta}^* - \hat{\beta}^* x_i)^2$, where $\hat{\theta}^*$ and $\hat{\beta}^*$ are weighted least-squares estimators of θ and β with known weights $w_i^* = 1/\sigma_i^2$, $i = 1, \ldots, k$, that is, the weighted least-squares estimators in the fixed effects meta-regression. So, the quadratic form Q_1 can also be seen as the residual sum of squares in the fixed effects meta-regression model. The MM estimator is given in its truncated form as

$$\hat{\sigma}_a^2 = \max \left\{ 0 \, ; \, \frac{Q_1 - (k - 2)}{F(\boldsymbol{w}^*, \boldsymbol{x})} \right\} \tag{10.7}$$

with

$$F(\boldsymbol{w}^*, \boldsymbol{x}) = \sum_{i=1}^{k} w_i^* - \frac{\sum w_i^{*2} \sum w_i^* \, x_i^2 - 2 \sum w_i^{*2} x_i \sum w_i^* x_i + \sum w_i^* \sum w_i^{*2} x_i^2}{\sum w_i^* \sum w_i^* \, x_i^2 - \left(\sum w_i^* \, x_i \right)^2}.$$

In practice, the usually unknown variances σ_i^2 have to be replaced by their estimates in Eq. (10.7).

The (approximate) REML estimator for σ_a^2 in model (10.1) is the solution of the estimating equation:

$$\hat{\sigma}_a^2 = \frac{\sum_{i=1}^{k} \hat{w}_i^2 \left\{ [k/(k-2)](Y_i - \hat{\theta} - \hat{\beta}x_i)^2 - \hat{\xi}_i \right\}}{\sum_{i=1}^{k} \hat{w}_i^2}. \tag{10.8}$$

This equation is iteratively solved using a starting value of σ_a^2, say $\sigma_a^2 = \sigma_{a0}^2$, on the right-hand side of Eq. (10.8). With the weights $\hat{w}_i = 1/(\sigma_{a0}^2 + \hat{\sigma}_i^2)$, the initial values of $\hat{\theta}$ and $\hat{\beta}$ are given. Then the right-hand side of Eq. (10.8) can be evaluated to yield a new value of $\hat{\sigma}_a^2$. This provides new weights $\hat{w}_i$ and leads to new estimates of θ and β and finally to a new value of $\hat{\sigma}_a^2$. The procedure continues until convergence under the restriction that $\hat{\sigma}_a^2$ is nonnegative.

The commonly used (large-sample) $1 - \alpha$ confidence intervals on the parameters θ and β are then given by

$$\hat{\theta} \pm \sqrt{\widehat{\mathrm{Var}}(\hat{\theta})}\, z_{\alpha/2} \tag{10.9}$$

and

$$\hat{\beta} \pm \sqrt{\widehat{\mathrm{Var}}(\hat{\beta})}\, z_{\alpha/2}, \tag{10.10}$$

where $\widehat{\mathrm{Var}}(\hat{\theta})$ and $\widehat{\mathrm{Var}}(\hat{\beta})$ are obtained by putting $\hat{w}_i$, $i = 1, \ldots, k$, in Eqs. (10.4) and (10.5), respectively, and $z_{\alpha/2}$ is the upper $\alpha/2$ cut-off point of the standard normal distribution.

Like in the random effects model of meta-analysis discussed in Chapter 7, the use of the standard normal distribution in Eqs. (10.9) and (10.10) is questionable, especially when the number of studies is small. Based on simulation results, Berkey et al. (1995) recommend the use of a t distribution with 4 degrees of freedom, where they consider the log relative risk as an outcome measure in the simulation.

Knapp and Hartung (2003) consider the quadratic form

$$Q_2 = \frac{1}{k-2} \sum_{i=1}^{k} w_i \, (Y_i - \tilde{\theta} - \tilde{\beta}\, x_i)^2, \quad k > 2. \tag{10.11}$$

This quadratic form can be seen as a mean sum of the weighted least-squares residuals with known variance components. Knapp and Hartung (2003) show that, under normality of Y_i, the quadratic form Q_2 from Eq. (10.11) is stochastically independent of the weighted least-squares estimators $\tilde{\theta}$ and $\tilde{\beta}$ and that $(k-2)\,Q_2$ is χ^2 distributed with $k-2$ degrees of freedom. Consequently, the expected value of Q_2 is equal to 1 for known variance components.

Hence, unbiased and nonnegative estimators of the variances of θ and β are given by

$$Q_2(\tilde{\theta}) = \frac{1}{k-2} \sum_{i=1}^{k} g_i \, (Y_i - \tilde{\theta} - \tilde{\beta}\, x_i)^2 \tag{10.12}$$

with $g_i = w_i / [\sum w_j - (\sum w_j x_j)^2 / \sum w_j x_j^2]$, $i = 1, \ldots, k$, and

$$Q_2(\tilde{\beta}) = \frac{1}{k-2} \sum_{i=1}^{k} h_i \, (Y_i - \tilde{\theta} - \tilde{\beta} x_i)^2 \qquad (10.13)$$

with $h_i = w_i / [\sum w_j x_j^2 - (\sum w_j x_j)^2 / \sum w_j]$, $i = 1, \ldots, k$.

Replacing the unknown variance components in Eqs. (10.12) and (10.13) by appropriate estimates, Knapp and Hartung (2003) propose the following approximate $1 - \alpha$ confidence intervals on θ and β:

$$\hat{\theta} \pm \sqrt{\hat{Q}_2(\hat{\theta})} \, t_{k-2,\alpha/2} \qquad (10.14)$$

and

$$\hat{\beta} \pm \sqrt{\hat{Q}_2(\hat{\beta})} \, t_{k-2,\alpha/2} \, , \qquad (10.15)$$

where $t_{k-2,\alpha/2}$ denotes the upper $\alpha/2$ cut-off point of the t distribution with $k - 2$ degrees of freedom.

Using either the MM estimator or the REML estimator of the between-trial variance, the confidence intervals (10.14) and (10.15) are smaller than the corresponding intervals (10.9) and (10.10) when the realized value of the quadratic form Q_2 from Eq. (10.11) is less than 1 given equal test distributions in both cases. Therefore, Knapp and Hartung (2003) consider an ad hoc modification of the variance estimates $\hat{Q}_2(\hat{\theta})$ and $\hat{Q}_2(\hat{\beta})$ in the limits of the confidence intervals (10.14) and (10.15) to the effect that they force the realized value of Q_2 to be at least 1. That is, the modified confidence intervals are given by

$$\hat{\theta} \pm \sqrt{\hat{Q}_2^*(\hat{\theta})} \, t_{k-2,\alpha/2} \qquad (10.16)$$

with

$$\hat{Q}_2^*(\hat{\theta}) = \frac{1}{\sum \hat{w}_i - (\sum \hat{w}_i x_i)^2 / \sum \hat{w}_i x_i^2} \max\left\{ 1 \, ; \, \frac{1}{k-2} \sum \hat{w}_i (Y_i - \hat{\theta} - \hat{\beta} x_i)^2 \right\}$$

and

$$\hat{\beta} \pm \sqrt{\hat{Q}_2^*(\hat{\beta})} \, t_{k-2,\alpha/2} \qquad (10.17)$$

with

$$\hat{Q}_2^*(\hat{\beta}) = \frac{1}{\sum \hat{w}_i x_i^2 - (\sum \hat{w}_i x_i)^2 / \sum \hat{w}_i} \max\left\{ 1 \, ; \, \frac{1}{k-2} \sum \hat{w}_i (Y_i - \hat{\theta} - \hat{\beta} x_i)^2 \right\} .$$

In a simulation study, Knapp and Hartung (2003) consider the log relative risk as outcome measure in a meta-regression setting. The main result of their simulation study is that the intervals (10.16) and (10.17) outperform the other corresponding intervals with respect to the nominal confidence coefficient.

10.2 MODEL WITH MORE THAN ONE COVARIATE

The extension of model (10.1) to the case with more than one covariate is given as

$$Y_i \sim N\left(\theta + x_i'\beta, \sigma_a^2 + \sigma_i^2\right), \quad i = 1\ldots, k,$$

where x_i is now a vector of covariates and β a vector of corresponding regression parameters. In matrix notation, the general random effects meta-regression for meta-analysis with $r - 1$ covariates can be described as

$$Y \sim N(X\gamma, \sigma_a^2 I_k + \Delta) \tag{10.18}$$

with $Y = (Y_1, \ldots, Y_k)'$, X the $(k \times r)$-dimensional known regressor matrix with rank$(X) = r < k - 1$, $\gamma = (\theta, \beta_1, \ldots, \beta_{r-1})'$ the unknown parameter vector of the fixed effects, σ_a^2 the between-trial variance, I_k the $(k \times k)$-dimensional identity matrix, and Δ a $(k \times k)$-dimensional diagonal matrix with entries σ_i^2, $i = 1, \ldots, k$, that is, Δ contains the within-trial variances. Note that the case of a factor with more than two levels can be included in model (10.18) by defining appropriate indicator variables equal to the number of factor levels minus 1.

The residual sum of squares in model (10.18) with $\sigma_a^2 = 0$ can be expressed as a quadratic form in Y and has the matrix representation

$$Q = Y'P'\Delta^{-1}PY \quad \text{with} \quad P = [I_k - X(X'\Delta^{-1}X)^{-1}X'\Delta^{-1}] \,.$$

Since $PX = 0$, the expected value of Q is given as

$$
\begin{aligned}
\mathrm{E}(Q) &= \text{trace}[P'\Delta^{-1}P\,\text{Cov}(Y)] \\
&= \text{trace}[P'\Delta^{-1}P\,\Delta] + \sigma_a^2\,\text{trace}[P'\Delta^{-1}P] \\
&= k - r + \sigma_a^2\,f(X, \Delta^{-1})
\end{aligned}
$$

with $f(X, \Delta^{-1}) = \text{trace}(\Delta^{-1}) - \text{trace}[(X'\Delta^{-1}X)^{-1}X'\Delta^{-2}X]$. Consequently, the MM estimator of σ_a^2 is given in its truncated form as

$$\hat{\sigma}_a^2 = \max\left\{ 0, \frac{Q - (k - r)}{f(X, \Delta^{-1})}\right\} \,.$$

The (approximate) REML can be determined by solving iteratively the equation

$$\hat{\sigma}_a^2 = \frac{\sum_{i=1}^{k} \hat{w}_i^2 \left\{ [k/(k-r)](y_i - \hat{\theta} - x_i'\hat{\beta})^2 - \hat{\sigma}_i^2\right\})}{\sum_{i=1}^{k} \hat{w}_i^2} \,.$$

Let $\hat{\Lambda} = \hat{\sigma}_a^2 I_k + \hat{\Delta}$ be the estimated covariance matrix; then the estimate of γ is given by

$$\hat{\gamma} = \left(X'\hat{\Lambda}^{-1}X\right)^{-1} X'\hat{\Lambda}^{-1}Y$$

with estimated covariance matrix

$$\widehat{\mathrm{Cov}}(\hat{\gamma}) = \left(X'\hat{\Lambda}^{-1}X\right)^{-1}.$$

With the estimated variances on the main diagonal of $\widehat{\mathrm{Cov}}(\hat{\gamma})$, confidence intervals and hypothesis tests on the fixed effects can be constructed in the usual manner. To carry forward the approach by Knapp and Hartung (2003) to the case of more than one covariate, let us consider the matrix

$$P_1 = I_k - X\left(X'\hat{\Lambda}^{-1}X\right)^{-1}X'\hat{\Lambda}^{-1}$$

and calculate the quadratic form

$$\hat{Q}_r = \frac{Y'P_1'\hat{\Lambda}^{-1}P_1Y}{k-r}.$$

The improved variance estimate of a fixed effect estimate is then given by multiplying the corresponding diagonal element in $\widehat{\mathrm{Cov}}(\hat{\gamma})$ with $\hat{Q}_r$. For constructing confidence intervals on the fixed effects the t distribution with $k-r$ degrees of freedom should be used.

For illustrating the methods presented above we consider the data of 13 trials from Colditz et al. (1994), also used in Berkey et al. (1995), van Houwelingen, Arends, and Stijnen (2002), and Knapp and Hartung (2003). In these 13 trials the effect of Bacillus Calmette-Guérin (BCG) vaccination has been investigated on the prevention of tuberculosis. Possible covariates that may explain the heterogeneity between the trials are latitude, year of study, and type of allocation. Three different methods of treatment allocation were used: alternate, random, or systematic. All the necessary data are put together in Table 10.1; see Section 18.8 for more information about the data and the research problem.

The effect size measure used here is the relative risk. The study results on the logarithmic scale along with the corresponding 95% confidence intervals are summarized in Table 10.2. Studies 8 and 12 have positive but nonsignificant log relative risk estimates, and studies 1, 5, and 13 negative but nonsignificant estimates. The remaining eight studies yield significant results in favor of the vaccination in preventing tuberculosis. Obviously, the study results are heterogeneous and the random effects approach of meta-analysis is the appropriate one.

First, ignoring covariates, the DerSimonian-Laird estimate of σ_a^2 is 0.304 and the REML estimate is 0.298. Both heterogeneity estimates lead to the estimate -0.700 of the overall log relative risk with 95% confidence interval $[-1.084, -0.317]$, a significant result in favor of the vaccination. Throughout this example, the estimates of the heterogeneity parameter using either the DerSimonian-Laird approach or the REML approach are pretty similar and do not influence the conclusions of the inference on further parameters. Therefore, we omit the results using the REML estimate of σ_a^2.

In the following, we provide analyses of the data in different random effects meta-regression models. For calculating confidence intervals we always use formulas

Table 10.1   Data on 13 trials on the prevention of tuberculosis using BCG vaccination

	Vaccinated		Not vaccinated				
Trial	Disease	No disease	Disease	No disease	Latitude	Year	Allocation
1	4	119	11	128	44	1948	Random
2	6	300	29	274	55	1949	Random
3	3	228	11	209	42	1960	Random
4	62	13,536	248	12,619	52	1977	Random
5	33	5,036	47	5,761	13	1973	Alternate
6	180	1,361	372	1,079	44	1953	Alternate
7	8	2,537	10	619	19	1973	Random
8	505	87,886	499	87,892	13	1980	Random
9	29	7,470	45	7,232	27*	1968	Random
10	17	1,699	65	1,600	42	1961	Systematic
11	186	50,448	414	27,197	18	1974	Systematic
12	5	2,493	3	2,338	33	1969	Systematic
13	27	16,886	29	17,825	33	1976	Systematic

*This was actually a negative number; we used the absolute value in the analysis.

Table 10.2   Results of the tuberculosis trials: estimates of log relative risk and corresponding 95% confidence intervals

Trial	Estimate	95% CI
1	−0.8164	[−1.8790, 0.2461]
2	−1.5224	[−2.3567, −0.6881]
3	−1.2383	[−2.4205, −0.0561]
4	−1.4355	[−1.7118, −1.1592]
5	−0.2131	[−0.6537, 0.2275]
6	−0.7847	[−0.9473, −0.6220]
7	−1.6085	[−2.5086, −0.7084]
8	0.0119	[−0.1114, 0.1352]
9	−0.4634	[−0.9255, −0.0012]
10	−1.3500	[−1.8731, −0.8269]
11	−0.3402	[−0.5582, −0.1222]
12	0.3871	[−0.9519, 1.7261]
13	−0.0161	[−0.5352, 0.5030]

(10.16) and (10.17) in case of one covariate and the corresponding intervals in case of more than one covariate.

The first covariate we consider is the latitude centered around its mean. The estimate of the heterogeneity parameter is 0.062 using Eq. (10.7) in the random effects meta-regression. This leads to an estimate of the overall log relative risk at the mean latitude of the trials of -0.708. The standard error is 0.1179 and, with 2.201, the upper 2.5 percentage point of a t variate with 11 df, the 95% confidence interval is $[-0.967, -0.448]$. The estimate of the slope parameter is $\hat{\beta} = -0.0286$ with 95% confidence interval $[-0.046, -0.011]$ given a standard error of 0.0079.

When we consider the year centered around its mean as a covariate, the estimate of the heterogeneity parameter is 0.297, which is only a small reduction of the between-trial variance compared to the random effects model without covariates. The estimate of the overall log relative risk at the mean year of the trials is -0.723 with standard error 0.176. The corresponding 95% confidence interval is $[-1.117, -0.342]$. The estimated slope parameter is 0.025 with 95% confidence interval $[-0.062, 0.012]$. Consequently, the year of the trial has no significant impact on the study results.

Considering both the covariates, latitude and year, each centered around its own mean in a random effects meta-regression, the estimate of the between-trial variance is 0.077. This estimate is larger than the estimate of the heterogeneity parameter in the model with latitude as the only covariate. The estimated log relative risk at mean latitude and mean year is -0.711 with standard error 0.123. With 2.228, the upper 2.5 percentage point of a t variate with 10 df, this leads to a 95% confidence interval of $[-1.000, -0.423]$. The estimate of the latitude parameter is -0.0285, nearly the same value as in the model with latitude as the only covariate, but now the standard error is larger, namely 0.0106. Larger standard error and larger critical value lead to the wider 95% confidence interval $[-0.052, -0.005]$. Still, the covariate is significant even in this model. The estimate of the year parameter is -0.0002 with 95% confidence interval $[-0.034, 0.034]$, clearly again a nonsignificant result.

When we consider the treatment allocation as covariate, note that the treatment allocation was random in seven studies, systematic in four studies, and alternate in only two studies. In the computation, we have used a coding with two indicator variables. The first indicator variable is $x_1 = 1$ when the allocation in the trial is random and $x_1 = 0$ otherwise. The second indicator variable is $x_2 = 1$ when the allocation is systematic and $x_2 = 0$ otherwise. Consequently, the estimate of the intercept is an estimate of the treatment effect for the trials with alternate treatment allocation and the estimates the two regression parameters are estimates of the difference of the trials with random and systematic treatment allocation, respectively, compared to the trials with alternate treatment allocation. In the present model, the estimate of the between-trial variance is 0.5452. That is nearly 80% larger than the estimate of the between-trial in the model ignoring any covariates. Note that this estimate does not depend on the choice of the indicator variables. Clearly, the treatment allocation does not help to explain between-trial variability and we omit further analysis.

Summarizing, the latitude is the most important covariate to explain heterogeneity in this example. The inclusion of this covariate in the meta-regression model boils down the between-trial variance to about 80%.

10.3 FURTHER EXTENSIONS AND APPLICATIONS

In the above sections we considered the random effects meta-regression model for explaining a certain of amount of heterogeneity between the study results using co-variates on the study level. However, the model as well as the described analysis in Sections 10.1 and 10.2 can be used in a variety of different applications in meta-analysis. Some of these applications are described in this section.

Witte and Victor (2004) consider meta-regression for combining results of clinical noninferiority trials where the results of either one of two different analysis sets are published. They use model (10.1) and the value of the covariate x_i indicates which of the two analysis sets has been used.

Hartung and Knapp (2005b) use a meta-regression approach for combining the results of groups with different means which includes the Witte and Victor approach as a special case. Suppose that the k studies can be divided in L groups, $L < k$, that is, $k = k_1 + k_2 + \cdots + k_L$, and k_ℓ is the number of studies in the ℓth group. Let $Y_{i,\ell}$, $i = 1, \ldots, k_\ell$, be an estimator of the treatment effect in the ith study and the ith study uniquely belongs to the ℓth group, $\ell = 1, \ldots, L$. Then, the mean of $Y_{i,\ell}$ is $\mu + \alpha_\ell$ and α_ℓ is the effect of the ℓth group. The random effects model in this case can be written as

$$Y_{i,\ell} \sim N(\mu + \alpha_\ell, \sigma_a^2 + \sigma_{i,\ell}^2), \quad i = 1, \ldots, k_\ell, \quad \ell = 1, \ldots, L.$$

Begg and Pilote (1991) consider the combination of results from controlled and uncontrolled studies. Let (X_i, Y_i), $i = 1, \ldots, n$, be pairs of estimators of the effect of treatments 1 and 2 from n comparative trials with $X_i \sim N(\theta_i, \sigma_{i,X}^2)$ and $Y_i \sim N(\theta_i + \delta, \sigma_{i,X}^2)$. The parameter δ stands for the baseline risk in the ith trial and δ is the effect of the treatment difference, which is assumed to be equal for all comparative trials. Let U_i, $i = n+1, \ldots, n+k$, be estimators of the effect of treatment 1 from k uncontrolled (or historical) trials with $U_i \sim N(\theta_i, \sigma_{i,U}^2)$ and let V_i, $i = n+k+1, \ldots, n+k+m$, be estimators of the effect of treatment 2 from m uncontrolled (or historical) trials with $V_i \sim N(\theta_i + \delta, \sigma_{i,V}^2)$. Similar to the random effects meta-analysis model (see Chapter 7), in which the treatment effects may vary from study to study, Begg and Pilote (1991) allow that the baseline effects θ_i may vary from study to study and assume $\theta_i \sim N(\mu, \sigma^2)$. These assumptions lead to the model

$$\begin{pmatrix} X \\ Y \\ U \\ V \end{pmatrix} \sim N \left[\begin{pmatrix} 1_n & 0 \\ 1_n & 1_n \\ 1_k & 0 \\ 1_m & 1_m \end{pmatrix} \begin{pmatrix} \mu \\ \delta \end{pmatrix}, \Sigma \right] \tag{10.19}$$

with

$$\Sigma = \begin{pmatrix} \mathrm{diag}(\sigma^2 + \sigma_{i,X}^2) & \sigma^2 I_n & 0 & 0 \\ \sigma^2 I_n & \mathrm{diag}(\sigma^2 + \sigma_{i,Y}^2) & 0 & 0 \\ 0 & 0 & \mathrm{diag}(\sigma^2 + \sigma_{i,U}^2) & 0 \\ 0 & 0 & 0 & \mathrm{diag}(\sigma^2 + \sigma_{i,V}^2) \end{pmatrix}$$

and $\boldsymbol{X} = (X_1,\ldots,X_n)'$, $\boldsymbol{Y} = (Y_1,\ldots,Y_n)'$, $\boldsymbol{U} = (U_1,\ldots,U_k)'$, and $\boldsymbol{V} = (V_1,\ldots,V_m)'$.

Begg and Pilote (1991) use maximum likelihood methods for analyzing model (10.19). Each study provides an estimator of the variability within the treatment groups and these estimators are treated as the known variances. Consequently, the variability of the baseline risk σ^2 is the only unknown covariance parameter. In a subsequent paper, Li and Begg (1994) consider weighted least-squares estimation of the fixed effects parameters and estimation of σ^2 following the lines of the DerSimonian-Laird estimator; see Chapter 7.

Begg and Pilote (1991) discuss two generalizations of model (10.19). In their first generalization, they assume also that the results of the uncontrolled studies may be biased due to selection or publication bias. Therefore, they introduce two further parameters, one for the bias of the uncontrolled studies of treatment 1 and a second one for the bias of the uncontrolled studies of treatment 2. Finally, Begg and Pilote (1991) consider the generalization that also the effect of the treatment difference may vary from study to study and introduce a further variance component. We omit the details.

CHAPTER 11

MULTIVARIATE META-ANALYSIS

In this chapter we discuss techniques for multivariate meta-analysis with some examples. It will be seen that the methods of multivariate meta-analysis can be applied quite generally, irrespective of the nature of effect of interest, be it based on means, proportions, odds ratio, or correlations. Moreover, in the context of multivariate synthesis of data, it is possible to study within-study differences between effects for different outcomes as well as different relations of potential predictors with study outcomes.

Multivariate data can arise in meta-analysis due to several reasons. First, the primary studies can be multivariate in nature because these studies may measure multiple outcomes for each subject and are typically known as multiple-endpoint studies. For example, a systematic review of prognostic marker MYCN in neuroblastoma seeks to extract two outcomes: log hazard ratio estimates for overall survival and disease-free survival (Riley et al., 2004). Berkey et al. (1998) reported results of five studies assessing the difference in a surgical and nonsurgical procedure for treating periodontal disease with two outcomes: improvement in probing depth and improvement in attachment level. It should however be noted that not all studies in a review would have the same outcomes. For example, studies of Scholastic Aptitude Tests (SATs)

Statistical Meta-Analysis with Applications. By Joachim Hartung, Guido Knapp, Bimal K. Sinha
Copyright © 2008 John Wiley & Sons, Inc.

do not all report math and verbal scores. In fact, only about half of the studies dealt with in Becker (1990) provided coaching results for both math and verbal!

Second, multivariate data may arise when primary studies involve several comparisons among groups based on a single outcome. As an example, Ryan, Blakeslee, and Furst (1986) studied the effects of practice on motor skill levels on the basis of a five-group design, four different kinds of practice groups and one no-practice group, thus leading to comparisons of multivariate data. These kinds of studies are usually known as multiple-treatment studies.

Meta-analysis of multivariate data can be accomplished in a number of ways. Each approach has its benefits and disadvantages, depending on the nature of outcomes and effect sizes. When meta-analysis of multivariate data is performed either by ignoring dependence or handling it inadequately or by trying to model it fully, some difficulties arise (Hedges and Olkin, 1985) in regard to a possible effect on Type I error rate and accuracy of probability statements made on the observed data. Moreover, ignoring dependence may affect the bias and precision in underlying estimation problems as well.

Treating multivariate data arising out of multiple outcomes as independent and hence creating a separate data record for each outcome and carrying out separate analyses, without linking these records, have been a practice in some multivariate meta-analysis studies. The reasons for this oversimplification are tradition, the increased complexity of the multivariate approach, and also a lack of proper understanding as to why and when a genuine multivariate meta-analysis is beneficial over separate univariate meta-analyses. A significant problem that may arise in this context by ignoring dependence is due to the fact that studies reporting more outcomes have in general more data records and hence should be appropriately weighted. The simple procedure of weighting each outcome of a study by the inverse of the count of outcomes within each study may not take into account dependence among the outcomes.

Rosenthal and Rubin (1986) argue that one can eliminate dependence in the data by first summarizing data within studies to produce one outcome, often by applying standard data reduction techniques, and then pooling estimates across studies. Obviously, there is some information loss associated with data reduction, especially when the results differ systematically across meaningfully different outcomes. In spite of this shortcoming, their procedure is outlined in Section 11.1.

Another suggestion to reduce dependence is due to Steinkamp and Maehr (1983) and Greenwald, Hedges, and Laine (1996). These authors recommend creation of independent subsets of data for analysis and carrying out separate analyses for each subset (construct or time point). Obviously, such an approach does not permit a comparison of results across the data subsets due to inherent dependence existing in the original data set and would be reasonable only if there is low intercorrelations within studies. These methods are not described in this book.

An accepted approach that acknowledges the issue and importance of dependence is to conduct appropriate sensitivity analyses, essentially by carrying out separate analyses with and without multiple outcomes per study (Greenhouse and Iyengar, 1994). Quite generally, one starts with analyzing data sets consisting of only one outcome per study and then keeps on adding the extra outcomes to the data set and analyzing afresh. If the results of the analyses appear similar, then the dependence due to multiple outcomes is not severe and can be ignored. This is however not pursued here any more.

It is clear from the previous discussion that the most complete and accurate study of multivariate meta-analysis needs to address the nature and magnitude of dependence in study outcomes. This is precisely where most studies fail because they do not provide the relevant information to handle the nature of dependence. Becker (1990), Chiu (1997), and Kim (1998) provide important examples of multiple outcome studies where information about some vital correlations are missing. Of course, as advocated by Little and Rubin (1987) and Piggott (1994), various data imputation schemes can be applied to insert estimates for missing correlations, and one can then carry out sensitivity analyses to examine a range of correlation values. This is also not pursued here.

The rest of the chapter is organized as follows. Following pioneering works of Hedges and Olkin (1985), Rosenthal and Rubin (1986), Raudenbush, Becker and Kalaian (1988), Gleser and Olkin (1994), Berkey, Anderson, and Hoaglin (1996), Timm (1999), and Becker (2000), we present in the following sections various meta-analytic procedures for combining studies with multiple effect sizes, taking into account possible intercorrelations of multiple outcomes within each study, be they multiple endpoints or multiple treatments. This is done primarily keeping in mind the measures of effect sizes based on standardized means as developed in Chapter 2.

We conclude this section with the important observation that Berkey et al. (1995, 1998) and Riley et al. (2007a,b) reported results of a bivariate random effects meta-analysis with a novel application involving an experiment on two outcomes related to improvement in probing depth and improvement in attachment level, each outcome being obtained as the difference between two procedures for treating periodontal disease: surgical and nonsurgical. Since this analysis is essentially Bayesian in nature, we report details of this example in Chapter 12. This example serves as an illustration of the point that often bivariate meta-analysis taking into account the correlation between the two outcomes leads to better inference than individual meta-analysis which ignores such correlation.

11.1 COMBINING MULTIPLE DEPENDENT VARIABLES FROM A SINGLE STUDY

The object of this section is to suggest procedures to define a single summary statistic for each study entering into a meta-analysis. This is based on incorporating the information from all possibly dependent effect sizes relevant to the hypothesis being tested for the single study under consideration. Obviously such a summary statistic can then be combined with similar independent statistics arising out of other studies by means of standard meta-analysis procedures requiring independence of effect sizes. Such procedures are already described in Chapter 4.

A popular procedure for summarizing the possibly dependent effect sizes arising from a single study is to use the mean effect size! While the mean effect size is very easy to compute, without requiring any knowledge of intercorrelations of the variables involved in the study, and may make sense to provide a representative per dependent variable effect size estimate, unless the dependent variables are almost perfectly correlated, the mean effect size provides too low an estimate compared to the one based on a composite variable. We refer to Rosenthal and Rubin (1986) for some examples to this effect. A typical example in the realm of education involves combining effect sizes of SAT-M and SAT-V scores (two dependent variables), each arising out of an experimental (coached) and a control (uncoached) group. This can be done for each study and then combined across studies.

A new procedure based on some assumptions leading to much more accurate and useful summaries can be obtained when the degrees of freedom of the component effect sizes as well as the intercorrelations among the dependent variables are available. The assumptions essentially require a large sample size and very few missing values of the dependent variables, and in case of assigning unequal weights to combine the measurements on the dependent variables, it is necessary that the weights are predetermined and also assigned before data examination.

To describe this procedure, suppose there are p dependent variables in a study, I denotes an index of the effect size of the study (in most cases this is related to the sample size), t_i denotes the value of a test statistic used for testing the significance of the effect of the independent variable on the ith dependent variable, λ_i is the a priori weight assigned to the ith dependent variable, and ρ denotes the intercorrelation among the p dependent variables in the study. Then, following Rosenthal and Rubin (1986), the combined or composite effect size e_c is defined as

$$e_c = \frac{\sum_{i=1}^{p} \lambda_i t_i / I}{\left[\rho \left(\sum_{i=1}^{p} \lambda_i\right)^2 + (1 - \rho) \sum_{i=1}^{p} \lambda_i^2\right]^{1/2}}. \tag{11.1}$$

In the above, t_i / I can be considered as the exclusive effect size of the ith dependent variable so that e_c can be expressed in terms of effect sizes, their weights, and ρ and interpreted as a suitably defined linear combination of the dependent effect sizes.

When the effect size is based on the standardized mean difference and taken as Glass's estimate (see Chapter 2), we can take I as $(n/2)^{1/2}$. However, if we use Cohen's estimate (see Chapter 2), we take I as $[(n - 1)/2]^{1/2}$. Here n is the sample size of the two groups being compared (independent and dependent) within a study and, as mentioned earlier in Chapter 2, with studies of unequal sample sizes, one can choose n as an average (harmonic mean) of the sample sizes.

On the other hand, if the effect size is based on a partial correlation r_i between the response variable and the ith dependent variable, t_i is defined as

$$t_i = \frac{r_i \sqrt{\nu}}{\sqrt{1 - r_i^2}},$$

where ν is the degree of freedom of the residual mean square. Then t_i's are combined as in e_c given above in Eq. (11.1), and an overall composite effect size expressed as a correlation is given by

$$r_c = \frac{e_c}{[e_c^2 + \nu/I^2]^{1/2}}.$$

Once e_c is defined as above, under a large-sample theory assumption, a test of significance of the composite effect size e_c can be easily tested based on t_c defined as

$$t_c = \frac{\sum_{i=1}^{p} \lambda_i t_i}{\left[\rho\left(\sum_{i=1}^{p} \lambda_i\right)^2 + (1-\rho)\left(\sum_{i=1}^{p} \lambda_i^2\right) + (1-\rho^2)\left(\sum_{i=1}^{p} \lambda_i^2 t_i^2 / 2\nu\right)\right]^{1/2}}.$$

Example 11.1. Let us consider an example from Rosenthal and Rubin (1986). Table 11.1 contains the results of a two-group experiment with four subjects in each condition and three dependent variables, A, B, and C. In the control group, the mean of

Table 11.1   Experimental results for three dependent variables

Subjects	Dependent variable		
	A	B	C
Control			
S_1	3	3	3
S_2	1	-1	-1
S_3	-1	-1	1
S_4	-1	1	-1
Experimental			
S_5	6	6	6
S_6	4	2	2
S_7	2	2	4
S_8	2	4	2

all the three dependent variables is 0.5 and the mean is 3.5 for all dependent variables in the treatment group. The intercorrelations among the three dependent variables are all 0.64 in this example. The effect size estimates are 0.67 when effect sizes are defined in terms of r, the correlation coefficient, and 1.81 when defined in terms of Cohen's d.

We refer to Rosenthal and Rubin (1986) for further discussions about choice of ρ, and details about the above results and for some more examples.

11.2   MODELING MULTIVARIATE EFFECT SIZES

Rather than combining dependent effect sizes arising out of a single study to define a single summary statistic as done in the previous section, here we describe a flexible and widely applicable procedure which allows suitable meaningful combinations of different sets of outcomes for each study. In essence, this is a procedure for modeling multivariate effect size data using a generalized least-squares regression approach. Our model uses a variance-covariance matrix for the effect size estimates to account for interdependence in outcomes and it also allows different outcomes to be measured across studies. Additionally, different predictor variables can be used in the suggested regression models to explain the variation in effect sizes for each outcome. It should be mentioned that Hedges and Olkin (1985) developed methods for analyzing vectors of effect sizes when all studies use the same outcome variables.

11.2.1   Multiple-endpoint studies

To fix ideas, suppose a series of k studies are performed to compare treatment and control means on one or more of p outcome variables. A standard example would be to compare the mean difference of coached and uncoached groups of students for their performance in SAT-M and SAT-V for a series of studies where some studies record performance in both SAT-M and SAT-V while some other studies record performance on only one of SAT-M and SAT-V. The studies may also differ in terms of some predictor variables such as duration and nature of the coaching treatment. An example of this type appears at the end of this section. The regression model proposed below can accommodate such flexibility.

In the notation of Chapter 2, referring to Glass's estimate Δ of an effect size based on means, let Δ_{ij} denote the standardized effect size of the jth outcome variable in the ith study, $j = 1, \ldots, p$, $i = 1, \ldots, k$. It may be recalled that based on original data from the ith study on the jth outcome variable, Δ_{ij} is computed as

$$\Delta_{ij} = \frac{\bar{Y}_{ij}^E - \bar{Y}_{ij}^C}{S_{ij}^C},$$

where $\bar{Y}_{ij}^E$ and $\bar{Y}_{ij}^C$ are the experimental and control group sample means on the jth outcome variable from the ith study and S_{ij}^C is the square root of the control group sample variance of the jth outcome variable from the ith study.

In this context one can also use Cohen's d_{ij} or its variation, namely, Hedges's g_{ij}, a biased estimate of the population effect size θ_{ij}, or even a first-order bias corrected estimate of θ_{ij} which is given by $g_{ij}^* = [1 - 3/(4N_i - 9)]\, g_{ij}$, where $N_i = n_i^E + n_i^C$, and n_i^E is the experimental group sample size and n_i^C is the control group sample size for the ith study.

Returning to Δ_{ij}, its large-sample variance is given by

$$\sigma^2(\Delta_{ij}) = \frac{1}{n_i^E} + \frac{1}{n_i^C} + \frac{\theta_{ij}^2}{2n_i^C}.$$

Moreover, the large-sample covariance between the estimated effect sizes Δ_{ij} and $\Delta_{ij'}$ based on measures j and j' from study i is given by (Gleser and Olkin, 1994)

$$\sigma(\Delta_{ij}, \Delta_{ij'}) = \rho_{ijj'} \left(\frac{1}{n_i^E} + \frac{1}{n_i^C} \right) + \frac{\theta_{ij}\theta_{ij'}\rho_{ijj'}^2}{2n_i^C},$$

where $\rho_{ijj'}$ is the population correlation between jth and j'th outcome variables in the ith study.

If one chooses to use Cohen's d_{ij} or Hedges's g_{ij} or a modification of Hedges's g_{ij}, namely g_{ij}^*, the large-sample variance of d_{ij} or g_{ij} or g_{ij}^*, which are the same, is given by

$$\sigma^2(d_{ij}) = \frac{1}{n_i^E} + \frac{1}{n_i^C} + \frac{\theta_{ij}^2}{2(n_i^E + n_i^C)}. \tag{11.2}$$

Moreover, the large-sample covariance between the estimated effect sizes d_{ij} and $d_{ij'}$ based on measures j and j' from study i is given by (Gleser and Olkin, 1994)

$$\sigma(d_{ij}, d_{ij'}) = \rho_{ijj'} \left(\frac{1}{n_i^E} + \frac{1}{n_i^C} \right) + \frac{\theta_{ij}\theta_{ij'}\rho_{ijj'}^2}{2(n_i^E + n_i^C)}, \tag{11.3}$$

where as before $\rho_{ijj'}$ is the population correlation between the jth and j'th outcome variables in the ith study. In general, the above variances and covariances will be unknown and can be estimated based on sample data. When correlations are found to be homogeneous across studies, following an idea of Hedges and Olkin (1985) which is essentially a variance-stabilizing transformation, a pooled correlation estimate can be used.

It should be noted that the above formulas of large-sample variances and covariances of estimated effect sizes are based on the assumption of homogeneous covariance matrices of experimental and control group measurements within studies. When complete homogeneity of these two types of matrices does not hold, a partial homogeneity in the sense of $\sigma_{jj}^C = \sigma_{jj}^E$ for $j = 1, \ldots, p$ may still hold. Obviously in this case what is required is a knowledge of the correlations of the p outcome variables in both the control and experimental groups. The large-sample covariance between Δ_{ij} and $\Delta_{ij'}$ is then recalculated as (Gleser and Olkin, 1994)

$$\sigma(\Delta_{ij}, \Delta_{ij'}) = \rho_{ijj'}^E \frac{1}{n_i^E} + \rho_{ijj'}^C \frac{1}{n_i^C} + \frac{\theta_{ij}\theta_{ij'}\rho_{ijj'}^E \rho_{ijj'}^C}{2n_i^C}.$$

In case no homogeneity assumption holds, the large-sample covariance between the estimated effect sizes Δ_{ij} and $\Delta_{ij'}$ is given by (Gleser and Olkin, 1994)

$$\sigma(\Delta_{ij}, \Delta_{ij'}) = \frac{1}{n_i^E} \rho_{ijj'}^E \tau_{ij}\tau_{ij'} + \frac{\rho_{ijj'}^C}{n_i^C} + \frac{\theta_{ij}\theta_{ij'}\rho_{ijj'}^E \rho_{ijj'}^C}{2n_i^C},$$

where $\tau_{ij}^2 = \sigma_{ijj}^E / \sigma_{ijj}^C$. Similar modifications of variances and covariances can be derived when one uses Cohen's d or Hedges's g.

In most cases the population variances and covariances will be unknown and are estimated based on sample data. Having constructed an estimated variance-covariance matrix of the estimated effect sizes for each study and noting that the order of the variance-covariance matrix can be unequal depending on what kind of outcome measures are available in each study, we are now in a position to formulate a model for variation in effect sizes. Basically, we model each g_{ij}^* as

$$g_{ij}^* = \theta_{ij} + e_{ij}, \tag{11.4}$$

where e_{ij}'s are error components such that their variances are given by Eq. (11.2) and their covariances are given by Eq. (11.3). If there are m_i outcome variables (out of a total of p outcome variables) recorded in the ith study, allowing flexibility in the number of outcome variables across studies, then the variance-covariance matrix of e_{ij}'s is of order $m_i \times m_i$ and we denote it by S_i.

We now collect all the outcome measures g_{ij}^*'s and represent them by g^* using a standard vector notation which is of order $M \times M$ where $M = m_1 + \cdots + m_k$. Similarly, we write θ and e for the vectors of population effect sizes and error components, respectively.

A test for the homogeneity of population effect sizes across studies for the jth outcome variable can then be carried out as follows. Assume that there are k_j studies out of k studies, providing information on the j outcome variable, and let us denote by $\mathcal{C}_j$ the index set of these k_j studies. Then a test for homogeneity of the population effect sizes belonging to $\mathcal{C}_j$ can be carried out based on a χ^2 test statistic with $k_j - 1$ df, given by

$$\chi_j^2 = \sum_{i \in \mathcal{C}_j} \frac{(g_{ij}^* - g_w^*)^2}{\hat{\sigma}^2(d_{ij})}, \tag{11.5}$$

where

$$g_w^* = \frac{\sum_{i \in \mathcal{C}_j} g_{ij}^* / \hat{\sigma}^2(d_{ij})}{\sum_{i \in \mathcal{C}_j} 1 / \hat{\sigma}^2(d_{ij})}. \tag{11.6}$$

The justification of the above test statistic in large samples follows from independence of the k_j studies.

To represent variation in effect sizes due to presence of some predictor variables, we can express θ as

$$\theta = X\beta, \tag{11.7}$$

where X is the design matrix of covariates or predictor variables and β is the vector of covariate effects. Combining model (11.4) and model (11.7), we can write in the notation of a standard linear model set-up

$$g^* = X\beta + e, \tag{11.8}$$

and well known results on estimation and tests of β can be easily applied. In particular, the significance of the model (11.8) can be easily tested as well as the significance of individual regression coefficients. It should however be noted that the variance-covariance matrix of e is an unknown block-diagonal matrix and needs to be estimated from the data.

Thus, an overall estimate of the vector β of covariate effects is given by

$$\hat{\beta} = (X'S^{-1}X)^{-1}X'S^{-1}g^*$$

with an estimated variance-covariance matrix as

$$\text{Cov}(\hat{\beta}) = \left(\boldsymbol{X}'\boldsymbol{S}^{-1}\boldsymbol{X}\right)^{-1},$$

where $\boldsymbol{S}$ is a block-diagonal matrix with (i, i)th entry as $\boldsymbol{S}_i$. Large-sample normal-theory-based inference for any linear combination of the elements of β can be carried out in the usual fashion (see Searle, 1971; Graybill, 1976). Finally, a test for homogeneity of population effect sizes across studies, whose validity makes meta-analysis or a combination of information from different studies meaningful, can be carried out based on the χ^2 statistic, defined as

$$\chi^2 = \boldsymbol{d}'\boldsymbol{S}^{-1}\boldsymbol{d} - \hat{\beta}'(\boldsymbol{X}'\boldsymbol{S}^{-1}\boldsymbol{X})\hat{\beta},$$

where $\boldsymbol{d}$ is the vector of Cohen's estimates of population effect sizes and rejecting the null hypothesis of homogeneity of population effect sizes when χ^2 exceeds the table value with df $= M - d$, where d is the dimension of β.

We conclude this section with an example taken from Raudenbush, Becker, and Kalaian (1988).

Example 11.2. Kalaian and Becker (1986) reported results on SAT coaching from 38 studies. A selection of six such studies appears in Table 11.2. There are two possible endpoints in these studies, SAT-M and SAT-V, and one treatment (coaching) and one control (noncoaching). It should be noted that not all studies provide reports on both the endpoints. Obviously, $m_1 = m_2 = m_3 = 2$, $m_4 = m_5 = m_6 = 1$, $p = 2$, and $k = 6$.

Table 11.2   Results of the SAT coaching studies

Study	Outcome measured	Sample size Coached (E)	Uncoached (C)	Effect size d
1	SAT-M	71	37	0.626
	SAT-V	71	37	0.129
2	SAT-M	225	193	0.269
	SAT-V	225	193	0.100
3	SAT-M	45	45	0.297
	SAT-V	45	45	0.238
4	SAT-V	28	22	0.453
5	SAT-V	39	40	0.178
6	SAT-M	145	129	0.229

Note: SAT-M = Scholastic Aptitude Test, math subtest; SAT-V = Scholastic Aptitude Test, verbal subtest.

There are nine estimated effect sizes in our example. Using the approximately unbiased version g^* of Hedges's estimate g, these are given by

$$\boldsymbol{g}^* = (0.626, 0.129, 0.269, 0.100, 0.297, 0.238, 0.453, 0.178, 0.229).$$

The estimated variance-covariance matrix of the estimated effect sizes are given in Table 11.3. Obviously, some covariances cannot be computed because of lack of data on both endpoints.

Table 11.3   Estimated variances and covariances in the SAT coaching studies

Study no.	Variance of SAT-M effect size	Variance of SAT-V effect size	Covariance between SAT-M and SAT-V effect sizes
1	0.043	0.041	0.028
2	0.010	0.010	0.006
3	0.045	0.045	0.030
4	—	0.083	—
5	—	0.051	—
6	0.015	—	—

Note: SAT-M = Scholastic Aptitude Test, math subtest; SAT-V = Scholastic Aptitude Test, verbal subtest.

To carry out a test for the homogeneity of SAT-M effects across studies, following Eqs. (11.5) and (11.6), we compute $g^*_{Mw} = 0.2985$ and $\chi^2_M = 2.90$ with 3 df, which is nonsignificant. Similarly, to test the homogeneity of SAT-V effects across studies, we compute $g^*_{Vw} = 0.1536$ and $\chi^2_V = 0.5523$ with 3 df, which is again nonsignificant. Hence we can conclude that the SAT-M and SAT-V effect sizes across studies are homogeneous.

Under the assumption of homogeneous SAT-M and SAT-V effects, in order to study if the effects of the covariate representing the number of hours of coaching is significant, we can write model (11.8) with X given by (see Raudenbush, Becker, and Kalaian, 1988, p. 116)

$$X = \begin{bmatrix} 1 & 0 & 12.0 & 0 \\ 0 & 1 & 0 & 12.0 \\ 1 & 0 & 12.0 & 0 \\ 0 & 1 & 0 & 7.5 \\ 1 & 0 & 30.0 & 0 \\ 0 & 1 & 0 & 30.0 \\ 0 & 1 & 0 & 7.5 \\ 0 & 1 & 0 & 10.0 \\ 1 & 0 & 21.0 & 0 \end{bmatrix}$$

and $\beta = (\theta_1, \theta_2, \eta_1, \eta_2)$. Here η_1 and η_2 represent the covariate coaching effects for SAT-M and SAT-V. Estimates of β and the estimated variance-covariance matrix are given by

$$\hat{\beta} = (0.467, 0.152, -0.009, -0.001) \tag{11.9}$$

and

$$\text{Cov}(\hat{\boldsymbol{\beta}}) = \begin{bmatrix} 0.0368 & 0.0158 & -0.0019 & -0.0001 \\ & 0.0178 & 0.0001 & -0.0001 \\ & & 0.0001 & 0.0004 \\ & & & 0.0001 \end{bmatrix}. \tag{11.10}$$

The significance of the two covariate coaching effects η_1 and η_2 can now be easily tested by computing $Z_1 = \hat{\eta}_1/\hat{\sigma}(\hat{\eta}_1) = (-0.01/0.01) = -1$ and $Z_2 = \hat{\eta}_2/\hat{\sigma}(\hat{\eta}_2) = (-0.001/0.01) = -0.1$, implying that both the covariate effects are nonsignificant. A similar computation shows that the main effects θ_1 and θ_2 are significant. We refer to Raudenbush, Becker, and Kalaian (1988) for details.

In the context of multiple-endpoint studies, Timm (1999) suggested that an alternative measure of an overall study effect size by combining the information in all the variables in a study can be provided by what is known as a noncentral parameter. For study i, such a measure can be defined as $\Delta_i^2 = \boldsymbol{\delta}_i' \boldsymbol{\Sigma}_i^{-1} \boldsymbol{\delta}_i$, where $\boldsymbol{\Sigma}_i$ is the population variance-covariance matrix for the ith study. As mentioned before, Δ_i^2 will be unknown in applications and can be estimated by $\hat{\Delta}_i^2 = \boldsymbol{d}_i' \boldsymbol{\Psi}_i^{-1} \boldsymbol{d}_i$, where $\boldsymbol{d}_i$ is an estimate of $\boldsymbol{\delta}_i$ and $\boldsymbol{\Psi}_i$ is an estimate of $\boldsymbol{S}_i$. Using well-known results from multivariate analysis (Timm, 1975; Anderson, 1984), the distribution of $\hat{\Delta}_i^2$ is given by a multiple of a noncentral F distribution whose first two moments can be readily computed (see Johnson and Kotz, 1970). A test for the significance of Δ_i^2 for study i can be based on a central F distribution. A test for the homogeneity of such overall effect size measures across all studies can be developed based on a multivariate F distribution. Once homogeneity is established, an overall effect size can be proposed and its significance can be tested based on a multivariate chi-square distribution. We refer to Timm (1999) for details.

11.2.2 Multiple-treatment studies

As mentioned earlier, this section deals with combining data or information from several studies where each study is designed to compare several treatments with a control. Most of the material here appears in Gleser and Olkin (1994). We denote the control group by C and treatment groups by $T_1, \ldots, T_m$. It should however be noted that not all studies will involve the same set of treatments, thus allowing for some flexibility in the design of experiments. An example at the end of this section will illustrate this point.

Denoting the means of control and treatment groups by $\mu_0, \mu_1, \ldots, \mu_m$ and the standard deviations of control and treatment groups by $\sigma_0, \sigma_1, \ldots, \sigma_m$, the population effect sizes are obviously defined by

$$\delta_i = \frac{\mu_i - \mu_0}{\sigma_0}, \ i = 1, \ldots, m.$$

Our object is to combine information from several studies, each providing information about the population effect sizes based on samples collected from control and treatment groups. For a given study, denoting by $\bar{Y}_0, \bar{Y}_1, \ldots, \bar{Y}_m$ the sample means of control and treatment groups and by $S_0, S_1, \ldots, S_m$ the sample standard deviations of control and treatment groups, the population effect sizes are estimated by

$$\hat{\delta}_i = d_i = \frac{\bar{Y}_i - \bar{Y}_0}{S_0}, \quad i = 1, \ldots, m.$$

It should be noted that it is the common control sample mean $\bar{Y}_0$ and the common control sample standard deviation S_0 appearing in all the estimated effect sizes that make the estimated effect sizes correlated. Under the assumption of large sample sizes, the variance of ith estimated effect size d_i is given by

$$\sigma^2(d_i) = \frac{1}{n_i} + \frac{1}{n_0} + \frac{\delta_i^2}{2n_0},$$

where n_i is the sample size of treatment i and n_0 is the control group sample size. The large-sample covariance between the estimated effect sizes d_i and d'_i is given by

$$\sigma(d_i, d'_i) = \frac{1}{n_0} + \frac{\delta_i \delta'_i}{2n_0}.$$

It should be noted that the above expressions of large-sample variances and co-variances are derived based on the assumption of homogeneity of variances, namely, $\sigma_0 = \sigma_1 = \cdots = \sigma_m$. However, when this assumption holds, population effect sizes δ_i can be more accurately estimated by using a pooled sample standard deviation s_p rather than just s_0 where

$$S_p^2 = \frac{(n_0 - 1)S_0^2 + \sum_{i=1}^m (n_i - 1)S_i^2}{n_0 + 1 + \sum_{i=1}^m (n_i - 1)}.$$

Denoting the modified effect size estimates by $d_i^* = (\bar{Y}_i - \bar{Y}_0)/S_p$, its large-sample variance is given by

$$\sigma(d_i^*) = \frac{1}{n_i} + \frac{1}{n_0} + \frac{\delta_i^2}{2n^*}$$

and the covariance between d_i^* and $d_i^{*'}$ is given by

$$\sigma(d_i^*, d_i^{*'}) = \frac{1}{n_0} + \frac{\delta_i \delta'_i}{2n^*},$$

where $n^* = n_0 + n_1 + \cdots + n_m$.

When the assumption of homogeneity of variances mentioned above does not hold, the large-sample variances of d_i are modified as

$$\sigma_{\text{mod}}^2(d_i) = \frac{\sigma_i^2}{n_i \sigma_0^2} + \frac{1}{n_0} + \frac{\delta_i^2}{2n_0}.$$

However, the expression for the large-sample covariance between d_i and d'_i remains the same as before.

Obviously, in practical applications, all the variances and covariances will be unknown because they involve population effect sizes δ_i and need to be estimated. It is done simply by replacing δ_i by d_i, σ_i by S_i, and σ_0 by S_0.

Having obtained from each study an $m \times 1$ vector of estimated effect sizes d_i along with its estimated variance-covariance matrix Ψ_i of order $m \times m$, $i = 1, \ldots, k$, we can proceed as in the previous section to formulate a linear regression model approach in order to combine the information from all k studies. It should however be noted that, depending on the nature of information obtained from the ith study, the dimension of the vector d_i and the estimated variance-covariance matrix Ψ_i may vary. We denote the dimension of d_i by $q_i \leq m$. Nevertheless, we can always choose to denote the dimensions by $m \times 1$ and $m \times m$, respectively, leaving blanks at places where there is no information from a study.

Writing $d' = (d_1', \ldots, d_k')$ and $\delta = (\delta_1, \ldots, \delta_k)'$, under the assumption of homogeneous population effect sizes across studies, we now have the linear model

$$d = X\delta + e, \tag{11.11}$$

where X is the associated design matrix which is readily obtained from the configuration of the study designs and e can be regarded as an error component which has mean 0 and a block-diagonal variance-covariance matrix Ψ whose elements corresponding to the ith block is Ψ_i and correspond to the estimated variances and covariances of the estimated effect sizes from study i. From the representation (11.11), applying standard results from linear models theory, we can readily get combined estimates of all the effect sizes δ and carry out relevant inference about them. Thus, an overall estimate of the vector of population effect sizes is given by

$$\hat{\delta} = (X'\Psi^{-1}X)^{-1}X'\Psi^{-1}d \tag{11.12}$$

with an estimated variance-covariance matrix as

$$\text{Cov}(\hat{\delta}) = (X'\Psi^{-1}X)^{-1}.$$

Large-sample normal-theory-based inference for any linear combination of the elements of δ can be carried out in the usual fashion (see Searle, 1971; Graybill, 1976). Finally, a test for homogeneity of population effect sizes across studies, whose validity makes meta-analysis or combination of information from different studies meaningful, can be carried out based on the χ^2 statistic, defined as

$$\chi^2 = d'\Psi^{-1}d - \hat{\delta}'(X'\Psi^{-1}X)^{-1}\hat{\delta}, \tag{11.13}$$

and rejecting the null hypothesis of homogeneity of population effect sizes when χ^2 exceeds the table value with df $= q_1 + \cdots + q_k - m$.

Example 11.3. We conclude this section with an example drawn from Gleser and Olkin (1994) in which there are six studies and five treatments are compared with a control. Data appear in Table 11.4, which shows that not all treatments appear in each study. Obviously, in this data set, $q_1 = 3$, $q_2 = 3$, $q_3 = 2$, $q_4 = 2$, $q_5 = 4$, $q_6 = 1$.

Table 11.4 Summary information for studies of the effect of exercise on systolic blood pressure

Study	C	E_1	E_2	E_3	E_4	E_5
			Sample sizes			
1	25	22	25	23	—	—
2	40	—	38	37	40	—
3	30	—	30	—	28	—
4	50	—	50	—	—	50
5	30	30	30	28	26	—
6	100	100	—	—	—	—
			Means			
1	150.96	144.14	139.92	139.32	—	—
2	149.94	—	141.23	137.36	136.44	—
3	152.45	—	140.80	—	136.14	—
4	149.49	—	140.69	—	—	135.39
5	150.36	144.55	140.32	138.34	134.69	—
6	150.19	145.62	—	—	—	—
			Standard deviation			
1	8.44	4.25	5.06	3.60	—	—
2	6.88	—	5.11	5.29	3.34	—
3	6.35	—	4.52	—	3.35	—
4	6.92	—	5.33	—	—	3.35
5	4.96	5.58	4.16	5.76	4.05	—
6	6.71	5.06	—	—	—	—

From study 1, we have the vector of estimated effect sizes as $(0.808, 1.308, 1.379, -, -)$ with estimated variance-covariance matrix as

$$
\hat{\mathbf{\Psi}}_1 = \begin{bmatrix} 0.0985 & 0.0611 & 0.0623 & - & - \\ & 0.1142 & 0.0761 & - & - \\ & & 0.1215 & - & - \\ & & & - & - \\ & & & & - \end{bmatrix}.
$$

From study 2, we have the vector of estimated effect sizes as $(-, 1.266, 1.828, 1.962, -)$ with estimated variance-covariance matrix as

$$
\hat{\mathbf{\Psi}}_2 = \begin{bmatrix} - & - & - & - & - \\ & 0.0713 & 0.0539 & 0.0561 & - \\ & & 0.0938 & 0.0698 & - \\ & & & 0.0981 & - \\ & & & & - \end{bmatrix}.
$$

From study 3, we have the vector of estimated effect sizes as $(-, 1.835, -, 2.568, -)$ with estimated variance-covariance matrix as

$$
\hat{\boldsymbol{\Psi}}_3 = \begin{bmatrix} - & - & - & - & - \\ & 0.1228 & - & 0.1119 & - \\ & & - & - & - \\ & & & 0.1790 & - \\ & & & & - \end{bmatrix}.
$$

From study 4, we have the vector of estimated effect sizes as $(-, 1.272, -, -, 2.038)$ with estimated variance-covariance matrix as

$$
\hat{\boldsymbol{\Psi}}_4 = \begin{bmatrix} - & - & - & - & - \\ & 0.0562 & - & - & 0.0459 \\ & & - & - & - \\ & & & - & - \\ & & & & 0.0815 \end{bmatrix}.
$$

From study 5, we have the vector of estimated effect sizes as $(1.171, 2.024, 2.423, 3.159, -)$ with estimated variance-covariance matrix as

$$
\hat{\boldsymbol{\Psi}}_5 = \begin{bmatrix} 0.0895 & 0.0729 & 0.0806 & 0.0950 & - \\ & 0.1350 & 0.1151 & 0.1394 & - \\ & & 0.1669 & 0.1609 & - \\ & & & 0.2381 & - \\ & & & & - \end{bmatrix}.
$$

From study 6, we have the vector of estimated effect sizes as $(0.681, -, -, -, -)$ with estimated variance-covariance matrix as

$$
\hat{\boldsymbol{\Psi}}_6 = \begin{bmatrix} 0.0223 & - & - & - & - \\ & - & - & - & - \\ & & - & - & - \\ & & & - & - \\ & & & & - \end{bmatrix}.
$$

Using Eq. (11.12), a combined estimate of the population effect sizes is obtained as

$$
\hat{\boldsymbol{\delta}} = (0.756, 1.398, 1.746, 2.146, 2.141)
$$

with its estimated variance-covariance matrix as

$$
\text{Cov}(\hat{\boldsymbol{\beta}}) = \begin{bmatrix} 0.0131 & 0.0038 & 0.0051 & 0.0048 & 0.0031 \\ 0.0038 & 0.0160 & 0.0113 & 0.0134 & 0.0131 \\ 0.0051 & 0.0113 & 0.0271 & 0.0172 & 0.0092 \\ 0.0048 & 0.0134 & 0.0172 & 0.0332 & 0.0109 \\ 0.0031 & 0.0131 & 0.0092 & 0.0109 & 0.0547 \end{bmatrix}.
$$

The value of χ^2 statistic defined in Eq. (11.13) turns out to be 10.102, which is smaller than the 5% table value of 18.30 with $q_1 + \cdots + q_6 - 5 = 10$ df. Hence, we can conclude that the homogeneity hypothesis cannot be rejected for the given data set.

CHAPTER 12

BAYESIAN META-ANALYSIS

Most statistical methods of meta-analysis focus on deriving and studying properties of a common estimated effect which is supposed to exist across all studies. However, when heterogeneity across studies is believed to exist, a meta-analyst ought to estimate the extent and sources of heterogeneity among studies. While fixed effects models discussed in this book under the assumption of homogeneous effects sizes continue to be the most common method of meta-analysis, the assumption of homogeneity given variability among studies due to varying research and evaluation protocols may be unrealistic. In such cases, a random effects model which avoids the homogeneity assumption, and models effects as random and coming from a distribution is recommended. The various study effects are believed to arise from a population and random effects models borrow strength across studies in providing estimates of both study-specific effects and underlying population effects.

Whether a fixed effects model or a random effects model, a Bayesian approach considers all parameters (population effect sizes for fixed effects models, in particular) as random and coming from a superpopulation with its own parameters. There are two standard approaches to estimate the parameters of the superpopulation: empirical Bayes and hierarchical Bayes. In the first, the parameters are estimated based on the available data from all studies, considering marginal distributions of sample study

Statistical Meta-Analysis with Applications. By Joachim Hartung, Guido Knapp, Bimal K. Sinha   **155**
Copyright © 2008 John Wiley & Sons, Inc.

effects and using well-known frequentist methods of estimating parameters such as the maximum likelihood or moment method. In the latter, prior distributions are placed on the parameters of the superpopulation in several layers (hierarchy) often using expert opinions. Obviously, as one moves upward in the hierarchy, less and less information is known about the parameters and the prior eventually becomes diffuse. When the parameters of the superpopulation are all estimated, it is possible to estimate study-specific effect sizes along with their standard errors.

There are several advantages for a Bayesian approach to meta-analysis. The Bayesian paradigm provides in a very natural way a method for data synthesis from all studies by incorporating model and parameter uncertainty. Moreover, a predictive distribution for future observations coming from any study, which may be a quantity of central interest to some decision makers, can be easily developed based on what have been already observed. The use of Bayesian hierarchical models often leads to more appropriate estimates of parameters compared to the asymptotic ones arising from maximum likelihood, especially in case of small sample sizes of component studies, which is typical in meta-analysis.

This chapter is designed as follows. A general Bayesian model for meta-analysis under normality with some examples is presented in Section 12.1. Further examples of Bayesian meta-analysis are discussed in Section 12.2. A unified Bayesian approach to meta-analysis is attempted in Section 12.3 with some further results on Bayesian meta-analysis in Section 12.4. An example is worked out in detail to explicitly show how the Bayesian methods work in applications.

12.1   A GENERAL BAYESIAN MODEL FOR META-ANALYSIS UNDER NORMALITY

In this section we provide a very general setting of a Bayesian model for meta-analysis under the usual assumption of normality. Consider k studies with the ith study reporting a study effect X_i and assume that $X_1, \ldots, X_k$ are statistically independent and $X_i \sim N(\theta_i, \sigma_i^2)$, $i = 1, \ldots, k$. Here θ_i's are the population effect sizes. The reader may recall the definitions of the various effect sizes and how these are estimated from the discussion in Chapter 2.

A Bayesian approach now assumes that θ_i's are independent with

$$\theta_i \sim N(\mu, \tau^2),$$

where μ represents the mean of the study effects and τ^2 represents the between-study variability. Obviously, marginally, $X_i \sim N(\mu, \tau^2 + \sigma_i^2)$. When τ^2 is known, μ is estimated by

$$\hat{\mu} = \frac{\sum_{i=1}^k (\tau^2 + \sigma_i^2)^{-1} X_i}{\sum_{i=1}^k (\tau^2 + \sigma_i^2)^{-1}}.$$

Here we have assumed that the variances σ_i^2's are either known or estimated based on sample data if these are unknown. When τ is unknown, there are standard approaches to estimate it (see Chapter 7). It may be noted that what we have described so far is essentially a random effects model.

A fully Bayesian approach would model the unknown parameters as

$$\mu \sim N(a, b), \quad \tau^2 \sim \text{IG}(c, d), \quad \sigma_i^2 \sim \text{IG}(u_i, v_i),$$

where IG stands for an inverse gamma distribution and a, b, c, d, u_i, v_i are known as hyperparameters and estimated following either an empirical Bayes approach or a hierarchical approach. Methods of Markov chain Monte Carlo and Gibbs sampling can be used in this context (Bernardo and Smith, 1993; Berger, 1985). Of course, whenever a diffuse information is available about a parameter, one can specify a large variance in the corresponding prior to take this into account. We refer to Abrams et al. (2000) for an application of the above methods to perform a meta-analysis of six studies on levels of long-term anxiety.

Quite generally, given a prior $\pi(\mu, \tau^2)$, the Bayesian approach is based on inference from the posterior distribution $\pi(\mu, \tau^2 | \boldsymbol{X})$, which is proportional to $L(\mu, \tau^2) \times \pi(\mu, \tau^2)$, where $L(\mu, \tau^2)$ denotes the likelihood for (μ, τ^2). It is rather common to assume an improper prior for μ and independence of μ and τ^2 in which case $\phi(\mu, \tau^2)$ is proportional to $\pi(\tau^2)$. The marginal posterior of τ^2, $\pi(\tau^2 | \text{data})$, then turns out to be proportional to $L_R(\tau^2) \times \pi(\tau^2)$, where $L_R(\tau^2)$, known as the restricted likelihood, is given, apart from a constant, by

$$L_R(\tau^2) = \left(\sum \frac{1}{\tau^2 + \sigma_i^2} \right)^{-1/2} \prod (\tau^2 + \sigma_i^2)^{-1/2} \exp \left\{ -\frac{1}{2} \sum \frac{[X_i - \mu^*(\tau^2)]^2}{\tau^2 + \sigma_i^2} \right\}.$$

Here

$$\mu^*(\tau^2) = \left(\sum \frac{X_i}{\tau^2 + \sigma_i^2} \right) \left(\sum \frac{1}{\tau^2 + \sigma_i^2} \right)^{-1}$$

is the weighted mean of study effects with weights proportional to the precision of each data point.

A rejection algorithm, as described in Pauler and Wakefield (2000), can then be used to generate samples on τ^2 from the above posterior. Once τ^2 values have been generated, it is straightforward to generate values of the average treatment effect μ and random effects θ_i because, conditional on τ^2,

$$\mu | \tau^2, \text{data} \sim N \left[\mu^*(\tau^2), \left(\sum \frac{1}{\tau^2 + \sigma_i^2} \right)^{-1} \right]$$

and

$$\theta_i | \mu, \tau^2, \text{data} \sim N \left(\frac{X_i\, w_i + \mu/\tau^2}{w_i + 1/\tau^2}, \frac{\tau^2}{1 + w_i \tau^2} \right),$$

where $w_i = 1/\sigma_i^2$.

It is also possible to easily extend the above model to include study-level covariates $\boldsymbol{z}_i' = (z_{i1}, \ldots, z_{ip})$ from the ith study for $p < k - 1$. The model for θ_i in this case changes to

$$\theta_i | \mu, \boldsymbol{\beta}, \tau^2 \sim N \left(\mu + \boldsymbol{z}_i' \boldsymbol{\beta}, \tau^2 \right),$$

where β is the vector of population regression coefficients. Assuming as before improper priors for $\gamma = (\mu, \beta)$, the restricted likelihood $L_R(\tau^2)$ in this case is given, apart from a constant, by

$$L_R(\tau^2) = \left| \sum (\tau^2 + \sigma_i^2)^{-1} z_i z_i' \right|^{-1/2} \prod (\tau^2 + \sigma_i^2)^{-1/2} D,$$

where

$$D = \exp \left\{ -\frac{1}{2} \sum \frac{[X_i - z_i' \gamma^*(\tau^2)]^2}{\tau^2 + \sigma_i^2} \right\}$$

and

$$\gamma^*(\tau^2) = \left[\sum (\tau^2 + \sigma_i^2)^{-1} z_i z_i' \right]^{-1} \sum (\tau^2 + \sigma_i^2)^{-1} X_i z_i.$$

As before, once posterior marginal values of τ^2 are generated from this distribution, the regression coefficients γ and random effects θ_i can be easily simulated by using the following facts:

$$\gamma | \tau^2, \text{data} \sim N \left(\gamma^*(\tau^2), \left[\sum (\tau^2 + \sigma_i^2)^{-1} z_i z_i' \right]^{-1} \right)$$

and

$$\theta_i | \tau^2, \text{data} \sim N \left(\frac{X_i w_i + z_i' \gamma / \tau^2}{w_i + 1/\tau^2}, \frac{\tau^2}{1 + w_i \tau^2} \right).$$

We now present one example from Pauler and Wakefield (2000) involving dentrifice data (see also Section 18.3) to explain the Bayesian analysis discussed above. We also refer to Pauler and Wakefield (2000) for two other examples involving anti-hypertension data and preeclampsia data.

The data set given in Table 12.1 represents the outcome measure $X = $ NaF$-$SMFP, the difference in changes from baseline in the decayed/missing/filled-surface dental index between sodium fluoride (NaF) and sodium monofluorophosphate (SMFP) at three years follow-up, from nine studies. We also present their associated precisions w's.

Choosing two forms of inverse gamma priors, IG$(0, 0.5)$ and IG$(0.5, 0.11)$, and using the likelihood $L_R(\tau^2)$, one can employ the rejection algorithm suggested in Pauler and Wakefield (2000) to generate the posterior distributions of τ^2 for the given data set. Pauler and Wakefield (2000) carried out this analysis and reported the following results:

IG$(0, 0.5)$ prior: posterior median of $\tau^2 = 0.28$ with 95% posterior distribution interval $(0.10, 1.12)$.

IG$(0.5, 0.11)$ prior: posterior median of $\tau^2 = 0.08$ with 95% posterior distribution interval $(0.03, 0.39)$.

Table 12.1 Treatment effects Y_i and precisions w_i for the dentifrice data set

Study	Y_i	w_i
1	−0.86	3.07
2	−0.33	3.25
3	−0.47	8.09
4	−0.50	15.88
5	0.28	3.43
6	−0.04	13.21
7	−0.80	1.63
8	−0.19	55.97
9	−0.49	12.92

Using

$$\mu | \tau^2, \text{data} \sim N\left[\mu^*(\tau^2), \left(\sum \frac{1}{\tau^2 + \sigma_i^2} \right)^{-1} \right],$$

one can generate values of μ for a given generated value of τ^2 and the data set and compute some measures of the posterior distribution of μ by averaging over the values of τ^2. The following summary statistics are reported in Pauler and Wakefield (2000):

IG$(0, 0.5)$ prior: posterior median of $\mu = -0.35$ with 95% posterior distribution interval $(-0.83, 0.12)$.

IG$(0.5, 0.11)$ prior: posterior median of $\mu = -0.33$ with 95% posterior distribution interval $(-0.66, -0.01)$.

It is clear from the above results that the posterior measures of μ are somewhat sensitive to the choice of the prior of τ^2. However, there exists a negative difference between the results of the two dental treatment plans.

12.2 FURTHER EXAMPLES OF BAYESIAN ANALYSES

In a novel application of Bayesian analysis which involves questions about benefits and risks of mammography of women based on six studies (Berry, 2000), a Poisson model is assumed for X_i and Y_i, which represent the number of breast cancer deaths in control and mammography groups in study i out of n_i and m_i life years (in thousands), respectively. To be specific, it is assumed that

$$X_i \sim \text{Poisson}(n_i \, \theta_i), \quad Y_i \sim \text{Poisson}(m_i \, \theta_i \, \rho_i),$$

where θ_i is the mean number of breast cancer deaths per thousand life years and ρ_i represents the relative risk between the control and the mammography group in study i.

Under the simplest assumption of total homogeneity of θ_i's and ρ_i's, being equal to θ_0 and ρ_0, respectively, a routine Bayesian analysis can be carried out under the prior independent distributional choice

$$\theta_0 \sim \text{LN}(\mu, \sigma^2), \quad \rho_0 \sim \text{LN}(\tau, \delta^2),$$

where LN stands for a lognormal distribution. The posterior distributions of θ_0 and ρ_0 are readily derived based on the above priors and likelihoods. The hyperparameters $\mu, \sigma^2, \tau, \delta^2$ can again be estimated either on the basis of empirical (data-based) evidence or by applying a hierarchical prior distribution. The posterior distribution of ρ_0 which captures the relative risk between control and mammography groups across studies is most relevant in this context.

Since the assumption of total homogeneity can hardly be tenable, allowing θ_i's to be different and assuming only the equality of ρ_i's, we can model θ_i's as

$$\theta_i \sim \text{LN}(\mu, \sigma^2)$$

and the hyperparameters μ and σ^2 are modeled as

$$\mu \sim N(\mu_0, \eta^2), \quad \sigma^2 \sim \text{IG}(\alpha, \beta).$$

The lognormal assumption

$$\theta_0 \sim \text{LN}(\mu, \sigma^2), \quad \rho_0 \sim \text{LN}(\tau, \delta^2)$$

allows the control rates and mammography rates to vary across trials although their ratios are held constant. This model is generally referred to as additively heterogeneous and interactively homogeneous with similarities as in Mantel and Haenszel (1959). The hyperparameters $\mu_0, \eta^2, \alpha, \beta, \tau, \delta^2$ can again be estimated based on either empirical evidence or hierarchical priors, and as before the posterior distribution of the common relative risk ρ_0 is the most relevant quantity in this context.

Lastly, it is possible to let ρ_i's vary in addition to θ_i's and one can use the distributions

$$\rho_i \sim \text{LN}(\tau, \delta^2), \quad \tau \sim \text{LN}(\tau_0, \delta_0^2), \quad \delta^2 \sim \text{IG}(p, q).$$

The above model allows control and mammography group rates as well as their ratios to vary and is the most flexible of all. The hyperparameters can be estimated based on the data or are assumed to be known from expert opinions, and the posterior distributions of ρ_i's as well as the posterior distribution of τ are relevant here.

Another Bayesian application which also appears in Berry (2000) involves independent binomial variables X_i and Y_i corresponding to control and treatment groups, respectively, in study i, where

$$X_i \sim B(n_i, p_i), \quad Y_i \sim B(m_i, q_i),$$

and the following log-linear models are assumed for p_i and q_i:

$$\ln \frac{p_i}{1 - p_i} = \theta_i, \quad \ln \frac{q_i}{1 - q_i} = \theta_i \, \rho_i,$$

suggesting that both additive and interactive heterogeneity are present. Incidentally, the parameter ρ is called the log odds ratio in this context (see Chapter 2). A Bayesian analysis is now performed by modeling θ_i's and ρ_i's as conditionally independent and assuming that

$$\theta_i \sim N(\mu, \sigma^2), \quad \rho_i \sim N(\tau, \delta^2).$$

The variability in the θ_i's accounts for control variation across studies while the variation in the ρ_i's takes into account possible treatment variation across studies. It is possible to estimate the four hyperparameters $\mu, \sigma^2, \tau, \delta^2$ based on empirical (data-based) evidence or by putting hierarchical priors on them. In the former case, the posterior distributions of ρ_i's are relevant while in the latter case the posterior distribution of τ is the most relevant.

We refer to Brophy and Joseph (2000) for an example dealing with an application of the above binomial model involving three studies. The studies are used to compare streptokinase and tissue-plasminogen activator to reduce mortality following an acute myocardial infarction.

The problem of combining information from studies which report outcomes in two distinct ways can indeed be quite challenging. An application of this type in which outcomes are reported on continuous variables for some medical outcomes in some studies and on binary variables on similar medical outcomes in some other studies appears in Dominici and Parmigiani (2000). A common approach in this situation is to dichotomize the continuous outcomes; however, a better approach is to do the other way around and assume that the binary responses are the results of dichotomizing some underlying but unobserved continuous variables. Using an appropriate Bayesian analysis, it is then possible to reconstruct the values of the unobserved continuous variables and one can then apply standard meta-analysis procedures to combine results of all the studies

To describe the main ideas, suppose there are k studies reporting continuous responses on a treatment and a control and m studies reporting only binary responses on the same treatment and control using points of dichotomy. Assume that the responses y_T from the treatment effect are normally distributed with mean θ_T and variance σ^2 and responses y_C from the control are normally distributed with mean θ_C and variance σ^2. Assume also that the binary responses x_T and x_C from treatment and control, respectively, are based on a common point of dichotomy α in the sense that

$$x_T \sim \text{Bernoulli}\left[\Phi\left(\frac{\alpha - \theta_T}{\sigma}\right)\right], \quad x_C \sim \text{Bernoulli}\left[\Phi\left(\frac{\alpha - \theta_C}{\sigma}\right)\right],$$

where Φ is the standard normal cdf and α is the point of dichotomy.

The joint likelihood based on data from all four types of studies (treatment: continuous, binary; control: continuous, binary) can then be written as

$$L(\theta_T, \theta_C, \sigma^2 | \text{data}) = L_1 \times L_2 \times L_3 \times L_4,$$

where

$$L_1 = \prod_{i=1}^{n_1} \frac{1}{\sigma} \phi \left(\frac{y_{Ti} - \theta_T}{\sigma} \right),$$

$$L_2 = \prod_{i=1}^{n_2} \frac{1}{\sigma} \phi \left(\frac{y_{Ci} - \theta_C}{\sigma} \right),$$

$$L_3 = \prod_{i=1}^{n_3} p_B \left[x_{Ti} | \Phi \left(\frac{\alpha - \theta_T}{\sigma} \right) \right],$$

$$L_4 = \prod_{i=1}^{n_4} p_B \left[x_{Ci} | \Phi \left(\frac{\alpha - \theta_C}{\sigma} \right) \right].$$

Here n_i's are the respective sample sizes and p_B stands for the Bernoulli probability.

It is indeed possible to use the above expression of the joint likelihood to derive suitable estimates of all the unknown parameters and study their properties from a likelihood perspective view. However, as is well known, deriving exact inference about the parameters of interest is quite difficult in this case unless of course one uses large-sample approximations.

It turns out, however, that using a Bayesian approach it is relatively easy to derive the joint and hence the marginal posteriors of all the relevant parameters. This approach proceeds by specifying the prior distributions of θ_T, θ_C, and σ^2 and are usually chosen as conjugate priors given by

$$\theta_T \sim N(\tau_1, \eta_1^2), \quad \theta_C \sim N(\tau_0, \eta_0^2), \quad \sigma^2 \sim IG(a, b),$$

where one can choose η_1^2 and η_0^2 to be very large to allow huge dispersion and IG stands for an inverse gamma distribution. It is then possible to study the posterior distributions of the basic parameters and, in particular, that of the effect size $\Delta = (\theta_T - \theta_C)/\sigma$ to draw suitable inferences. The hyperparameters τ's and η's can be either assumed to be known (from past experience or expert opinion) or estimated based on an empirical Bayes approach or one can specify a hierarchical prior on them. Of course, as is evident from this kind of Bayesian analysis, one needs to freely use MCMC and Gibbs sampler to generate posterior distributions and posterior moments of the parameters. We refer to Dominici and Parmigiani (2000) for details along with an example involving a study of efficacy of calcium channel blocking agents for migraine headache.

As mentioned in the previous chapter, following Berkey et al. (1995, 1998) and Riley et al. (2007a), we now provide a novel application of a bivariate random effects meta-analysis. In this motivating example, the experimenter collects data on two outcomes related to improvement in probing depth (PD) and improvement in attachment level (AL), each outcome being obtained as the difference between two procedures for treating periodontal disease: surgical and nonsurgical. Bivariate fixed effects meta-analysis procedures taking into account the dependence between the two outcomes described in the previous chapter are not appropriate in this example because the relevant tests of homogeneity of univariate effect sizes lead to rejection (Berkey et al., 1998). To use random effects meta-analysis procedures, we have a choice of using either two separate univariate random effects models or a single bivariate random effects meta-analysis model. We describe below our analysis from both of these perspectives.

To fix notation, let Y_{ij} denote the summary statistic from study $i = 1, \ldots, n$ on outcome $j = 1, 2$ and assume that θ_{ij} denotes the underlying true values of the effect sizes. We also assume normality of both Y_{ij} and θ_{ij}.

Under independent univariate random effects meta-analysis (URMA), we assume the following distributional models:

$$\text{Outcome 1: } Y_{i1} \sim N(\theta_{i1}, s_{i1}^2), \quad \theta_{i1} \sim N(\beta_1, \tau_1^2).$$

$$\text{Outcome 2: } Y_{i2} \sim N(\theta_{i2}, s_{i2}^2), \quad \theta_{i2} \sim N(\beta_2, \tau_2^2).$$

Note that there are no correlation terms linking the two outcomes. Following the general discussion of Bayesian analysis, the pooled estimate for outcome j can be written as

$$\hat{\beta}_j = \sum_{i=1}^n \frac{Y_{ij}}{s_{ij}^2 + \hat{\tau}_j^2} \left(\sum_{i=1}^n \frac{1}{s_{ij}^2 + \hat{\tau}_j^2} \right)^{-1}$$

with its estimated variance as

$$\widehat{\text{Var}}(\hat{\beta}_j) = \left(\sum_{i=1}^n \frac{1}{s_{ij}^2 + \hat{\tau}_j^2} \right)^{-1}.$$

It should be noted that the methods to estimate the so-called between-treatment variability τ^2 have been described earlier.

Under a bivariate random effects meta-analysis (BRMA), we consider the bivariate normal distribution of the underlying random variables as follows:

$$\left(\begin{array}{c} Y_{i1} \\ Y_{i2} \end{array} \right) \sim N \left[\left(\begin{array}{c} \theta_{i1} \\ \theta_{i2} \end{array} \right), \delta_i \right], \quad \delta_i = \left(\begin{array}{cc} s_{i1}^2 & \lambda_i \\ \lambda_i & s_{i2}^2 \end{array} \right),$$

$$\left(\begin{array}{c} \theta_{i1} \\ \theta_{i2} \end{array} \right) \sim N \left[\left(\begin{array}{c} \beta_1 \\ \beta_2 \end{array} \right), \Delta \right], \quad \Delta = \left(\begin{array}{cc} \tau_1^2 & \tau_{12} \\ \tau_{12} & \tau_2^2 \end{array} \right).$$

It may be noted that the above model follows from a general Bayesian framework using summary statistics and δ_i and Δ are, respectively, the within-study and between-study covariance matrices. The inclusion of the terms λ_i and τ_{12} makes the distinction between univariate and bivariate meta-analysis models. Naturally when these parameters are 0, the two models coincide. We assume the elements of δ_i to be known and those of Δ to be unknown and must be estimated from the data. One can use the standard SAS Proc Mixed in conjunction with restricted iterative generalized least squares (RIGLS) for this purpose. Analytic expressions for the estimates of β_1 and β_2 along with their estimated variances and covariance appear in Riley et al. (2007a). We refer the interested reader to this excellent paper for details.

The Berkey et al. (1998) data set and its URMA and BRMA analyses, as performed by Riley et al. (2007a), are given in Tables 12.2 and 12.3.

Table 12.2 Details of meta-analysis data set ('Berkey data')

Study	Outcome	Y_{ij}	s_{ij}^2	λ_i
1	PD	0.47	0.0075	0.0030
1	AL	-0.32	0.0077	
2	PD	0.20	0.0057	0.0009
2	AL	-0.60	0.0008	
3	PD	0.40	0.0021	0.0007
3	Al	-0.12	0.0014	
4	PD	0.26	0.0029	0.0009
4	AL	-0.31	0.0015	
5	PD	0.56	0.0148	0.0072
5	AL	-0.39	0.0304	

Table 12.3 Details of URMA and BRMA meta-analysis of 'Berkey data'

Outcome	PD		AL		
	$\hat{\beta}_i$ (s.e)		$\hat{\beta}_2$ (s.e)		
Model	[95% CI]	$\hat{\tau}_1^2$	[95% CI]	$\hat{\tau}_2^2$	$\hat{\tau}_{12}$
URMA	0.361 (0.0592)	0.0119	-0.346 (0.0885)	0.0331	—
	[0.196,0.525]		[-0.591,-0.100]		
BRMA	0.353 (0.0589)	0.0117	-0.339 (0.0879)	0.0327	0.0119
	[0.190,0.517]		[-0.583,-0.095]		

12.3 A UNIFIED BAYESIAN APPROACH TO META-ANALYSIS

Statistical meta-analysis may often involve nonstandard data structures and assumptions associated with the studies to be combined. Thus, each study may have its own measure of effect size and precision along with design covariates and within-study predictors. Here, following DuMouchel and Normand (2000), we present a unified modeling approach to meta-analysis, integrating fixed, random, and mixed effect models as well as Bayesian hierarchical models.

Assume that there are k studies and the ith study results in an effect size Y_i with its mean μ_i and variance s_i^2, which is known. One can think of s_i^2 as the estimated variance of Y_i based on large samples (see Chapter 2 for various measures of effect sizes and their estimated variances). Also, assume that the characteristics of the ith study can be denoted by the vector of covariates $x_i = (x_{i1}, \ldots, x_{iJ})'$, $i = 1, \ldots, k$.

Before conducting the meta-analysis, we should recall that there are at least three sources of variation which may exist in the results of the k studies. First, sampling errors (population variances σ_i^2) occurring within a study may vary across the k studies. Second, actual treatment effects may vary across studies, often leading to random effect models. Third, a treatment effect within a study may vary across its subgroups defined by study design covariates such as investigator differences and uncontrolled conditions. Naturally these sources of variation are not mutually exclusive in nature.

Under a fixed effects model, it is assumed that the k studies provide summary information about a common effect across studies, that is, each summary statistic provides an estimate of the same underlying parameter μ (say). As mentioned in a previous chapter, it is indeed desirable that one performs a test for homogeneity of the population effect sizes $\mu_1, \ldots, \mu_k$ to make sure that this is indeed the case before performing a meta-analysis. Thus, in our notation, Y_i can be modeled as $N(\mu, \sigma_i^2)$ under the homogeneity assumption, where μ is the common effect. In case study design covariates are present, this can be taken into account by designating $E(Y_i) = \mu_i = \boldsymbol{x}_i'\boldsymbol{\beta}$.

In case interstudy variation is believed to be present, a random effects approach is undertaken to allow existence of such a variance component τ^2 (say), and we model $E(Y_i) = \mu_i$ as $N(\mu, \tau^2)$. We refer to Chapter 7 for a detailed discussion on this model and related materials for estimation of τ^2.

A unified approach using the concept of a hierarchical Bayes linear model which integrates fixed effects and random effects models into one framework can be given as follows. We model in a hierarchy $Y_i \sim N(\mu_i, s_i^2)$, $\mu_i \sim N(\boldsymbol{x}_i'\boldsymbol{\beta}, \tau^2)$, and $\boldsymbol{\beta} \sim N(\boldsymbol{b}, \boldsymbol{D})$ with $\tau \sim \pi(\tau)$. In case of no covariates, we model $\mu_i \sim N(\mu, \tau^2)$ and $\mu \sim N(b, d^2)$. The Bayesian specification is completed by assigning suitable prior distributions to μ, $\boldsymbol{\beta}$, and τ as above under the assumption of independence of μ, $\boldsymbol{\beta}$, and τ. In the absence of specific prior information on $\boldsymbol{\beta}$, one can use what is known as a diffuse prior for $\boldsymbol{\beta}$ by allowing the diagonal elements of $\boldsymbol{D}$ to approach ∞. The same is true of d, which can be made to tend to ∞ if a priori no value of μ is preferred over other values. Clearly it is rather important to specify a prior for τ with some caution. A prior for τ with a small variation would almost lead to a fixed effects model while one with a large variation means the model is far from being a fixed effects model.

Keeping the above points in mind, DuMouchel and Normand (2000) proposed the prior $\pi(\tau) = s_0/(s_0 + \tau)^2$, where $s_0^2 = k/[\sum_{i=1}^{k} s_i^{-2}]$ is the harmonic mean of the sampling variances. As observed by these authors, this distribution is highly dispersed because both τ and τ^{-1} have infinite means.

Having specified the priors of all parameters as above, once the data have been observed, the Bayesian analysis proceeds by computing the posterior distributions of the relevant parameters. In this context, one can first derive the marginal posterior of τ and then the conditional posteriors of $\boldsymbol{\beta}$, μ_i, and μ, as appropriate, conditional on τ. We should also mention that typically the posterior means and variances of the parameters are computed and reported.

We describe below the various results on posteriors. We refer to DuMouchel and Normand (2000) for details.

1. In case of no covariates, the posterior mean and variance of μ conditional on τ:

$$\begin{aligned}
\mathrm{E}(\mu|\boldsymbol{Y},\tau) &= \mu^*(\tau) = \frac{\sum Y_i(s_i^2 + \tau^2)^{-1}}{\sum(s_i^2 + \tau^2)^{-1}}, \\
\mathrm{Var}(\mu|\boldsymbol{Y},\tau) &= \mu^{**}(\tau) = \frac{1}{\sum(s_i^2 + \tau^2)^{-1}}.
\end{aligned}$$

2. In case of no covariates, the posterior mean and variance of μ_i conditional on τ:

$$\begin{aligned}
\mathrm{E}(\mu_i|\boldsymbol{Y},\tau) &= [1 - B_i(\tau)]\, Y_i + B_i\, \mu^*(\tau), \\
\mathrm{Var}(\mu_i|\boldsymbol{Y},\tau) &= B_i(\tau)\, [\tau^2 + B_i(\tau)\, \mu^{**}(\tau)],
\end{aligned}$$

where $B_i(\tau) = s_i^2/(s_i^2 + \tau^2)$ is known as the shrinkage factor.

3. In case of presence of covariates, the posterior mean and covariance of $\boldsymbol{\beta}$ conditional on τ:

$$\begin{aligned}
\mathrm{E}(\boldsymbol{\beta}|\boldsymbol{Y},\tau) &= \boldsymbol{\beta}^*(\tau) = [\boldsymbol{X}'\boldsymbol{W}(\tau)\boldsymbol{X} + \boldsymbol{D}^{-1}]^{-1}(\boldsymbol{X}'\boldsymbol{W}(\tau)\boldsymbol{Y} + \boldsymbol{D}^{-1}\boldsymbol{b}), \\
\mathrm{Cov}(\boldsymbol{\beta}|\boldsymbol{Y},\tau) &= \boldsymbol{\beta}^{**}(\tau) = [\boldsymbol{X}'\boldsymbol{W}(\tau)\,\boldsymbol{X} + \boldsymbol{D}^{-1}]^{-1},
\end{aligned}$$

where $\boldsymbol{W}(\tau) = [\mathrm{diag}(s_1^2, \ldots, s_k^2) + \tau^2\, \boldsymbol{I_k}]^{-1}$.

Of course, when the information on $\boldsymbol{\beta}$ is diffuse, $\boldsymbol{\beta}^*(\tau)$ and $\boldsymbol{\beta}^{**}(\tau)$ reduce to

$$\boldsymbol{\beta}^*(\tau) = [\boldsymbol{X}'\boldsymbol{W}(\tau)\boldsymbol{X}]^{-1}(\boldsymbol{X}'\boldsymbol{W}(\tau)\boldsymbol{Y})$$

and

$$\boldsymbol{\beta}^{**}(\tau) = [\boldsymbol{X}'\boldsymbol{W}(\tau)\boldsymbol{X}]^{-1}.$$

Here $\boldsymbol{X}' = [\boldsymbol{x}_1 : \boldsymbol{x}_2 : \cdots : \boldsymbol{x}_k]$.

4. In case of presence of covariates, the posterior mean and covariance of μ_i conditional on τ:

$$\begin{aligned}
\mathrm{E}(\mu_i|\boldsymbol{Y},\tau) &= \mu_i^*(\tau) = Y_i[1 - B_i(\tau)] + B_i(\tau)\boldsymbol{x}_i'\boldsymbol{\beta}^*(\tau), \\
\mathrm{Var}(\mu_i|\boldsymbol{Y},\tau) &= B_i(\tau)[\tau^2 + B_i(\tau)\boldsymbol{x}_i'\boldsymbol{\beta}^{**}(\tau)\boldsymbol{x}_i].
\end{aligned}$$

5. To compute the unconditional mean and variance of various quantities listed above, it is necessary to integrate with respect to the marginal posterior of τ given $\boldsymbol{Y}$. In the case of presence of covariates with diffuse prior information, once the parameters $\boldsymbol{\beta}$ are integrated out, the resulting log-likelihood $\ln L(\tau|\boldsymbol{Y})$ can be expressed, apart from constants, as

$$-2\ln L(\tau|\boldsymbol{Y}) = \sum \ln(\tau^2 + s_i^2) + \ln[\det(\boldsymbol{X}'\boldsymbol{W}_\tau\boldsymbol{X})] + S_\tau^2,$$

where

$$W_\tau = \mathrm{diag}[(\tau^2 + s_1^2)^{-1}, \ldots, (\tau^2 + s_k^2)^{-1}],$$
$$S_\tau^2 = \sum [Y_i - x_i'\beta(\tau)]^2 / (\tau^2 + s_i^2),$$

and

$$\beta(\tau) = (X'W_\tau X)^{-1} X'W_\tau Y.$$

It may be noted that the REML estimate of τ is based on the above log-likelihood (see Chapter 7).

The above likelihood $L(\tau|Y)$ combined with the prior $\pi(\tau)$ provides the marginal posterior distribution $\pi(\tau|Y)$ of τ, given the data Y, which is used to compute the unconditional mean and variance of the quantities listed under 1–4 above, often using Gauss-Hermite integration methods.

12.4 FURTHER RESULTS ON BAYESIAN META-ANALYSIS

A different type of Bayesian analysis in the context of examining possible association between estrogen exposure and endometrial cancer is reported in Larose (2000). This is based on 17 published studies reporting the effect size log relative risk of contracting cancer for users of estrogen at various duration levels compared to never-users. We refer to Chapter 2 for definition and properties of this effect size.

Denoting by y_i the vector of sample means of log relative risk observed at several duration levels, d_i the known duration vector of midpoints of the intervals corresponding to each duration level in the ith study, and S_i the diagonal matrix of sample standard errors, within-study dependence is then modeled as

$$y_i|d_i, \beta_i, S_i, \Sigma_i \sim N(d_i\beta_i, S_i\Sigma_i S_i), \tag{12.1}$$

where the scalar β_i represents the unknown exposure-response slope arising from the ith study, which is to be estimated. Obviously, the dependence of the elements of the vector y_i arising from the ith study is captured by Σ_i.

A Bayesian formulation now proceeds by assuming the following:

(i) $\beta_i|\mu, \sigma^2 \sim N[\mu, \sigma^2]$.

(ii) $\Sigma_i^{-1} \sim \mathrm{Wishart}(\nu_i, R_0)$.

(iii) $\mu \sim N[0, V]$ and $\sigma^2 \sim \mathrm{IG}(b, c)$.

In the above, the hyperparameters μ and σ^2 denote, respectively, the underlying mean slope and the between-study variation. Typically, R_0, V, b, and c are chosen so that the priors are diffuse. One now computes the posteriors of the various parameters, given the data vectors and duration vectors, by deriving the marginal posteriors of β_i and conditional posteriors of Σ_i from the complete Bayesian model (likelihood multiplied by priors). It turns out that the conditional posterior of Σ_i is again inverted Wishart with $\nu_i + 1$ df and precision matrix

$$C = [(\boldsymbol{y}_i - \boldsymbol{d}_i\beta_i)(\boldsymbol{y}_i - \boldsymbol{d}_i\beta_i)' + \boldsymbol{R_0}^{-1}]^{-1}.$$

Standard Gibbs sampling using MCMC can be used to generate data from the posteriors.

We now present an example from Larose (2000) to discuss this application. To study a possible link between duration of estrogen exposure and development of endometrial cancer among women, Table 12.4 provides results of 17 studies on exposure-response information. Midpoints in the table represent midpoints of exposure duration classified into several groups. Log relative risks are computed by comparing two groups of women, those using estrogen at different duration levels and those who never use it. We refer to Chapters 2 and 9 for formulas to compute log relative risks and their standard errors.

It is generally believed that the longer the duration, the larger is the risk, suggesting a linear relationship of log relative risk with exposure. For study i, we denote by $\boldsymbol{y}_i$ the vector of log relative risks. We model $\boldsymbol{y}_i$ as having the mean vector $\boldsymbol{d}_i\beta_i$ where β_i represents the unknown exposure-response slope for study i and $\boldsymbol{d}_i$ denotes the vector of the midpoints of exposure duration times. Since the relative risk estimates within a study use the same reference group (never users of estrogen), the components of $\boldsymbol{y}_i$ are correlated and we assume that Σ_i represents the variance-covariance matrix of $\boldsymbol{y}_i$. We mention that the standard errors reported in Table 12.4 for different studies provide estimates of the diagonal elements of such covariance matrices. Denoting by $\boldsymbol{S}_i$ the diagonal matrix of standard errors from study i, we assume that Σ_i is calibrated by $\boldsymbol{S}_i$ in the sense that the variance-covariance matrix of $\boldsymbol{y}_i$ is given by $\boldsymbol{S}_i\Sigma_i\boldsymbol{S}_i$.

To complete the Bayesian approach to modeling, we assume the following:

(i) $\boldsymbol{y}_i \sim N[\boldsymbol{d}_i\beta_i, \boldsymbol{S}_i\Sigma_i\boldsymbol{S}_i]$.

(ii) $\beta_i|\mu, \sigma^2 \sim N[\mu, \sigma^2]$.

(iii) $\mu \sim N[0, V]$.

(iv) $\sigma^2 \sim \text{IG}(0.001, 1000)$.

(v) $\Sigma_i^{-1}|\nu_i, \boldsymbol{R} \sim \text{Wishart}(\nu_i, R)$.

Here the hyperparameters V, ν_i, and $\boldsymbol{R}$ are chosen so that the resultant prior is diffuse. Based on the above model and data given in Table 12.4, it is possible to write down the likelihood and compute the joint and hence marginal/conditional posteriors of μ, σ^2, and individual study slopes β_i by applying the usual MCMC technique. Some important features of these posteriors are given in Table 12.5.

It follows from the posterior distribution of μ that there is evidence that the mean slope across all studies is positive, a significant exposure-response relationship uncovered by meta-analysis! The between-study variability as shown in the posterior distribution of σ^2 is also nonneglible. Lastly, the posterior distributions of individual slope parameters reveal that some of them are nonsignificant because the associated 95% posterior intervals contain the value 0! For details, we refer to Larose (2000).

Table 12.4 Duration midpoints, log relative risks, and standard errors

Study	Mid-points	Log RR	s.e.	Study	Mid-points	Log RR	s.e.
Antunes	0.5	0.79	0.24	Mack	0.5	1.03	0.22
	3.0	1.06	0.19		3.0	1.50	0.10
	6.0	2.71	0.37		6.5	2.23	0.26
Brinton	2.5	0.34	0.25		9.6	2.17	0.11
	6.0	1.79	0.15	McDonald	0.25	-0.45	0.24
Buring	0.5	0.15	0.11		0.75	1.15	0.46
	2.5	0.69	0.12		2.0	0.86	0.55
	7.0	1.86	0.15		3.6	1.78	0.29
	12.0	2.03	0.34	Paganini-Hill	1.0	1.65	0.52
Gray	2.0	0.18	0.26		5.0	1.95	0.52
	7.0	1.41	0.66		11.0	1.39	0.52
	12.0	2.45	1.11		18.0	3.00	0.52
Hoogerland	0.25	0.18	0.22	Shapiro	0.5	-0.11	0.13
	0.75	0.59	0.21		2.5	1.06	0.07
	2.0	1.16	0.15		7.0	1.72	0.08
	4.0	1.36	0.22		12.0	2.30	0.09
	7.5	1.22	0.19	Spengler	0.3	0.34	0.33
	12.0	1.90	0.59		1.25	0.96	0.22
Hulka	1.75	-0.22	0.12		3.5	0.79	0.32
	4.2	1.41	0.24		6.0	2.15	0.25
Jelovsek	1.75	0.34	0.20	Stavracky	1.0	-0.36	0.18
	4.0	0.34	0.59		3.0	0.00	0.12
	7.5	1.57	0.31		7.0	0.53	0.13
	12.0	0.96	0.19		12.0	1.86	0.25
Kelsey	0.5	0.10	0.11	Weiss	1.5	0.18	0.81
	1.75	0.00	0.30		3.5	1.69	0.45
	3.75	1.06	0.14		6.0	1.55	0.24
	6.25	1.46	0.18		9.0	2.46	0.28
	8.75	2.10	0.19		12.5	3.19	0.44
	12.0	0.99	0.15		17.0	2.32	0.39
Levi	2.5	0.53	0.06		24.0	2.12	1.31
	6.0	1.44	0.09	Ziel	2.0	1.53	0.18
					14.0	2.22	0.13

Table 12.5 Posterior statistics for the overall mean slope μ, between-study variance σ^2, and individual study slopes β_i, $i = 1, \ldots, 17$

Parameter	2.5th Percentile	Median	97.5th Percentile	Mean	SD
Overall mean slope μ	0.013	0.220	0.442	0.222	0.106
Between-study var σ^2	0.028	0.104	0.759	0.174	0.257
1. Antunes	0.124	0.398	0.664	0.387	0.142
2. Brinton	−0.004	0.263	0.535	0.258	0.140
3. Buring	0.069	0.195	0.330	0.196	0.069
4. Gray	0.088	0.195	0.334	0.197	0.061
5. Hoogerland	0.069	0.171	0.310	0.180	0.062
6. Hulka	−0.113	0.257	0.602	0.252	0.177
7. Jelovsek	−0.007	0.106	0.281	0.109	0.059
8. Kelsey	0.059	0.166	0.266	0.160	0.045
9. Levi	−0.039	0.243	0.537	0.244	0.141
10. Mack	0.087	0.290	0.460	0.281	0.098
11. McDonald	0.063	0.366	1.137	0.390	0.230
12. Paganini-Hill	0.084	0.174	0.260	0.173	0.045
13. Shapiro	0.048	0.211	0.365	0.202	0.068
14. Spengler	0.026	0.325	0.571	0.300	0.122
15. Stavracky	−0.003	0.134	0.259	0.132	0.068
16. Weiss	0.078	0.154	0.188	0.148	0.029
17. Ziel	0.055	0.176	0.316	0.176	0.067

CHAPTER 13

PUBLICATION BIAS

As mentioned in the introduction, if a meta-analyst is restricted only to the published studies, then there is a risk that it will lead to biased conclusions because there may be many nonsignificant studies which are often unpublished and hence are ignored, and it is quite possible that their combined effect, significant and nonsignificant studies together, may change the overall conclusion. Publication bias thus results from ignoring unavailable nonsignificant studies, and this is the familiar file-drawer problem. In this chapter, which is patterned after Rosenthal (1979) and Begg (1994), we describe some statistical methods to identify the presence of publication bias and how to deal with it in case it is present.

A general principle is that one ought to perform a preliminary analysis to assess the chances that publication bias could be playing a role in the selection of studies before the component studies are assembled for meta-analysis purposes. This assessment can be done informally by using what is known as a funnel graph, which is merely a plot of the sample size (sometimes the standard error) versus the effect size of the k studies (Light and Pillemer, 1984). If no bias is present, this plot would look like a funnel, with the spout pointing up. This is because there will be a broad spread of points for the highly variable small studies (due to a small sample size) at the

Statistical Meta-Analysis with Applications. By Joachim Hartung, Guido Knapp, Bimal K. Sinha
Copyright © 2008 John Wiley & Sons, Inc.

bottom and decreasing spread as the sample size increases, with the indication that publication bias is unlikely to be a factor for this meta-analysis.

For illustration, let us consider the data sets in Tables 13.1 and 13.2. Table 13.1 contains the results from 20 validity studies where the correlation between student ratings of the instructor and student achievement is examined; see Cohen (1983). The effect size is the correlation coefficient r and the measure of precision is the sample size n.

Table 13.1   Validity studies correlating student ratings of the instructor with student achievement

Study	n	r	P-value
1	10	0.68	0.0153
2	20	0.56	0.0051
3	13	0.23	0.2248
4	22	0.64	0.0007
5	28	0.49	0.0041
6	12	−0.04	0.5491
7	12	0.49	0.0529
8	36	0.33	0.0247
9	19	0.58	0.0046
10	12	0.18	0.2878
11	36	−0.11	0.7385
12	75	0.27	0.0096
13	33	0.26	0.0720
14	121	0.40	< 0.0000
15	37	0.49	0.0010
16	14	0.51	0.0312
17	40	0.40	0.0053
18	16	0.34	0.0988
19	14	0.42	0.0674
20	20	0.16	0.2502

In Table 13.2, we have taken a data set from Raudenbush and Bryk (1985), in which the results of 19 studies are reported studying the effects of teacher expectancy on pupil IQ. The effect size is Cohen's d (see Chapter 2), and the inverse of the reported standard error can be used as the measure of precision.

Referring to the data set from Table 13.1, the validity correlation studies, and the resulting graph, in Figure 13.1, we observe a funnel graph consistent with the pattern mentioned above. On the other hand, for the data set from Table 13.2, the teacher expectancy studies, and the associated graph (Figure 13.2), the contrast is clear. The large studies at the top (with small standard errors) are clustered around the null value while the small studies at the bottom (with large standard errors) show a positive effect, suggesting that there could be a number of small studies with positive effects, which might remain unpublished. We refer to Begg (1994) for details.

Table 13.2   Studies of the effects of teacher expectancy on pupil IQ

Study	Cohen's d	Standard Error	P-value
1	0.03	0.125	0.4052
2	0.12	0.147	0.2072
3	−0.14	0.167	0.7991
4	1.18	0.373	0.0008
5	0.26	0.369	0.2405
6	−0.06	0.103	0.7199
7	−0.02	0.103	0.5770
8	−0.32	0.220	0.9271
9	0.27	0.164	0.0498
10	0.80	0.251	0.0007
11	0.54	0.302	0.0369
12	0.18	0.223	0.2098
13	−0.02	0.289	0.5276
14	0.23	0.290	0.2139
15	−0.18	0.159	0.8712
16	−0.06	0.167	0.6403
17	0.30	0.139	0.0155
18	0.07	0.094	0.2282
19	−0.07	0.174	0.6563

There are two general strategies to deal with publication bias: sampling methods and analytic methods. Sampling methods are designed to eliminate publication bias as far as possible by directly addressing the manner in which the studies are selected for inclusion in the meta-analysis and attempting by all reasonable means to get hold of relevant unpublished studies on the topic. This method, which has been advocated by Peto and his colleagues at Oxford (see Collins et al., 1987), strongly suggests following up on published abstracts on the particular topic and contacting leading researchers in the field for leads on relevant studies being conducted worldwide with the hope that such an attempt would reveal many or some hitherto unpublished nonsignificant articles. The criticism of this method is that accuracy of some of these sought-after studies may be questionable and also the quality of some of these studies may not be acceptable.

The second method, the well-known file-drawer method (Rosenthal, 1979), is designed to provide a simple qualification on a summary P-value from a meta-analysis. Assume that the meta-analysis of k available studies leads to a significant result, that is, the combination of k P-values by one of the methods described earlier leads to rejection of H_0. Recall the method of computation of the P-values described in Chapter 3 and also that small P-values lead to a significance of the null hypothesis, that is, rejection of H_0. We are then wondering if a set of k_0 nonsignificant studies, which remain unpublished and hence unknown to us, would have made a difference

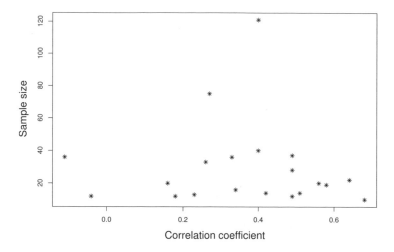

Figure 13.1   Funnel plot for validity correlation studies

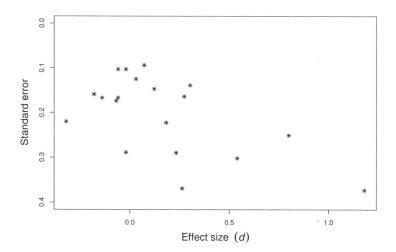

Figure 13.2   Funnel plot for teacher expectancy studies

in the overall conclusion, that is, would have made rejection of H_0 on the basis of all the $k + k_0$ studies impossible. The file-drawer method provides a technique to get some idea about k_0. Once such a value of k_0 is determined, we then use our judgment to see if so many nonsignificant studies on the particular problem under consideration could possibly exist!

To describe the file-drawer method, suppose we have used Stouffer et al.'s (1949) inverse normal method to combine the k P-values. This method suggests that we first convert the individual P-values $P_1, \ldots, P_k$ of the k published studies to normal

Z scores, $Z_1, \ldots, Z_k$, defined by

$$Z_i = \Phi^{-1}(P_i), \quad i = 1, \ldots, k,$$

and then use the overall Z defined by

$$Z = \frac{1}{\sqrt{k}} \sum_{i=1}^{k} Z_i$$

to test the significance of H_0. Since Z behaves like $N(0, 1)$ under H_0 and H_0 is rejected for small values of Z, the assumed rejection of H_0 at the significance level α essentially implies that $Z < -z_\alpha$, or, $|Z| > z_\alpha$. To determine a plausible value of k_0, we assume that the average observed effect of the k_0 unpublished (or unavailable) studies is 0, that is, the sum of the Z scores corresponding to these k_0 studies is 0. Under this assumption, even if these k_0 studies were available, the value of the combined sum of all the Z_i's remains the same as before (i.e., $\sum_{i-1}^{k} Z_i = \sum_{i=1}^{k+k_0} Z_i$). Therefore, this combined sum would have led to the acceptance of H_0, thus reversing our original conclusion, if

$$\frac{1}{\sqrt{k + k_0}} \left| \sum_{i=1}^{k} Z_i \right| < z_\alpha,$$

which happens if

$$k_0 > -k + \frac{\left(\sum_{i=1}^{k} Z_i \right)^2}{(z_\alpha)^2}. \tag{13.1}$$

The above equation provides us with an expression about the number k_0 of unpublished studies with nonsignificant conclusions which, when combined with the results of k published studies, would have made a difference in the overall conclusion. The rationale behind the method is that, considering the relevant research domain, if k_0 is judged to be sufficiently large, it is unlikely that so many unpublished studies exist, and hence we can conclude that the significance of the observed studies is not affected by publication bias.

The determination of the value k_0 in Eq. (13.1) heavily relies on the assumption that the average observed effect of the k_0 unpublished (or unavailable) studies is 0, that is, the sum of the Z scores corresponding to these k_0 studies is 0. Relaxing this assumption to $P_{k+1} = P_{k+2} = \cdots = P_{k+k_0} = \tilde{P}$, we can write $Z_{k+1} = Z_{k+2} = \cdots = Z_{k+k_0} = \tilde{Z}$. If the k_0 unpublished studies were available, the Z value would be given by

$$Z = \frac{1}{\sqrt{k + k_0}} \left\{ \sum_{i=1}^{k} Z_i + \sum_{i=k+1}^{k+k_0} Z_i \right\} = \frac{1}{\sqrt{k + k_0}} \left\{ \left(\sum_{i=1}^{k} Z_i \right) + k_0 \tilde{Z} \right\}.$$

Suppose that, based on the published P-values $P_1, P_2, \ldots, P_k$, the hypothesis H_0 was rejected. Then the conclusion based on a combination of $k + k_0$ P-values would be reversed if

$$\frac{1}{\sqrt{k + k_0}} \left\{ \left(\sum_{i=1}^{k} Z_i \right) + k_0 \tilde{Z} \right\} \geq -z_\alpha. \tag{13.2}$$

It is indeed possible to determine k_0^*, the smallest value of k_0 which satisfies Eq. (13.2), and use our judgment to verify if that could be a possibility.

We have descried above the file-drawer method based on Stouffer et al.'s (1949) way of combination of P-values. It is quite possible to derive similar conditions on k_0 for other combination methods as well. We describe below two such methods.

Under Tippett's method, if we observe just the published P-values $P_1, P_2, \ldots, P_k$, then the overall test of H_0 versus H_1 would reject H_0 at significance level α if

$$\min(P_1, P_2, \ldots, P_k) < 1 - (1 - \alpha)^{1/k}. \tag{13.3}$$

Now suppose that based on the published P-values $P_1, P_2, \ldots, P_k$ the hypothesis H_0 was rejected. Then the P-values $P_{k+1}, P_{k+2}, \ldots, P_{k+k_0}$ would reverse the original decision and hence lead to an overall conclusion of nonsignificance if and only if

$$\min(P_1, P_2, \ldots, P_k, P_{k+1}, P_{k+2}, \ldots, P_{k+k_0}) \geq 1 - (1 - \alpha)^{1/(k+k_0)}. \tag{13.4}$$

Now since the P-values $P_{k+1}, P_{k+2}, \ldots, P_{k+k_0}$ correspond to unpublished and nonsignificant studies, we may assume that all of these P-values are large, which would naturally imply

$$\min(P_1, P_2, \ldots, P_k, P_{k+1}, P_{k+2}, \ldots, P_{k+k_0}) = \min(P_1, P_2, \ldots, P_k). \tag{13.5}$$

Looking at Eqs. (13.3) and (13.4) we see that the original decision of significance would be reversed if and only if

$$\min(P_1, P_2, \ldots, P_k) \geq 1 - (1 - \alpha)^{1/(k+k_0)},$$

which occurs if and only if

$$k_0 \geq \frac{\ln[1 - \alpha)}{\ln(1 - \min(P_1, P_2, \ldots, P_k)]} - k. \tag{13.6}$$

From the above equation it follows that

$$k_0^* = \left\lceil \frac{\ln(1 - \alpha)}{\ln[1 - \min(P_1, P_2, \ldots, P_k)]} - k \right\rceil. \tag{13.7}$$

Note that under Tippett's method k_0^* does not depend on the values of the unpublished P-values as long as these unpublished P-values are large enough so that Eq. (13.5) holds, that is, even a certain number of significant unpublished studies could change the overall conclusion.

Under Fisher's method, if we observe just the published P-values $P_1, P_2, \ldots, P_k$, then the overall test of H_0 versus H_1 would reject H_0 at significance level α if and only if

$$-2 \sum_{i=1}^{k} \ln P_i > \chi_{\alpha, 2k}^2,$$

where $\chi^2_{\alpha,2k}$ is the upper α percentile of the chi-square distribution with $2k$ degrees of freedom. Now suppose that based on the published P-values $P_1, P_2, \ldots, P_k$ the hypothesis H_0 was rejected. Then the P-values $P_{k+1}, P_{k+2}, \ldots, P_{k+k_0}$ would reverse the original decision and hence lead to an overall conclusion of nonsignificance if and only if

$$-2 \sum_{i=1}^{k+k_0} \ln P_i \leq \chi^2_{\alpha,2(k+k_0)}.$$

To simplify things let us assume as before that

$$P_{k+1} = P_{k+2} = \cdots = P_{k+k_0} = \tilde{P}$$

so that

$$-2 \sum_{i=1}^{k+k_0} \ln P_i = -2 \sum_{i=1}^{k} \ln P_i - 2 \sum_{i=k+1}^{k+k_0} \ln P_i = -2 \left(\sum_{i-1}^{k} \ln P_i \right) - 2k_0 \ln \tilde{P}.$$

Hence we would reverse the original decision and conclude nonsignificance if and only if

$$-2 \left(\sum_{i=1}^{k} \ln P_i \right) - 2k_0 \ln \tilde{P} \leq \chi^2_{\alpha,2(k+k_0)}. \tag{13.8}$$

Then k_0^* is given by the smallest value of k_0 which satisfies Eq. (13.8). This value can easily be computed numerically. We now apply the above methods to two examples.

Example 13.1. We can apply the file-drawer method to the data set dealing with teacher expectancy studies; see Table 13.2. The individual Z scores are computed by dividing the effect sizes by the corresponding standard errors, details of which appear in Chapter 4. This leads to $\sum_{i=1}^{19} Z_i = 11.017$, which yields $Z = 2.527$, a significant value at the 5% level. Using Eq. (13.1) we find that $k_0 \geq 26$. This means if there are at least 26 unpublished nonsignificant studies, then the conclusion obtained by ignoring them would have been wrong. The plausibility of the existence of so many unpublished studies is of course a judgment call and would depend on the search technique used by the meta-analyst. Using Fisher's method with $\tilde{P} = 0.5$, at least 21 nonsignificant results would change the overall conclusion. For $\tilde{P} = 0.4$, ignoring at least 44 unpublished studies, the overall result obtained would have been wrong. Increasing $\tilde{P}$ to 0.6, then 10 unpublished studies using Stouffer's method and 15 studies using Fisher's method would change the overall conclusion if the P-values were available. Irrespective of the true P-values of the nonpublished studies, as long as Eq. (13.5) is fulfilled, 53 studies would change the overall result into nonsignificance with Tippett's method.

Example 13.2. We can also apply this method to the data set dealing with validity correlation studies; see Table 13.1. In this case the individual Z scores are computed from P-values, which in turn are obtained from the t values. This leads to $\sum_{i=1}^{20} Z_i = 36.632$, which yields $Z = 8.191$, a highly significant value at the 5%

level. Again, using the formula given above, we find that $k_0 \geq 476$. This means if there are at least 476 unpublished nonsignificant studies, then the conclusion obtained by ignoring them would have been wrong. Using Tippett's method, an additional 18,706 unpublished studies are necessary to change the overall result into nonsignificance as long as the P-values of the unpublished studies fulfill Eq. (13.5). Using Fisher's method with $\tilde{P} = 0.5$, 129 studies would change the overall conclusion to nonsignificance. For $\tilde{P} = 0.4$, 339 studies would be necessary and for $\tilde{P} \leq 0.35$, an infinite number of studies would not change the overall result.

The plausibility of the existence of so many unpublished nonsignificant studies seems very remote, and we can therefore conclude that publication bias is unlikely to make a difference in this problem.

If the meta-analysis of k available studies leads to a nonsignificant conclusion, then of course the issue of publication bias does not arise!

The advantage of the file-drawer method is that it is very simple and easily interpretable. A disadvantage is the assumption that the results of the missing studies are centered on the null hypothesis.

Several methods have been suggested in the literature which translate the graphical approach of the funnel plot into a statistical model. In the statistical model, the associations between study size (or other measures of precision) and estimated treatment effects are examined. Begg and Mazumdar (1994) proposed an adjusted rank correlation method to examine the association between the effect estimates and their variances (or, equivalently, their standard errors). This correlation test is based on Kendall's tau. Egger et al. (1997) introduced a linear regression approach in which the standardized effect size, say $T/\hat{\sigma}(T)$, is regressed onto a measure of precision, for example, $1/\hat{\sigma}(T)$. For k studies, the statistical model is given as

$$\frac{T_i}{\hat{\sigma}(T_i)} = \beta_0 + \beta_1 \, \frac{1}{\hat{\sigma}(T)} + e_i, \; i = 1, \ldots, k, \tag{13.9}$$

with e_i a normally distributed random error with mean 0 and variance σ^2. The null hypothesis of no publication bias is stated as $H_0 : \beta_1 = 0$, that is, there is no association between the precision $1/\hat{\sigma}(T_i)$ and the standardized effect size. The test statistic $\hat{\beta}_1/\hat{\sigma}(\hat{\beta}_1)$ is compared to the t distribution with $k - 2$ df to obtain a P-value. Usually the test is assessed at the 10% level of significance because of the usually small number of studies in a meta-analysis.

More sophisticated methods for adjusting the meta-analysis for publication bias have been developed using weighted distribution theory (Patil and Rao, 1977) and a Bayesian data augmentation approach (Givens, Smith, and Tweedie, 1997). These methods lead to a much more complicated analysis and are omitted. We also refer to Iyengar and Greenhouse (1988) for some related results.

## CHAPTER 14

RECOVERY OF INTERBLOCK INFORMATION

In this chapter we provide a different kind of application of meta-analysis which arises in the context of analysis of data obtained from specially designed experiments.

In block designs with fixed treatment effects and no interaction, it is a well-known (and an easily verifiable) fact that the usual least-squares estimator of the treatment effects, computed assuming that the block effects are fixed, continues to provide an unbiased estimator of the treatment effects even when the block effects are random. This least-squares estimator of the treatment effects is referred to as the intrablock estimator since it is based on contrasts among the observations within the blocks, thereby eliminating the block effects. Similarly, the usual F test (known as the intrablock F test) can always be used to test the equality of the treatment effects irrespective of whether the block effects are fixed effects or random effects. However, when the block effects are random as opposed to being fixed and are independently and identically distributed as normal, additional information is available for inference concerning the treatment effects. Such information is referred to as interblock information and this information is based on the sum of the observations in each block. An important problem in this context is that of suitably combining the intrablock and interblock information to obtain a combined estimator of the treatment effects or to obtain a combined test for the equality of the treatment effects. Such a problem of

Statistical Meta-Analysis with Applications. By Joachim Hartung, Guido Knapp, Bimal K. Sinha   **179**
Copyright © 2008 John Wiley & Sons, Inc.

obtaining a combined estimator was first addressed by Yates (1939, 1940) for certain special designs and later by Rao (1947) for general incomplete block designs. Since then, there has been considerable research activity on the problem of combining the intrablock and interblock information about the treatment effects. We refer to Shah (1975, 1992) for a review of these results. This problem is very much in the spirit of statistical meta-analysis.

In spite of the fairly extensive literature on the problem of obtaining a combined estimator, the problem of deriving a combined test has received very little attention. An obvious way of combining the intrablock and interblock F tests is by using Fisher's procedure described in Chapter 3, namely, by combining the two individual P-values via the sum of the log P-values multiplied by the factor -2. The null distribution of the statistic so obtained is a chi-squared distribution with 4 degrees of freedom, since the individual P-values are independent. Thus the combined test is very easy to implement. However, it is obvious that this procedure of combining P-values ignores the underlying structure of the problem.

Some tests that do take into account the underlying structure of the problem are proposed in Feingold (1985, 1988). However, Feingold's tests are not exact and are applicable only for testing whether a single contrast among the treatment effects is zero. The first satisfactory solution to the problem of combining the intrablock and interblock F tests appears to be due to Cohen and Sackrowitz (1989). These authors derived a simple and exact combined test for balanced incomplete block designs (BIBDs). Through simulation, they also showed that their test was superior to the usual intrablock F test. Their results were generalized and extended by Mathew, Sinha, and Zhou (1993) and Zhou and Mathew (1993) by proposing and comparing a variety of exact tests and also by considering designs other than BIBDs.

It turns out that the problem of combining interblock and intrablock F tests also arises in random effects models, that is, when, in addition to the block effects, the treatment effects are also independent identically distributed normal random variables, distributed independently of the block effects and the experimental error terms, and the problem is to test the significance of the treatment variance component. We provide a brief description of some of these results in this chapter and refer to the excellent textbook by Khuri, Mathew, and Sinha (1998) for details. A technical tool used in this chapter is invariance.

14.1 NOTATION AND TEST STATISTICS

Consider a block design for comparing v treatments in b blocks of k plots each and let y_{ij} denote the observation from the ith plot in the jth block. When the blocks and treatments do not interact, which is the set-up we are considering in this chapter, we have the following two-way classification model for the observations y_{ij}'s:

$$y_{ij} = \mu + \sum_{s=1}^{v} \delta_{ij}^s \tau_s + \beta_j + e_{ij}, \; i = 1, 2, \ldots, k; \; j = 1, 2, \ldots, b, \qquad (14.1)$$

where μ is a general mean, τ_s is the effect due to the sth treatment, β_j is the effect due to the jth block, e_{ij} is the experimental error term, and δ_{ij}^s takes the value 1 if the sth treatment occurs in the ith plot of the jth block and 0 otherwise. Writing $\boldsymbol{y} = (y_{11}, \dots, y_{1k}, y_{21}, \dots, y_{2k}, \dots, y_{b1}, \dots, y_{bk})'$, $\boldsymbol{\tau} = (\tau_1, \dots, \tau_v)'$, and $\boldsymbol{\beta} = (\beta_1, \dots, \beta_b)'$, model (14.1) can be written as

$$\boldsymbol{y} = \mu \boldsymbol{1}_{bk} + \boldsymbol{X}_1 \boldsymbol{\tau} + (\boldsymbol{I}_b \otimes \boldsymbol{1}_k)\boldsymbol{\beta} + \boldsymbol{e}, \tag{14.2}$$

where $\boldsymbol{e}$ is defined similarly to $\boldsymbol{y}$, $\boldsymbol{X}_1$ is an appropriate design matrix (with the δ_{ij}^s's as entries), and $\otimes$ denotes Kronecker product. We assume that $\boldsymbol{\tau}$ is a vector of fixed effects satisfying $\sum_{s=1}^v \tau_s = 0$, $\boldsymbol{\beta}$ is a vector of random effects, and $\boldsymbol{\beta}$ and $\boldsymbol{e}$ are independently distributed with

$$\boldsymbol{\beta} \sim N\left(\boldsymbol{0}, \sigma_\beta^2 \boldsymbol{I}_b\right) \quad \text{and} \quad \boldsymbol{e} \sim N\left(\boldsymbol{0}, \sigma_e^2 \boldsymbol{I}_{bk}\right). \tag{14.3}$$

We now give the expressions for certain estimators and sums of squares under model (14.1), where assumption (14.3) is satisfied. Derivations of these quantities are omitted here, since they are available in standard books on analysis of variance.

Let $n_{sj} = \sum_{i=1}^k \delta_{ij}^s$. Then n_{sj} is clearly the number of times the sth treatment occurs in the jth block and $\boldsymbol{N} = (n_{sj})$ is the $v \times b$ incidence matrix of the design. It is readily verified that

$$\boldsymbol{N} = \boldsymbol{X}_1'(\boldsymbol{I}_b \otimes \boldsymbol{1}_k). \tag{14.4}$$

Let T_s and B_j denote the sum of the observations corresponding to the sth treatment and the jth block, respectively. Write $\boldsymbol{T} = (T_1, \dots, T_v)'$ and $\boldsymbol{B} = (B_1, \dots, B_b)'$. Then

$$\boldsymbol{q}_1 = \boldsymbol{T} - \frac{1}{k}\boldsymbol{N}\boldsymbol{B} \tag{14.5}$$

is referred to as the vector of adjusted treatment totals. Let r_s be the number of times the sth treatment occurs in the design and define

$$\boldsymbol{C}_1 = \text{diag}(r_1, \dots, r_v) - \frac{1}{k}\boldsymbol{N}\boldsymbol{N}'. \tag{14.6}$$

Then

$$\boldsymbol{q}_1 \sim N(\boldsymbol{C}_1\boldsymbol{\tau}, \sigma_e^2\boldsymbol{C}_1). \tag{14.7}$$

The random vector $\boldsymbol{q}_1$ is an intrablock quantity, since each component of $\boldsymbol{q}_1$ can be written as a linear combination of contrasts among observations within blocks. When the τ_i's are fixed effects, the estimator of $\boldsymbol{\tau}$ based on $\boldsymbol{q}_1$ is referred to as its intrablock estimator. It is well known that for the estimability of all the treatment contrasts based on intrablock information, we must have $\text{rank}(\boldsymbol{C}_1) = v - 1$. We assume that this rank condition holds, since this condition is also necessary in order that we can test the equality of all the treatment effects. If s_1^2 denotes the intrablock error sum of squares [i.e., the error sum of squares based on model (14.1) when $\boldsymbol{\beta}$ is a vector of fixed effects], we then have

$$s_1^2 \sim \sigma^2 \chi_{bk-b-v+1}^2. \tag{14.8}$$

Let

$$F_1 = \frac{q_1' C_1^- q_1/(v-1)}{s_1^2/(bk-b-v+1)}. \tag{14.9}$$

Then F_1 is the intrablock F ratio for testing the equality of the treatment effects. Recall that for any matrix A, A^- denotes a generalized inverse.

From model (14.1) we get the following model for B_j, the sum of the observations from the jth block,

$$B_j = k\mu + \sum_{s=1}^{v} n_{sj}\tau_s + g_j, \tag{14.10}$$

where $g_j = k\beta_j + \sum_{i=1}^{k} e_{ij}$. Writing $\boldsymbol{g} = (g_1, g_2, \ldots, g_b)'$, Eq. (14.10) can be expressed as

$$\boldsymbol{B} = k\mu \mathbf{1}_b + \boldsymbol{N}'\boldsymbol{\tau} + \boldsymbol{g} \tag{14.11}$$

with

$$\boldsymbol{g} \sim N\left(\mathbf{0}, k\,(k\,\sigma_\beta^2 + \sigma_e^2)\boldsymbol{I}_b\right). \tag{14.12}$$

Interblock information is the information regarding the treatment effects that can be obtained using $\boldsymbol{B}$ based on model (14.11). It is easy to verify that under the distributional assumption (14.3), $\boldsymbol{B}$ is distributed independently of q_1 and s_1^2. Define

$$q_2 = N\left(\boldsymbol{I}_b - \frac{1}{b}\mathbf{1}_b\mathbf{1}_b'\right)\boldsymbol{B}, \quad \boldsymbol{C}_2 = N\left(\boldsymbol{I}_b - \frac{1}{b}\mathbf{1}_b\mathbf{1}_b'\right)\boldsymbol{N}'. \tag{14.13}$$

Then,

$$q_2 \sim N\left(\boldsymbol{C}_2\boldsymbol{\tau}, k(k\sigma_\beta^2 + \sigma_e^2)\boldsymbol{C}_2\right). \tag{14.14}$$

In order to be able to estimate all the treatment contrasts using $\boldsymbol{B}$, we need the condition $\text{rank}(\boldsymbol{C}_2) = v - 1$, which will be assumed in this chapter. Note that this condition implies $b \geq v$. If s_2^2 is the error sum of squares based on model (14.11), then

$$s_2^2 \sim k(k\sigma_\beta^2 + \sigma_e^2)\chi_{b-v}^2. \tag{14.15}$$

Let

$$F_2 = \frac{q_2' C_2^- q_2/(v-1)}{s_2^2/(b-v)}. \tag{14.16}$$

Then F_2 is referred to as the interblock F ratio for testing the equality of the treatment effects. Note that when $b = v$, s_2^2 and the F ratio F_2 are nonexistent, even though the treatment contrasts can be estimated using q_2 in Eq. (14.13). Our meta-analysis in this section will be based on the quantities q_1, s_1^2, q_2, and s_2^2 having the distributions as specified, respectively, in Eqs. (14.7), (14.8), (14.14), and (14.15). These quantities are all independently distributed. Note that in order to obtain the expressions for the above quantities and to arrive at their distributions, we have explicitly used the assumption of equal block sizes.

Assuming that $\text{rank}(\boldsymbol{C}_1) = \text{rank}(\boldsymbol{C}_2) = v - 1$ and $b > v$, the problem we shall address is that of combining the F tests based on F_1 and F_2 in order to test the equality of the treatment effects. It will also be of interest to see whether q_2 can be used in this testing problem when $b = v$, that is, when s_2^2 and F_2 are nonexistent. When the block design is a BIBD, this problem is analyzed in detail in Section 14.2 and we have derived and compared several tests.

We refer to Khuri, Mathew, and Sinha (1998) for related results for a general incomplete block design with equal block sizes and also for the situation when the treatment effects are random, distributed independently and identically as normal.

14.2 BIBD WITH FIXED TREATMENT EFFECTS

Consider a BIBD with parameters v, b, r, k, and λ, where v, b, and k are as in the previous section and r and λ, respectively, denote the number of times each treatment is replicated and the number of blocks in which every pair of treatments occur together. Using the facts that the incidence matrix N of a BIBD satisfies $NN' = (r - \lambda)I_v + \lambda 1_v 1_v'$ and $N1_b = r1_v$, the matrices C_1 and C_2 simplify to

$$C_1 = \frac{\lambda v}{k}\left(I_v - \frac{1}{v}1_v 1_v'\right), \quad C_2 = (r - \lambda)\left(I_v - \frac{1}{v}1_v 1_v'\right). \tag{14.17}$$

Note that C_2 is a multiple of C_1 and the matrix $I_v - (1/v)1_v 1_v'$ that occurs in both C_1 and C_2 is a symmetric idempotent matrix of rank $v - 1$ satisfying

$$\left(I_v - \frac{1}{v}1_v 1_v'\right)1_v = 0.$$

These facts will be used in the analysis that follows. Let O be any $v \times v$ orthogonal matrix whose last column is the vector $(1/\sqrt{v})1_v$. Then we can write $O = [O_1 : (1/\sqrt{v})1_v]$, where O_1 is a $v \times (v - 1)$ matrix denoting the first $v - 1$ columns of O. The orthogonality of O gives $O_1'O_1 = I_{v-1}$ and $O_1'1_v = 0$. Consequently,

$$O'\left(I_v - \frac{1}{v}1_v 1_v'\right)O = \text{diag}(I_{v-1}, 0).$$

Hence

$$O'C_1O = \frac{\lambda v}{k}\text{diag}(I_{v-1}, 0), \quad O'C_2O = (r - \lambda)\text{diag}(I_{v-1}, 0). \tag{14.18}$$

In view of Eq. (14.18), we have

$$O'q_1 \sim N\left[\frac{\lambda v}{k}\text{diag}(I_{v-1}, 0)\, O'\tau, \sigma_e^2\, \frac{\lambda v}{k}\text{diag}(I_{v-1}, 0)\right]$$

and

$$O'q_2 \sim N\left[(r - \lambda)\text{diag}(I_{v-1}, 0)\, O'\tau, k\,(k\,\sigma_\beta^2 + \sigma_e^2)\,(r - \lambda)\text{diag}(I_{v-1}, 0)\right],$$

where q_1 and q_2 are as in Eqs. (14.5) and (14.13), respectively. Define

$$x_1 = \frac{k}{\lambda v}O_1'q_1, \quad x_2 = \frac{1}{(r - \lambda)}O_1'q_2, \quad \tau^* = O_1'\tau, \tag{14.19}$$

and let s_1^2 and s_2^2 be as in Eqs. (14.8) and (14.15), respectively. We then have the canonical form

$$
\begin{aligned}
\boldsymbol{x}_1 &\sim N\left(\boldsymbol{\tau}^*, \frac{k}{\lambda v}\,\sigma_e^2 \boldsymbol{I}_{v-1}\right), \quad \boldsymbol{x}_2 \sim N\left(\boldsymbol{\tau}^*, \frac{k}{(r-\lambda)}(k\sigma_\beta^2 + \sigma_e^2)\boldsymbol{I}_{v-1}\right), \\
s_1^2 &\sim \sigma_e^2\,\chi_{bk-b-v+1}^2, \qquad\qquad s_2^2 \sim k\,(k\sigma_\beta^2 + \sigma_e^2)\,\chi_{b-v}^2.
\end{aligned}
$$

$$(14.20)$$

Note that since $\boldsymbol{O}_1'\boldsymbol{1}_v = \boldsymbol{0}$, $\boldsymbol{\tau}^*$ in model (14.20) is a $(v-1) \times 1$ vector of treatment contrasts and the equality of the treatment effects is equivalent to $\boldsymbol{\tau}^* = \boldsymbol{0}$. The F ratios F_1 and F_2 in Eqs. (14.9) and (14.16) simplify to

$$
\begin{aligned}
F_1 &= \frac{[k/(\lambda v)]\,\boldsymbol{q}_1'\boldsymbol{q}_1/(v-1)}{s_1^2/(bk-b-v+1)} = \frac{(\lambda v/k)\,\boldsymbol{x}_1'\boldsymbol{x}_1/(v-1)}{s_1^2/(bk-b-v+1)}, \\
F_2 &= \frac{[1/(r-\lambda)]\,\boldsymbol{q}_2'\boldsymbol{q}_2/(v-1)}{s_2^2/(b-v)} = \frac{(r-\lambda)\,\boldsymbol{x}_2'\boldsymbol{x}_2/(v-1)}{s_2^2/(b-v)}.
\end{aligned}
$$

Note that if $b = v$, that is, for a symmetrical BIBD, s_2^2 and F_2 are nonexistent. We shall first consider the case $b > v$. The situation $b = v$ will be considered later.

14.2.1   Combined tests when $b > v$

We shall work with the canonical form (14.20) since it is easy to identify a group that leaves the testing problem invariant. The tests that we shall derive can be easily expressed in terms of the original variables. In terms of model (14.20), the testing problem is H_0: $\boldsymbol{\tau}^* = \boldsymbol{0}$. Consider the group $\mathcal{G} = \{g = (\boldsymbol{\Gamma}, c):$ $\boldsymbol{\Gamma}$ is a $p \times p$ orthogonal matrix and c is a positive scalar$\}$, whose action on $(\boldsymbol{x}_1, \boldsymbol{x}_2, s_1^2, s_2^2)$ is given by

$$
g(\boldsymbol{x}_1, \boldsymbol{x}_2, s_1^2, s_2^2) = \left(c\boldsymbol{\Gamma}\boldsymbol{x}_1, c\boldsymbol{\Gamma}\boldsymbol{x}_2, c^2 s_1^2, c^2 s_2^2\right). \tag{14.21}
$$

It is clear that the testing problem H_0: $\boldsymbol{\tau}^* = \boldsymbol{0}$ in model (14.20) is invariant under the above group action. In order to derive invariant tests, we shall first compute a maximal invariant statistic. Recall that a maximal invariant statistic, say D, under the group action (14.21) is a statistic satisfying two conditions: (i) D is invariant under the group action (14.21) and (ii) any statistic that is invariant under the group action (14.21) must be a function of D. A maximal invariant parameter is similarly defined. A maximal invariant statistic and a maximal invariant parameter under the group action (14.21) are given in the following lemma whose proof is omitted. See Khuri, Mathew, and Sinha (1998) for details.

Lemma 14.1. Consider model (14.20) and the testing problem H_0: $\boldsymbol{\tau}^* = \boldsymbol{0}$. Let

$$
U = \frac{U_1}{U_2} \quad \text{and} \quad R = \frac{\boldsymbol{x}_1'\boldsymbol{x}_2}{\|\boldsymbol{x}_1\|\,\|\boldsymbol{x}_2\|} \tag{14.22}
$$

with

$$
U_1 = \frac{\lambda v}{k}\boldsymbol{x}_1'\boldsymbol{x}_1 + s_1^2 \quad \text{and} \quad U_2 = \frac{1}{k}\left[(r-\lambda)\boldsymbol{x}_2'\boldsymbol{x}_2 + s_2^2\right].
$$

Then a maximal invariant statistic, say D, under group action (14.21) is given by

$$D = (F_1, F_2, R, U),$$ (14.23)

where F_1 and F_2 are the F ratios given in Eq. (14.21) and R and U are given in Eq. (14.22). Furthermore, a maximal invariant parameter is

$$\left[\frac{\boldsymbol{\tau}^{*\prime} \boldsymbol{\tau}^*}{\sigma_e^2}, \frac{\sigma_e^2 + k\sigma_\beta^2}{\sigma_e^2} \right].$$

Obviously, a maximal invariant statistic can be expressed in other forms using functions of x_1, x_2, s_1^2, and s_2^2, different from those in D given in Eq. (14.23). The reason for expressing the maximal invariant as in Eq. (14.23) is that the tests we shall describe below are directly in terms of F_1, F_2, R, and U. Note that under H_0: $\boldsymbol{\tau}^* = \mathbf{0}$, $U_1 / \{(v-1) + (bk - b - v + 1)\}$ and $U_2 / \{(v-1) + (b-1)\}$ are unbiased estimators of σ_e^2 and $\sigma_e^2 + k\sigma_\beta^2$. This is a property that we shall eventually use. The following lemma establishes some properties of the quantities F_1, F_2, R, U_1, and U_2. Again, its proof is omitted. See Khuri, Mathew, and Sinha (1998) for details.

Lemma 14.2. Let F_1, F_2, R, U_1, and U_2 be as in Eqs. (14.21) and (14.22). Then, under H_0: $\boldsymbol{\tau}^* = \mathbf{0}$,
(a) U_1 and U_2 are complete and sufficient for σ_e^2 and σ_β^2 and
(b) F_1, F_2, R, U_1, and U_2 are mutually independent.

The statistic R defined in Eq. (14.22), which is a part of the maximal invariant statistic D in Eq. (14.23), plays a major role in some of the tests that we shall propose below. The reason for this is that the test that rejects H_0: $\boldsymbol{\tau}^* = \mathbf{0}$ for large values of R is a valid and meaningful one-sided test. This is implied by the properties $E(R|H_0 : \boldsymbol{\tau}^* = \mathbf{0}) = 0$ and $E(R|H_1 : \boldsymbol{\tau}^* \neq \mathbf{0}) > 0$. The first property follows trivially from the definition of R in Eq. (14.22) since x_1 and x_2, and hence R, are distributed symmetrically around zero under H_0: $\boldsymbol{\tau}^* = \mathbf{0}$. For a proof of the second property, see Khuri, Mathew, and Sinha (1998). From the definition of R, it is also clear that the null distribution of R is the same as that of the ordinary product moment correlation under independence in samples of sizes $v - 1$ from a bivariate normal population with mean zero. Recall that under H_0: $\boldsymbol{\tau}^* = \mathbf{0}$, R is independent of F_1 and F_2 (see Lemma 14.2). Thus there are three independent tests, one each based on F_1, F_2, and R, for testing H_0: $\boldsymbol{\tau}^* = \mathbf{0}$ in model (14.20). We shall now explore various methods for combining these tests.

Fisher's (1932) idea of combining independent tests is to suitably combine the P-values of the tests; see Chapter 3.

Let P_1, P_2, and P_3 denote the P-values of the tests that reject H_0: $\boldsymbol{\tau}^* = \mathbf{0}$ for large values of F_1, F_2, and R. Define

$$Z_i = -\ln P_i \; (i = 1, 2, 3), \quad Z = \sum_{i=1}^{2} Z_i, \quad Z^* = \sum_{i=1}^{3} Z_i.$$ (14.24)

Since we reject H_0: $\boldsymbol{\tau}^* = \mathbf{0}$ for small values of the P_i's, large values of Z and Z^* indicate evidence against H_0. Furthermore, using the fact that P_i's have independent uniform distributions under H_0, it can be easily shown that, under H_0, $2Z$ has a chi-squared distribution with 4 degrees of freedom and $2Z^*$ has a chi-squared distribution with 6 degrees of freedom. Here, Z and Z^* are the test statistics resulting from Fisher's idea of combining tests. We thus have the following rejection regions Φ_1 and Φ_2 of the size α tests based on Z and Z^*:

$$\Phi_1 : 2Z > \chi^2_{4,\alpha}, \quad \Phi_2 : 2Z^* > \chi^2_{6,\alpha}, \tag{14.25}$$

where $\chi^2_{m,\alpha}$ is the upper α cut-off point of the chi-squared distribution with m df. The test based on Φ_1 combines those based on F_1 and F_2; the one based on Φ_2 combines those based on F_1, F_2, and R.

A drawback of the tests based on Φ_1 and Φ_2 is that they put equal weights to the individual tests. From model (14.20), it is intuitively clear that a combined test should attach a smaller weight to F_2 as σ^2_β gets larger. One way of achieving this is by taking a weighted combination of the Z_i's defined in Eq. (14.24) with weights that suitably reflect the magnitude of σ^2_β relative to σ^2_e. Since these variances are unknown, one has to use estimated weights. Thus, let

$$\theta^2 = \frac{\sigma^2_e}{k\,\sigma^2_\beta + \sigma^2_e} \tag{14.26}$$

and let $\hat{\theta}^2$ be an estimator of θ^2. Define

$$\gamma_1 = \frac{1}{1 + \hat{\theta}^2}, \ \gamma_2 = 1 - \gamma_1,$$

$$\delta_1 = \frac{1}{(1+\hat{\theta}^2)^2}, \ \delta_2 = \frac{\hat{\theta}^4}{(1+\hat{\theta}^2)^2}, \ \delta_3 = \frac{2\,\hat{\theta}^2}{(1+\hat{\theta}^2)^2}, \tag{14.27}$$

$$W = \sum_{i=1}^{2} \gamma_i\, Z_i, \ W^* = \sum_{i=1}^{3} \delta_i\, Z_i.$$

Several choices of $\hat{\theta}^2$ are possible for computing the γ_i's and the δ_i's. Cohen and Sackrowitz (1989) recommended the following choice for $\hat{\theta}^2$:

$$\hat{\theta}^2_{(1)} = \min\left\{\frac{U_1}{U_2}, 1\right\}. \tag{14.28}$$

As pointed out earlier, under H_0: $\tau^* = 0$, unbiased estimators of σ^2_e and $\sigma^2_e + k\sigma^2_\beta$ are, respectively, given by $\hat{\sigma}^2_e = U_1/(bk - b)$ and $k\hat{\sigma}^2_\beta + \hat{\sigma}^2_e = U_2/(b - 1)$. Note that since $\theta^2 \leq 1$, a natural estimator of θ^2 is $\hat{\theta}^2_{(2)}$ given by

$$\hat{\theta}^2_{(2)} = \min\left\{\frac{\hat{\sigma}^2_e}{k\hat{\sigma}^2_\beta + \hat{\sigma}^2_e}, 1\right\}. \tag{14.29}$$

We note that the estimators of θ^2 given above are functions of only U_1 and U_2. This fact is crucial in the proof of the following theorem, which appears in Khuri, Mathew, and Sinha (1998).

Theorem 14.1. Let W and W^* be as defined in Eq. (14.27). Furthermore, let $\hat{\theta}^2$ be a function of U_1 and U_2 defined in Eq. (14.22). Then, Φ_3 and Φ_4, the critical regions of the size α tests that reject H_0: $\boldsymbol{\tau}^* = \mathbf{0}$ for large values of W and W^*, respectively, are given by

$$\Phi_3 : \quad \frac{\gamma_1 e^{-W/\gamma_1} - \gamma_2 e^{-W/\gamma_2}}{2\gamma_1 - 1} \leq \alpha,$$

$$\Phi_4 : \quad \sum_{i=1}^{3} \frac{\delta_i e^{-W^*/\delta_i}}{\prod_{j=1; j\neq i}^{3}(\delta_j - \delta_i)} \leq \alpha. \tag{14.30}$$

Note that the test based on the critical region Φ_4 combines the tests based on F_1, F_2, and R. Another way of combining these three tests was suggested by Cohen and Sackrowitz (1989). Their test is obtained by modifying Φ_3 and is given in the following theorem.

Theorem 14.2. Consider the critical region Φ_5 given by

$$\Phi_5 : \quad \frac{\gamma_1 e^{-W/\gamma_1} - \gamma_2 e^{-W/\gamma_2}}{2\gamma_1 - 1} \leq \alpha(1 + R), \tag{14.31}$$

where R is given in Eq. (14.22) and α satisfies $0 < \alpha < 1/2$. Then Φ_5 is the critical region of a size α test for testing H_0: $\boldsymbol{\tau}^* = \mathbf{0}$ in model (14.20).

14.2.2 Combined tests when $b = v$

In a BIBD with $b = v$, that is, a symmetrical BIBD, the interblock error sum of squares s_2^2 in Eq. (14.15) is nonexistent and, consequently, the interblock F ratio F_2 in Eq. (14.16) is not available. The canonical form (14.20) now reduces to

$$\boldsymbol{x}_1 \sim N\left(\boldsymbol{\tau}^*, \frac{k}{\lambda v}\sigma_e^2 \boldsymbol{I}_{v-1}\right), \quad \boldsymbol{x}_2 \sim N\left(\boldsymbol{\tau}^*, \frac{k}{(r-\lambda)}(k\sigma_\beta^2 + \sigma_e^2)\boldsymbol{I}_{v-1}\right),$$

$$s_1^2 \sim \sigma_e^2 \chi_{vk-2v+1}^2, \tag{14.32}$$

where the above quantities are as defined in model (14.20) and we have used $b = v$ in order to express the degrees of freedom associated with s_1^2. For testing H_0: $\boldsymbol{\tau}^* = \mathbf{0}$ in model (14.32), we shall now derive and compare several tests. This is similar to what was done in Section 14.2.1. In this context, an interesting observation is that even though F_2 is nonexistent and an estimator of $k\sigma_\beta^2 + \sigma_e^2$ is not available, $\boldsymbol{x}_2$ can still be used to test H_0 through the quantity R given in Eq. (14.22). The choice of the following three critical regions should be obvious from our discussion in Section 14.2.1:

$$\Psi_1 : \quad 2Z_1 \geq \chi_{\alpha,2}^2,$$

$$\Psi_2 : \quad 2(Z_1 + Z_3) \geq \chi_{\alpha,4}^2,$$

$$\Psi_3 : \quad e^{-Z_1} \leq \alpha(1 + R),$$

where Z_1 and Z_3 are as given in Eq. (14.24). We should point out that Ψ_3 is also derived in Zhang (1992). There is another additional test Ψ_4 which is not discussed here.

Simulated powers of the four tests $\Psi_1 - \Psi_4$ described above appear in Khuri, Mathew, and Sinha (1998) and are given in Table 14.1 for a symmetrical BIBD with $b = v = 16$ and $k = 6$. The simulations were carried out using $\alpha = 0.05$ and $\sigma_e^2 = 1$. The numerical results in Table 14.1 indicate that we should prefer the test Ψ_3 in this testing problem.

Table 14.1   Simulated powers (based on 100,000 simulations) of the tests $\Psi_1 - \Psi_4$ for testing the equality of the treatment effects in a symmetrical BIBD with $v = b = 16$ and $k = 6$ ($\alpha = 0.05$ and $\sigma_e^2 = 1$)

$\sigma_e^2 + k\sigma_\beta^2$	$\tau^{*\prime}\tau^*$	Ψ_1	Ψ_2	Ψ_3	Ψ_4
1	0.0	0.0509	0.0502	0.0509	0.0496
	0.1	0.0623	0.0613	0.0628	0.0609
	0.4	0.0997	0.1008	0.1030	0.1001
	1.0	0.1984	0.2070	0.2123	0.2030
	4.0	0.7717	0.8073	0.8043	0.7723
2	0.0	0.0509	0.0502	0.0509	0.0496
	0.1	0.0623	0.0602	0.0625	0.0596
	0.4	0.0997	0.0953	0.1019	0.0927
	1.0	0.1984	0.1891	0.2081	0.1783
	4.0	0.7717	0.7617	0.7949	0.6799
4	0.0	0.0509	0.0502	0.0509	0.0497
	0.1	0.0623	0.0595	0.0623	0.0587
	0.4	0.0997	0.0914	0.1011	0.0879
	1.0	0.1984	0.1772	0.2050	0.1621
	4.0	0.7717	0.7269	0.7869	0.6031

14.2.3   A numerical example

We shall now apply the results in Section 14.2.1 to a numerical example taken from Lentner and Bishop (1986, pp. 428–429). The example deals with comparing the effects of six diets on the weight gains of domestic rabbits using litters as blocks. The litter effects are assumed to be random. The data given in Table 14.2 are the weight gains (in ounces) for rabbits from 10 litters. In the table, the six treatments, that is, the six diets, are denoted by t_i ($i = 1, 2, \ldots, 6$) and the weight gains are given within parentheses. Note that the design is a BIBD with $b = 10$, $v = 6$, $r = 5$, $k = 3$, and $\lambda = 2$.

Table 14.2 Weight gains (in ounces) of domestic rabbits from 10 litters based on six diets t_i, $i = 1, 2, \ldots, 6$

Litters	Treatments and observations		
1	t_6 (42.2)	t_2 (32.6)	t_3 (35.2)
2	t_3 (40.9)	t_1 (40.1)	t_2 (38.1)
3	t_3 (34.6)	t_6 (34.3)	t_4 (37.5)
4	t_1 (44.9)	t_5 (40.8)	t_3 (43.9)
5	t_5 (32.0)	t_3 (40.9)	t_4 (37.3)
6	t_2 (37.3)	t_6 (42.8)	t_5 (40.5)
7	t_4 (37.9)	t_1 (45.2)	t_2 (40.6)
8	t_1 (44.0)	t_5 (38.5)	t_6 (51.9)
9	t_4 (27.5)	t_2 (30.6)	t_5 (20.6)
10	t_6 (41.7)	t_4 (42.3)	t_1 (37.3)

We have applied the test Φ_5 in this example; see Eq. (14.31). Direct computations using the expressions in Section 14.2.1 give

$$F_1 = 3.14, \qquad F_2 = 0.3172,$$
$$P_1 = 0.04, \qquad P_2 = 0.70,$$
$$Z_1 = 3.2189, \qquad Z_2 = 0.3425,$$

$$U_1 = 309.46, \quad U_2 = 2796.90, \quad R = 0.25,$$

$$\hat{\theta}^2_{(1)} = \min\left\{\frac{U_1}{U_2}, 1\right\} = 0.1106,$$

$$\gamma_1 = \frac{1}{1 + \hat{\theta}^2_{(1)}} = 0.90, \quad \gamma_2 = 1 - \gamma_1 = 0.10,$$

and

$$W = \gamma_1 Z_1 + \gamma_2 Z_2 = 2.93.$$

From Eq. (14.31), the rejection region Φ_5 simplifies to

$$\Phi_5 : 0.0433 \leq \alpha \times 1.25,$$

which holds for $\alpha = 0.05$. Thus, for $\alpha = 0.05$, the test based on Φ_5 rejects the null hypothesis of equality of the six treatment effects. We therefore conclude that there are significant differences among the six diets.

CHAPTER 15

COMBINATION OF POLLS

The basic motivation of this chapter, which is taken from Dasgupta and Sinha (2006), essentially arises from an attempt to understand various poll results conducted by several competing agencies and to meaningfully combine such results. As an example, consider the 1996 U.S. presidential election poll results, which are reproduced in Table 15.1 and were reported in leading newspapers back then, regarding several presidential candidates.

Table 15.1   Gallup poll results, August 18–20, 1996

Poll	President Clinton	Robert Dole	Others
ABC-*Washington Post*	44	40	16
Newsweek	44	42	14
CNN-Gallup	48	41	11
CBS-*New York Times*	50	39	11

Statistical Meta-Analysis with Applications. By Joachim Hartung, Guido Knapp, Bimal K. Sinha   **191**
Copyright © 2008 John Wiley & Sons, Inc.

It is clear that depending on which poll one looks at, the conclusion in terms of margin of variation can be different, sometimes widely. Similar phenomena exist in various other contexts, such as results of a series of studies comparing different brands of cereals, TV ratings, ratings of athletes by different judges, and so on. In studies of this type, one is bound to observe different levels of margin of variation between two suitably selected leading candidates, and one often wonders how much variation between polls would be considered as normal, that is, can be attributed to chance! Clearly, such a question would not arise had there been only one study, and in such a situation one could apply standard statistical techniques to estimate the margin of difference as well as test relevant hypotheses about the margin of difference. In the presence of several independent studies all with a common goal, what is needed is a data fusion or data synthesis technique, which can be used to meaningfully combine results of all the studies in order to come up with efficient inference regarding parameters of interest. It is the purpose of this chapter to describe appropriate statistical methods to deal with the above problems.

A general mathematical formulation of the problem involving k candidates and m polls (judges) is given in Section 15.1. This section also provides a solution to the problem posed earlier, namely, how much variation between two selected candidates can be expected as normal.

The major issue of combining polls is addressed in Section 15.2. Section 15.2.1 is devoted to estimation of the difference θ between the true proportions P_1 and P_2 of two selected candidates. Section 15.2.2 deals with providing a confidence interval for θ, and lastly Section 15.2.3 is concerned with a test for the significance of θ. Throughout, whenever applicable, we have discussed relevant asymptotics with applications.

We have also discussed the special case of two candidates (i.e., $k = 2$) and noted that often this leads to amazingly simple results.

15.1   FORMULATION OF THE PROBLEM

Assume that m independent polls are conducted to study the effectiveness of k candidates, and the results presented in Table 15.2 are obtained.

Table 15.2   General set-up

Study	Subject 1	Subject 2	$\cdots$	Subject k	Total
1	X_{11}	X_{12}	$\cdots$	X_{1k}	n_1
2	X_{21}	X_{22}	$\cdots$	X_{2k}	n_2
$\vdots$	$\vdots$	$\vdots$	$\ddots$	$\vdots$	$\vdots$
m	X_{m1}	X_{m2}	$\cdots$	X_{mk}	n_m
Total	$X_{.1}$	$X_{.2}$	$\cdots$	$X_{.k}$	N

Denoting by X_{ij} the number of votes received by the jth candidate (subject) in the ith poll (study), so that $\sum_{j=1}^{k} X_{ij} = n_i$, $i = 1, \ldots, m$, it follows readily that $X_{i1}, \ldots, X_{ik}$ follows a multinomial distribution with the parameters n_i and $P_{i1}, \ldots, P_{ik}$ with $\sum_{j=1}^{k} P_{ij} = 1$ for all i. The underlying probability structure is thus essentially m independent multinomials each with k classes and possibly unequal sample sizes $n_1, \ldots, n_m$. Here P_{ij} denotes the chance that a response in the ith study belongs to the jth subject. Clearly, an unbiased estimate of P_{ij} is provided by $p_{ij} = X_{ij}/n_i$, $i = 1, \ldots, m$, $j = 1, \ldots, k$. Moreover, it is well known that

$$
\begin{aligned}
\mathrm{E}(p_{ij}) &= P_{ij}, \\
\mathrm{Var}(p_{ij}) &= \frac{P_{ij}(1 - P_{ij})}{n_i}, \\
\mathrm{Cov}(p_{ij}, p_{ij'}) &= -\frac{P_{ij} P_{ij'}}{n_i}, j \neq j'.
\end{aligned}
\tag{15.1}
$$

Although there are k candidates, quite often we are interested in only two of them, namely, the two leading candidates, such as a sitting candidate and a close runner-up. Assuming without any loss of generality that we are interested in candidates 1 and 2, poll i reports an unbiased estimate of the difference between P_{i1} and P_{i2} as $p_{i1} - p_{i2} = Y_i$, say, for $i = 1, \ldots, m$. Obviously, $Y_1, \ldots, Y_m$ are independent but not identically distributed random variables. A measure of variation among the polls can then be taken as $Z_m = Y_{(m)} - Y_{(1)}$, where $Y_{(m)} = \max(Y_1, \ldots, Y_m)$ and $Y_{(1)} = \min(Y_1, \ldots, Y_m)$.

We now address the question of how much variation one should expect as normal. Obviously, any such measure would require us to compute at least the mean and the variance of Z_m. An exact computation of these quantities seems to be extremely complicated, and we therefore take recourse to asymptotics, which is quite reasonable since the sample sizes of the m polls are typically large in practical applications. We also assume that $P_{1j} = \cdots P_{mj} = P_j$, $j = 1, \ldots, k$, the unknown true values in the entire population. This is justified because the voters usually have a definite opinion about the candidates no matter who is conducting the gallup poll, thus making meta-analysis viable and useful. Using Eq. (15.1), we then get

$$
\mathrm{E}(Y_i) = P_1 - P_2, \quad \mathrm{Var}(Y_i) = \frac{P_1 + P_2 - (P_1 - P_2)^2}{n_i}.
\tag{15.2}
$$

Hence, under the assumption of a large sample size, we get

$$
\sqrt{n_i}\,[Y_i - (P_1 - P_2)] \sim N\left[0, P_1 + P_2 - (P_1 - P_2)^2\right].
$$

Let us write $\theta = P_1 - P_2$ and $\sigma_i^2 = \left[P_1 + P_2 - (P_1 - P_2)^2\right]/n_i$. In view of independence and uniform integrability of the Y_i's, for m fixed, we readily get

$$
\mathrm{E}(Y_{(m)}) \approx \mathrm{E}(W_m), \quad \mathrm{E}(Y_{(1)}) \approx \mathrm{E}(W_1),
$$

where W_m is a random variable with the cdf

$$
F_m(w) = \prod_{i=1}^{m} \Phi\left(\frac{w - \theta}{\sigma_i}\right)
$$

and W_1 is a random variable having the cdf

$$F_1(w) = 1 - \prod_{i=1}^{m} \bar{\Phi}\left(\frac{w - \theta}{\sigma_i}\right),$$

where $\Phi(\cdot)$ is the standard normal cdf and $\bar{\Phi}(\cdot) = 1 - \Phi(\cdot)$. Moreover,

$$
\begin{aligned}
\mathrm{Var}(Y_{(m)}) &\approx \mathrm{Var}(W_m), \\
\mathrm{Var}(Y_{(1)}) &\approx \mathrm{Var}(W_1), \\
\mathrm{Cov}(Y_{(m)}, Y_{(1)}) &\approx \mathrm{Cov}(W_m, W_1).
\end{aligned}
$$

By arguing probabilistically, the above expectations, namely, $\mathrm{E}(W_m)$ and $\mathrm{E}(W_1)$, can be computed without much difficulty for m up to 4 and are given below.

$$
\begin{aligned}
\mathrm{E}(W_m | m = 2) =\ & P_1 - P_2 \\
& + \left[\left(\frac{1}{2\pi}\right)\{P_1 + P_2 - (P_1 - P_2)^2\}\left(\frac{1}{n_1} + \frac{1}{n_2}\right)\right]^{1/2}, \\
\mathrm{E}(W_1 | m = 2) =\ & P_1 - P_2 \\
& - \left[\left(\frac{1}{2\pi}\right)\{P_1 + P_2 - (P_1 - P_2)^2\}\left(\frac{1}{n_1} + \frac{1}{n_2}\right)\right]^{1/2}, \\
\mathrm{E}(W_m | m = 3) =\ & P_1 - P_2 + \left[\left(\frac{1}{8\pi}\right)\{P_1 + P_2 - (P_1 - P_2)^2\}\right]^{1/2} \\
& \times \left(\left[\frac{1}{n_1} + \frac{1}{n_2}\right]^{1/2} + \left[\frac{1}{n_1} + \frac{1}{n_3}\right]^{1/2} + \left[\frac{1}{n_2} + \frac{1}{n_3}\right]^{1/2}\right), \\
\mathrm{E}(W_1 | m = 3) =\ & P_1 - P_2 - \left[\left(\frac{1}{8\pi}\right)\{P_1 + P_2 - (P_1 - P_2)^2\}\right]^{1/2} \\
& \times \left(\left[\frac{1}{n_1} + \frac{1}{n_2}\right]^{1/2} + \left[\frac{1}{n_1} + \frac{1}{n_3}\right]^{1/2} + \left[\frac{1}{n_2} + \frac{1}{n_3}\right]^{1/2}\right), \\
\mathrm{E}(W_m | m = 4) =\ & P_1 - P_2 + \left[\left(\frac{1}{2\pi}\right)\{P_1 + P_2 - (P_1 - P_2)^2\}\right]^{1/2} \\
& \times \sum_{i}\sum_{j\neq i}\sum_{k<l_{k,l\neq j,i}} \sqrt{\frac{n_j}{n_i(n_i + n_j)}} \\
& \times \left\{\frac{1}{4} + \frac{1}{2\pi}\sin^{-1}\sqrt{\frac{n_k n_l}{(n_i + n_k)(n_i + n_l)}}\right\},
\end{aligned}
$$

$$E(W_1|m=4) = P_1 - P_2 - \left[\left(\frac{1}{2\pi}\right)\{P_1 + P_2 - (P_1 - P_2)^2\}\right]^{1/2}$$

$$\times \sum_i \sum_{j\neq i} \sum_{k<l}{}_{k,l\neq j,i} \sqrt{\frac{n_j}{n_i(n_i+n_j)}}$$

$$\times \left\{\frac{1}{4} + \frac{1}{2\pi}\sin^{-1}\sqrt{\frac{n_k n_l}{(n_i+n_k)(n_i+n_l)}}\right\}.$$

Returning to the original problem, for large sample sizes, we then get the following:

$$E[Y_{(m)} - Y_{(1)}|m=2] \approx \left[\left(\frac{2}{\pi}\right)\{P_1 + P_2 - (P_1 - P_2)^2\}\left(\frac{1}{n_1}+\frac{1}{n_2}\right)\right]^{1/2},$$

$$E[Y_{(m)} - Y_{(1)}|m=3] \approx \left[\left(\frac{1}{2\pi}\right)\{P_1 + P_2 - (P_1 - P_2)^2\}\right]^{1/2}$$

$$\times \left(\left[\frac{1}{n_1}+\frac{1}{n_2}\right]^{1/2} + \left[\frac{1}{n_1}+\frac{1}{n_3}\right]^{1/2} + \left[\frac{1}{n_2}+\frac{1}{n_3}\right]^{1/2}\right),$$

$$E[Y_{(m)} - Y_{(1)}|m=4] \approx \left[\frac{2}{\pi}\{P_1 + P_2 - (P_1 - P_2)^2\}\right]^{1/2}$$

$$\times \sum_i \sum_{j\neq i} \sum_{k<l}{}_{k,l\neq j,i} \sqrt{\frac{n_j}{n_i(n_i+n_j)}} \qquad (15.3)$$

$$\times \left\{\frac{1}{4} + \frac{1}{2\pi}\sin^{-1}\sqrt{\frac{n_k n_l}{(n_i+n_k)(n_i+n_l)}}\right\}.$$

Table 15.3 provides the values of $E[Y_{(m)} - Y_{(1)}]$ for $m = 2, 3, 4$ and for various values of P_1 and P_2 when n_i's are equal.

Table 15.3   Values of $E[Y_{(m)} - Y_{(1)}]$

m	n	$P_1 = 0.40,$ $P_2 = 0.35$	$P_1 = 0.50,$ $P_2 = 0.40$	$P_1 = 0.60,$ $P_2 = 0.30$
2	$n_1 = n_2 = 500$	0.04514	0.04754	0.04399
	$n_1 = n_2 = 600$	0.04120	0.04340	0.04016
	$n_1 = n_2 = 700$	0.03815	0.04018	0.03718
3	$n_1 = n_2 = n_3 = 500$	0.06770	0.07131	0.06599
	$n_1 = n_2 = n_3 = 600$	0.06180	0.06510	0.06024
	$n_1 = n_2 = n_3 = 700$	0.05722	0.06027	0.05577
4	$n_1 = n_2 = n_3 = n_4 = 500$	0.09027	0.09508	0.08798
	$n_1 = n_2 = n_3 = n_4 = 600$	0.08241	0.08679	0.08032
	$n_1 = n_2 = n_3 = n_4 = 700$	0.07629	0.08036	0.07436

Example 15.1. Returning to the data in Table 15.1, we find that $m = 4$, $n_1 = n_2 = n_3 = n_4 = 100$, $Y_1 = 4\%$, $Y_2 = 2\%$, $Y_3 = 7\%$, and $Y_4 = 11\%$ so that $Y_{(4)} = 11\%$ and $Y_{(1)} = 2\%$, giving $Y_{(4)} - Y_{(1)} = 9\%$. To check if this amount of variation between polls is normal, we note from Eq. (15.3) that $E[Y_{(4)} - Y_{(1)}] \approx 0.2133$ when $P_1 + P_2 = 0.9$, $P_1 - P_2 = 0.08$. Thus we can conclude that, under this scenario, what we have observed can be treated as below normal. Again, if $P_1 + P_2 = 0.9$ and $P_1 - P_2 = 0.4$, then $E[Y_{(4)} - Y_{(1)}] \approx 0.1941$, which again suggests that the observed difference can be regarded as below normal. On the other hand, if $P_1 = 0.95$ and $P_2 = 0.05$, then $E[Y_{(4)} - Y_{(1)}] \approx 0.098$, implying that the observed difference can be taken as normal.

Assume $k = 2$ so that $P_1 + P_2 = 1$. In this case, it is interesting to observe that $E(Y_{(m)} - Y_{(1)})$ is a maximum when $P_1 = P_2$, and the above formulas simplify to the following:

$$E[Y_{(m)} - Y_{(1)}|m = 2] = \left[\left(\frac{2}{\pi}\right)\left(\frac{1}{n_1} + \frac{1}{n_2}\right)\right]^{1/2},$$

$$E[Y_{(m)} - Y_{(1)}|m = 3] = \left[\left(\frac{1}{2\pi}\right)\right]^{1/2}\left(\left[\frac{1}{n_1} + \frac{1}{n_2}\right]^{1/2} + \left[\frac{1}{n_1} + \frac{1}{n_3}\right]^{1/2}\right.$$
$$\left. + \left[\frac{1}{n_2} + \frac{1}{n_3}\right]^{1/2}\right),$$

$$E[Y_{(m)} - Y_{(1)}|m = 4] = \left[\frac{2}{\pi}\right]^{1/2}\sum_i\sum_{j\neq i}\sum_{k<l_{k,l\neq j,i}}\sqrt{\frac{n_j}{n_i(n_i + n_j)}}$$
$$\times \left\{\frac{1}{4} + \frac{1}{2\pi}\sin^{-1}\sqrt{\frac{n_k n_l}{(n_i + n_k)(n_i + n_l)}}\right\}.$$

15.2   META-ANALYSIS OF POLLS

We now describe various meta-analysis procedures to estimate θ, provide a confidence interval for θ, and test hypotheses about θ.

15.2.1   Estimation of θ

In this section we discuss the important issue of how to combine the results of independent polls to arrive at some meaningful conclusions. To fix ideas, referring to Table 15.2, we address the problem of combining independent estimates $p_{i1} - p_{i2}$ of $\theta = P_1 - P_2$ based on a sample of size n_i for $i = 1, \ldots, m$. As already noted, we have assumed that the differences $P_{i1} - P_{i2}$ are the same for all i, and the parameter θ stands for the common population difference. Basically, there are two standard ways of combining the $(p_{i1} - p_{i2})$'s to arrive at a pooled estimate of θ. The first, popularly known as the commentators's estimate, is given by

$$\hat{\theta}_C = \sum_{i=1}^{m} \frac{p_{i1} - p_{i2}}{m}, \tag{15.4}$$

while the second, which is essentially the uniformly minimum variance unbiased estimate (UMVUE) and also the maximum likelihood estimate (MLE) based on all the data, is given by

$$\hat{\theta}_{MLE} = \frac{\sum_{i=1}^{m} n_i(p_{i1} - p_{i2})}{\sum_{i=1}^{m} n_i}. \tag{15.5}$$

It may be noted that the two estimates $\hat{\theta}_C$ and $\hat{\theta}_{MLE}$ coincide when the sample sizes are all equal. Also, the computation of $\hat{\theta}_C$ does not directly require knowledge of the sample sizes and so can be readily used (by the commentators!). Using Eq. (15.2) and independence of the m studies, we get

$$\mathrm{E}(\dot{\theta}_C) = \theta, \quad \mathrm{Var}(\dot{\theta}_C) = \frac{(P_1 + P_2 - \theta^2)(\sum_{i=1}^{m} 1/n_i)}{m^2} \tag{15.6}$$

and

$$\mathrm{E}(\hat{\theta}_{MLE}) = \theta, \quad \mathrm{Var}(\hat{\theta}_{MLE}) = \frac{P_1 + P_2 - \theta^2}{\sum_{i=1}^{m} n_i}. \tag{15.7}$$

It is therefore easy to verify that the efficiency (E) of $\hat{\theta}_C$ with respect to $\hat{\theta}_{MLE}$, as measured by the ratio of their variances, is given by

$$E = \frac{m^2}{(\sum_{i=1}^{m} n_i)(\sum_{i=1}^{m} 1/n_i)}, \tag{15.8}$$

which is always less than 1 by the well-known arithmetic mean–harmonic mean (AM-HM) inequality. Hence the MLE $\hat{\theta}_{MLE}$ is always preferred to $\hat{\theta}_C$.

For large m, by the strong law of large numbers (SLLN), one can approximate E by $E \approx 1/[E(n)E(1/n)]$. Thus, assuming that n_i is uniform over $[a, b]$, we readily get $E = [2(b-a)]/[(a+b)(\ln b - \ln a)]$. In particular, choosing $[a, b] = [675, 1200]$, we get $E \approx 0.97$, which is very high. Table 15.4 provides values of E for $m = 2, 3, 4$ and various values of n_i.

Table 15.4 Values of E

m	n	E
2	$n_1 = 500, n_2 = 600$	0.9917
3	$n_1 = 400, n_2 = 500, n_3 = 600$	0.9730
4	$n_1 = 300, n_2 = 400, n_3 = 500, n_4 = 600$	0.9357

15.2.2 Confidence interval for θ

A more challenging and informative answer to provide in this context is a confidence interval for θ. This can be done on the basis of one of the following two point estimates of θ:

$$\bar{d} = \hat{\theta}_C = \sum_{i=1}^{m} \frac{p_{i1} - p_{i2}}{m} \tag{15.9}$$

and

$$\hat{d} = \hat{\theta}_{\text{MLE}} = \frac{\sum_{i=1}^{m} n_i(p_{i1} - p_{i2})}{\sum_{i=1}^{m} n_i}. \tag{15.10}$$

The exact distributions of the above two estimates again are quite difficult, and asymptotics seem to be the only recourse. One can think of two kinds of asymptotics in this context: (i) m fixed and each n_i tends to ∞ and (ii) each n_i is taken as fixed while m tends to ∞. It turns out, however, that under either type of asymptotic, the same result holds, and we get [see Eqs. (15.6) and (15.7)],

$$\frac{m(\bar{d} - \theta)}{\sqrt{\sum_{i=1}^{m} 1/n_i}} \sim N\left[0, P_1 + P_2 - (P_1 - P_2)^2\right] \tag{15.11}$$

and

$$(\hat{d} - \theta)\sqrt{\sum_{i=1}^{m} n_i} \sim N\left[0, P_1 + P_2 - (P_1 - P_2)^2\right]. \tag{15.12}$$

It should be noted that the use of $\bar{d}$ for inference purposes for θ requires that we know the sample sizes n_i's (just as for the use of $\hat{d}$) although computation of $\bar{d}$ does not require any direct knowledge of the sample sizes. From Eqs. (15.11) and (15.12), we find that $P_1 + P_2$ appears as a nuisance parameter for drawing inference about $P_1 - P_2$ unless $k = 2$, in which case $P_1 + P_2 = 1$. For $k = 2$, a two-sided confidence interval for θ based on $\hat{d}$ is easily obtained from the probability statement:

$$1 - \alpha = \Pr\left(|\hat{d} - \theta| < z_{\alpha/2}\sqrt{\frac{1 - \theta^2}{\sum_{i=1}^{m} n_i}}\right), \tag{15.13}$$

where $1 - \alpha$ is the level of confidence and $z_{\alpha/2}$ is the upper $\alpha/2$ cut-off point from a standard normal distribution. A straightforward computation yields the confidence bounds of θ as

$$\text{LB} = \frac{N\hat{d} - z_{\alpha/2}\left[N + z_{\alpha/2}^2 - N\hat{d}^2\right]^{1/2}}{N + z_{\alpha/2}^2},$$

$$\text{UB} = \frac{N\hat{d} + z_{\alpha/2}\left[N + z_{\alpha/2}^2 - N\hat{d}^2\right]^{1/2}}{N + z_{\alpha/2}^2},$$

where $N = \sum_{i=1}^{m} n_i$. Analogously, for $k = 2$, a two-sided confidence interval for θ based on $\bar{d}$ is obtained from the probability statement:

$$1 - \alpha = \Pr\left(m|\bar{d} - \theta| < z_{\alpha/2} \sqrt{(1 - \theta^2) \sum_{i=1}^{m} \frac{1}{n_i}} \right). \qquad (15.14)$$

This yields the confidence bounds of θ as

$$\text{LB} = \frac{\bar{d}\, m^2 N^* - z_{\alpha/2} \left[z_{\alpha/2}^2 + m^2 N^* - m^2 N^* (\bar{d})^2 \right]^{1/2}}{m^2 N^* + z_{\alpha/2}^2},$$

$$\text{UB} = \frac{\bar{d}\, m^2 N^* + z_{\alpha/2} \left[z_{\alpha/2}^2 + m^2 N^* - m^2 N^* (\bar{d})^2 \right]^{1/2}}{m^2 N^* + z_{\alpha/2}^2},$$

where $N^* = 1/[\sum_{i=1}^{m} 1/n_i]$.

Example 15.2. For the polling data in Table 15.1, we compute

$$\hat{d} = \frac{186 - 162}{400} = 0.06.$$

Taking $\alpha = 0.05$ so that $z_{\alpha/2} = 1.96$, we find that

$$\text{LB} = -0.038 \quad \text{and} \quad \text{UB} = 0.157.$$

Hence, a 95% confidence interval for θ based on $\hat{d}$ is given by $-0.038 < \theta < 0.157$. Of course, in this data set, $\hat{d} = \bar{d}$, so that the two methods provide identical confidence intervals. Finally, since this interval contains 0, we accept the null hypothesis $H_0 : \theta = 0$.

For $k > 2$, since $P_1 + P_2 < 1$, we get the same inequality as above, given in Eqs. (15.13) and (15.14), with confidence level $\geq 1 - \alpha$. Of course, any known upper bound η of $P_1 + P_2$ can also be used. Alternatively, instead of replacing $P_1 + P_2$ by an upper bound, we can estimate it based on the data by $p_1 + p_2$, where

$$p_1 = \frac{\sum_{i=1}^{m} n_i\, p_{i1}}{\sum_{i=1}^{m} n_i}, \quad p_2 = \frac{\sum_{i=1}^{m} n_i\, p_{i2}}{\sum_{i=1}^{m} n_i}.$$

Then, in large samples, by Slutsky's theorem (see Rao, 1973)

$$\frac{m[(\bar{d} - \theta)]}{[(\sum_{i=1}^{m} 1/n_i)(p_1 + p_2 - \theta^2)]^{1/2}} \sim N(0, 1)$$

and

$$\frac{(\hat{d} - \theta)\sqrt{\sum_{i=1}^{m} n_i}}{(p_1 + p_2 - \theta^2)^{1/2}} \sim N(0, 1).$$

The above two results can be readily used to provide an approximate $100(1-\alpha)\%$ confidence interval for θ. These are given below:

$$\text{LB} \quad = \quad \frac{N\hat{d} - z_{\alpha/2}\left[(p_1 + p_2)(N + z_{\alpha/2}^2) - N\hat{d}^2\right]^{1/2}}{N + z_{\alpha/2}^2},$$

$$\text{UB} \quad = \quad \frac{N\hat{d} + z_{\alpha/2}\left[(p_1 + p_2)(N + z_{\alpha/2}^2) - N\hat{d}^2\right]^{1/2}}{N + z_{\alpha/2}^2}$$

and

$$\text{LB} \quad = \quad \frac{\bar{d}\, m^2 N^* - z_{\alpha/2}\left[(p_1 + p_2)(z_{\alpha/2}^2 + m^2 N^*) - m^2 N^* (\bar{d})^2\right]^{1/2}}{m^2 N^* + z_{\alpha/2}^2},$$

$$\tag{15.15}$$

$$\text{UB} \quad = \quad \frac{\bar{d}\, m^2 N^* + z_{\alpha/2}\left[(p_1 + p_2)(z_{\alpha/2}^2 + m^2 N^*) - m^2 N^* (\bar{d})^2\right]^{1/2}}{m^2 N^* + z_{\alpha/2}^2}.$$

Obviously, one can also use the variance-stabilizing transformation in the above two cases.

Example 15.3. For the data in Table 15.1, we compute $p_1 = 186/400 = 0.465$ and $p_2 = 162/400 = 0.405$, and hence, using interval (15.15), we readily obtain the 95% confidence interval for θ as $[-0.031, 0.150]$.

15.2.3 Hypothesis testing for θ

We now discuss the problem of hypothesis testing about the difference $\theta = P_1 - P_2$ based on all the data given in Table 15.2. Let us consider the problem of testing

$$H_0 : \theta \leq \delta \quad \text{versus} \quad H_1 : \theta > \delta,$$

where $\delta \geq 0$ is a given constant. Clearly, for $k = 2$, this is a trivial problem of testing hypotheses about a single binomial proportion and is well known. In the following, we deal with the case when $k > 2$.

One can consider two classical tests in this context, namely, an intuitive test which rejects H_0 when $p_1 - p_2$, an estimate of θ, is large, and the likelihood ratio test (LRT), which rejects H_0 when

$$\lambda = \frac{\sup_{\theta \leq \delta} P_1^{X.1} \cdots P_k^{X.k}}{\sup_{\text{unrestricted}} P_1^{X.1} \cdots P_k^{X.k}}$$

is small. As to the choice of $p_1 - p_2$, we can choose either $\bar{d}$ or $\hat{d}$, described in Eqs. (15.9) and (15.10), respectively. In any event, the intuitive test can be carried out using standard asymptotic theory and by suitably standardizing $p_1 - p_2$ so that the test rejects H_0 when $p_1 - p_2 > c$, where c satisfies

$$
\begin{aligned}
\alpha &= \sup_{\theta \leq \delta} \Pr \left(\frac{N^{**}\{(p_1 - p_2) - \theta\}}{\sqrt{P_1 + P_2 - \theta^2}} > \frac{N^{**}(c - \theta)}{\sqrt{P_1 + P_2 - \theta^2}} \right) \\
&= \sup_{\theta \leq \delta} \Pr \left(N(0,1) > \frac{N^{**}(c - \theta)}{\sqrt{P_1 + P_2 - \theta^2}} \right),
\end{aligned}
$$

where N^{**} is a suitable normalizing constant. In the above, α is the level of the test. It can be shown that the supremum of the above probability occurs when $P_1 = (1+\delta)/2$, $P_2 = (1 - \delta)/2$, so that the above equation reduces to

$$
\alpha = \Pr \left(N(0,1) > \frac{N^{**}(c - \delta)}{\sqrt{1 - \delta^2}} \right).
$$

Hence, c is readily obtained as

$$
c = \delta + \frac{z_\alpha \left(1 - \delta^2\right)^{1/2}}{N^{**}}. \tag{15.16}
$$

It may be noted from Eqs. (15.11) and (15.12) that when $\bar{d}$ is used in place of $p_1 - p_2$, we take $N^{**} = m[N^*]^{1/2}$, while if $\hat{d}$ is used in place of $p_1 - p_2$, we take $N^{**} = N^{1/2}$. Recall that $N = \sum_{i=1}^m n_i$ and $N^* = 1/[\sum_{i=1}^m 1/n_i]$.

Example 15.4. For the data in Table 15.1, to test

$$
H_0 : P_1 - P_2 \leq 0 \quad \text{versus} \quad H_1 : P_1 - P_2 > 0
$$

at level 0.05, note from Eq. (15.16) that $c = 1.64/N^{**}$. Using $\hat{d} = 0.06$ and $N = 400$, we get $N^{**} = 20$ so that $c = 0.082$. We therefore accept the null hypothesis H_0.

The LRT, on the other hand, is in general highly nontrivial because of the computations involved in the numerator of λ, and we do not pursue it here.

CHAPTER 16

VOTE COUNTING PROCEDURES

We now describe the method of vote counting procedures which is used when we have scanty or incomplete information from the studies to be combined for statistical meta-analysis. This chapter, which contains standard materials on this topic, is mostly based on Hedges and Olkin (1985) and Cooper and Hedges (1994). Some new results are also added at the end. The nature of data from primary research sources which are available to a meta-analyst generally falls into three broad categories: (i) complete information (e.g., raw data, summary statistics) that can be used to calculate relevant effect size estimates such as means, proportions, correlations, and test statistic values; (ii) results of hypothesis tests for population effect sizes about statistically significant or nonsignificant relations; and (iii) information about the direction of relevant outcomes (i.e., conclusions of significant tests) without their actual values (i.e., without the actual values of the test statistics).

Vote counting procedures are useful for the second and third types of data, that is, when complete information about the results of primary studies are not available in the sense that effect size estimates cannot be calculated. In such situations often the information from a primary source is in the form of a report of the decision obtained from a significance test (i.e., significant positive relation or nonsignificant positive relation) or in the form of a direction (positive or negative) of the effect without regard

Statistical Meta-Analysis with Applications. By Joachim Hartung, Guido Knapp, Bimal K. Sinha
Copyright © 2008 John Wiley & Sons, Inc.

to its statistical significance. In other words, all is known is whether a test statistic exceeds a certain critical value at a given significance level (such as $\alpha^* = 0.05$) or if an estimated effect size is positive or negative, which amounts to the observation that the test statistic exceeds the special critical value at significance level $\alpha^* = 0.5$. Actual values of the test statistics are not available.

To fix ideas, recall that often a meta-analyst is interested in determining whether a relation exists between an independent variable and a dependent variable for each study, that is, whether the effect size is zero for each study. Let $T_1, \ldots, T_k$ be independent estimates from k studies of the corresponding population effect sizes $\theta_1, \ldots, \theta_k$ (i.e., difference of two means, difference/ratio of two proportions, difference of two correlations, or z-values). Under the assumption that the population effect sizes are equal, that is, $\theta_1 = \cdots = \theta_k = \theta$, the appropriate null and alternative hypotheses are $H_0 : \theta = 0$ (no relation) against $H_1 : \theta > 0$ (relation exists). The test rejects H_0 if an estimate T of the common effect size θ, when standardized, exceeds the one-sided critical value ψ_α. Typically, in large samples, one invokes the large-sample approximation of the distribution of T, resulting in the normal distribution of T, and we can then use $\psi_\alpha = z_\alpha$, the cut-off point from a standard normal distribution. On the other hand, if a $100(1 - \alpha)\%$ level confidence interval for θ is desired, it is usually provided by

$$T - \psi_{\alpha/2}\,\hat\sigma(T) \leq \theta \leq T + \psi_{\alpha/2}\,\hat\sigma(T),$$

where $\hat\sigma(T)$ is the (estimated, if necessary) standard error of T. Quite generally, the standard error $\sigma(\theta)$ of T will be a function of θ and can be estimated by $\hat\sigma(T)$, and a normal approximation can be used in large samples. We refer to Chapter 4 for details.

When the individual estimates $T_1, \ldots, T_k$ as well as their (estimated) standard errors $\hat\sigma(T_1), \ldots, \hat\sigma(T_k)$ are available, the solutions to these testing and confidence interval problems are trivial (as discussed in previous lectures). However, the essential feature of a vote counting procedure is that the values of $T_1, \ldots, T_k$ are not observed, and hence none of the estimated standard errors of the T_i's are available. What is known to us is not the exact values of the T_i's, but just the number of them which are positive or how many of them exceed the one-sided critical value ψ_{α^*}. The question then arises if we can test $H_0 : \theta = 0$ or estimate the common effect size θ based on just this very incomplete information.

The sign test, which is the oldest of all nonparametric tests, can be used to test the hypothesis that the effect sizes from a collection of k independent studies are all zero when only the signs of estimated effect sizes from the primary sources are known. If the population effect sizes are all zero, the probability of getting a positive result for the estimated effect size is 0.5. If, on the other hand, the treatment has an effect, the probability of getting a positive result for the estimated effect size is greater than 0.5. Hence, the appropriate null and alternative hypotheses can be described as

$$H_0 : \pi = 0.5 \quad \text{versus} \quad H_1 : \pi > 0.5, \tag{16.1}$$

where π is the probability of a positive effect size in the population. The test can be carried out in the usual fashion based on a binomial distribution and rejects H_0 if X/k exceeds the desired level of significance, where X is the number of studies out of a total of k studies with positive estimated effect sizes.

Example 16.1. Suppose that a meta-analyst finds exactly 10 positive results in 15 independent studies. The estimate of π is $p = 10/15 = 0.67$, and the corresponding tail area from the binomial table is 0.1509. Thus, we would fail to reject H_0 at the 0.05 overall significance level or even at the 0.10 overall significance level. On the other hand, if exactly 12 of the 15 studies had positive results, the tail area would become 0.0176, and we would reject H_0 at the 0.05 overall level of significance.

The main criticism against the sign test is that it does not take into account the sample sizes of the different studies, which are likely to be unequal, and also it does not provide an estimate of the underlying common effect size θ or provide a confidence interval for the common effect size. Under the simplifying assumption that each study in a collection of k independent studies has an identical sample size n, we now describe a procedure to establish a point estimate as well as a confidence interval for the common effect size θ based on a knowledge of the number of positive results. If a study involves an experimental (E) as well as a control (C) group, we assume that the sample sizes for each such group are the same, that is, $n_i^E = n_i^C = n$ for all k studies. In case k studies have different sample sizes, we may use an average value, namely,

$$\bar{n} = \left[\frac{\sqrt{n_1} + \cdots + \sqrt{n_k}}{k} \right]^2. \tag{16.2}$$

Based on a knowledge of the signs of T_i's, an unbiased estimate of π is given by $p = X/k$, where X is the number of positive T_i's. It is also well known that a $100(1 - \alpha)\%$ level approximate confidence interval for π (based on the normal approximation) is given by

$$[\pi_L, \pi_U] = \left[p - z_{\alpha/2} \sqrt{\frac{p(1 - p)}{k}}, p + z_{\alpha/2} \sqrt{\frac{p(1 - p)}{k}} \right], \tag{16.3}$$

where $z_{\alpha/2}$ is the two-sided critical value of the standard normal distribution. A second method uses the fact that

$$z^2 = \frac{k(p - \pi)^2}{\pi(1 - \pi)}$$

has an approximate chi-square distribution with 1 df, which leads to the two-sided interval

$$[\pi_L, \pi_U] = \left[\frac{(2p + b) - \sqrt{b^2 + 4bp(1 - p)}}{2(1 + b)}, \frac{(2p + b) + \sqrt{b^2 + 4bp(1 - p)}}{2(1 + b)} \right], \tag{16.4}$$

where $b = \chi_{1,\alpha}^2/k$ and $\chi_{1,\alpha}^2$ is the upper $100\alpha\%$ point of the chi-square distribution with 1 df.

Once a two-sided confidence interval $[\pi_L, \pi_U]$ has been obtained for π, a two-sided confidence interval for θ can be constructed by using the relation

$$
\begin{aligned}
\pi &= \Pr[T > \psi_\alpha] \\
&= \Pr\left[\frac{T - \theta}{S_\theta} > \frac{\psi_\alpha - \theta}{S_\theta}\right] \\
&\approx 1 - \Phi\left(\frac{\psi_\alpha - \theta}{S_\theta}\right)
\end{aligned}
$$

where $\Phi(\cdot)$ is the standard normal cdf. Solving the above equation yields

$$
\theta = \psi_\alpha - S(\theta)\Phi^{-1}(1 - \pi), \tag{16.5}
$$

which provides a relation between the effect size θ and the population proportion π of a positive effect size. A point estimate of θ is then obtained by replacing π by $p = X/k$ in the above equation and solving for θ. To obtain a two-sided confidence interval for θ, we substitute π_L and π_U for π and solve for the two bounds for θ.

Example 16.2. Let us consider the case when an effect size is measured by the standardized mean difference given by

$$
\theta_i = \frac{\mu_i^E - \mu_i^C}{\sigma_i}, \quad i = 1, \ldots, k,
$$

where μ_i^E is the population mean for the experimental group in the ith study, μ_i^C is the population mean for the control group in the ith study, and σ_i is the population standard deviation in the ith study, which is assumed to be the same for the experimental and the control groups. The corresponding estimates T_i's are given by (Hedges's g)

$$
T_i = \frac{\bar{Y}_i^E - \bar{Y}_i^C}{S_i}, \quad i = 1, \ldots, k, \tag{16.6}
$$

where $\bar{Y}_i^E$ is the sample mean for the experimental group in the ith study, $\bar{Y}_i^C$ is the sample mean for the control group in the ith study, and S_i is the pooled within-group sample standard deviation in the ith study. In large samples, the approximate variance $S_i(\theta_i)$ of T_i is given by

$$
\sigma^2(T_i) = S_i(\theta_i) \approx \frac{2}{n} + \frac{\theta_i^2}{4n},
$$

where n denotes the common sample size for all the studies. Equation (16.5) in this case then reduces to

$$
\theta = \psi_\alpha - \left[\frac{2}{n} + \frac{\theta^2}{4n}\right]\Phi^{-1}(1 - \pi). \tag{16.7}
$$

Let us consider a real data example from Raudenbush and Bryk (1985). The data are given in Table 16.1.

Table 16.1 Studies of the effects of teacher expectancy on pupil IQ

Study	n^E	n^C	$\bar{n}$	d
1	77	339	208.0	0.03
2	60	198	129.0	0.12
3	72	72	72.0	−0.14
4	11	22	16.5	1.18
5	11	22	16.5	0.26
6	129	348	238.5	−0.06
7	110	636	373.0	−0.02
8	26	99	62.5	−0.32
9	75	74	74.5	0.27
10	32	32	32.0	0.80
11	22	22	22.0	0.54
12	43	38	40.5	0.18
13	24	24	24.0	−0.02
14	19	32	25.5	0.23
15	80	79	79.5	−0.18
16	72	72	72.0	−0.06
17	65	255	160.0	0.30
18	233	224	228.5	0.07
19	65	67	66.0	−0.07

n^E = experimental group sample size, n^C = control group sample size,
$\bar{n} = (n^E + n^C)/2$ = mean group sample size.

For this data set, n is approximated as 84, using the mean group sample sizes $\bar{n}$ in Eq. (16.2), and the estimate of π based on the proportion of positive results is $p = 11/19 = 0.579$. Solving for θ, using $\psi_\alpha = 0$, we obtain $\hat{\theta} = 0.032$, which is the proposed point estimate of the population effect size. To obtain a 95% confidence interval for θ, we note that the confidence interval for π based on the Eq. (16.3) is $[0.357, 0.801]$ and that based on Eq. (16.4) is $[0.363, 0.769]$, which is slightly narrower. Using these latter values in Eq. (16.7), we find that the 95% confidence interval for θ is given by $[-0.056, 0.121]$. Since this confidence interval contains the value 0, we conclude that we can accept the null hypothesis that the population effect size is 0 for all the studies.

For the same data set, we can also obtain a point estimate and a confidence interval for θ based on the proportion of significant positive results. Since 3 of the 19 studies result in statistically significant values at $\alpha = 0.05$, with the corresponding value of $\psi_\alpha = 1.64$, our estimate of π is $p = 3/19 = 0.158$, and this results in the point estimate of θ as $\hat{\theta} = 0.013$. Again, the confidence interval for π based on the normal theory is obtained as $[-0.006, 0.322]$ and based on the chi-square distribution is given by $[0.055, 0.376]$. Using the latter bounds and Eq. (16.7), we obtain the 95%

confidence bounds for θ as $[0.032, 0.212]$. Since this interval does not contain 0, we can conclude that the common effect size θ is significantly greater than 0.

Example 16.3. We next consider the situation when both the variables X and Y are continuous, and a measure of effect size is provided by the correlation coefficient ρ. Typically, the population correlation coefficients $\rho_1, \ldots, \rho_k$ of the k studies are estimated by the sample correlation coefficients $r_1, \ldots, r_k$, which represent the θ_i's and the T_i's, respectively.

It is well known that, in large samples, $\mathrm{Var}(r_i) \approx (1 - \rho_i^2)^2/(n - 1)$, where n is the sample size. We thus have all the ingredients to apply formula (16.5) to any specific problem.

As an example, we consider the data set from Cohen (1983) on validity studies correlating student ratings of the instruction with student achievement. The relevant data are given in Table 16.2.

Table 16.2   Validity studies correlating student ratings of the instructor with student achievement

Study	n	r	Study	n	r
1	10	0.68	11	36	−0.11
2	20	0.56	12	75	0.27
3	13	0.23	13	33	0.26
4	22	0.64	14	121	0.40
5	28	0.49	15	37	0.49
6	12	−0.04	16	14	0.51
7	12	0.49	17	40	0.40
8	36	0.33	18	16	0.34
9	19	0.58	19	14	0.42
10	12	0.18	20	20	0.16

Suppose we wish to obtain a point estimate and a confidence interval for ρ, the assumed common population correlation, based on the proportion of positive results. Obviously, here $p = 18/20 = 0.9$, and, using Eq. (16.2), $\bar{n} = 26$. Taking $\psi_\alpha = 0$, we then get $\hat{\rho} = 0.264$ as the point estimate of ρ. The 95% approximate two-sided confidence interval for ρ based on the normal theory is given by $[0.769, 1.031]$ while that based on the chi-square theory is obtained as $[0.699, 0.972]$. Using the latter, the confidence bounds for ρ turn out as $[0.107, 0.381]$. Because this interval does not contain the value 0, we can conclude that there is a positive correlation between student ratings of the instructor and student achievement.

For the same data set, we can proceed to obtain point estimates and confidence bounds for ρ based on only significantly positive results. Taking $\alpha = 0.05$, so that $\psi_\alpha = 1.64$, and noting that $p = 12/20 = 0.6$, we obtain the point estimate of ρ as $\hat{\rho} = 0.372$. Similarly, using the chi-square-based confidence interval for π, namely, $[0.387, 0.781]$, the bounds for ρ are obtained as $[0.271, 0.464]$, leading to the same conclusion.

We now present a new and exact result pertaining to the estimation of the effect size θ when the sample sizes are unequal and these are not replaced by an average sample size! As before, we assume that the effect sizes $T_1, T_2, \ldots, T_k$ are not observed, and instead we observe $Z_1, Z_2, \ldots, Z_k$, where

$$
Z_i = \left\{ \begin{array}{ll} 1, & T_i > 0, \\ 0, & T_i \leq 0. \end{array} \right.
$$

Our goal then is to draw inference upon θ using the data $Z_1, Z_2, \ldots, Z_k$. Let $\sigma_i^2(\theta, n_i)$ denote the variance of T_i. Note that even though $T_1, T_2, \ldots, T_k$ are not observed, we typically know how they were computed (i.e., for each i we know whether T_i is a sample correlation, Cohen's d, Hedges's g, Glass's Δ, etc.) and so we at least have an approximate expression for $\sigma_i^2(\theta, n_i)$ for each i. Note that $\sigma_i^2(\theta, n_i)$ depends on θ and on n_i. Now $Z_1, Z_2, \ldots, Z_k$ are independent random variables such that $Z_i \sim \text{Bernoulli}(\pi_i)$, where

$$
\begin{aligned}
\pi_i &= \Pr[T_i > 0] \\
&= \Pr\left[\frac{T_i - \theta}{\sigma_i(\theta, n_i)} > \frac{-\theta}{\sigma_i(\theta, n_i)} \right] \\
&= 1 - \Pr\left[\frac{T_i - \theta}{\sigma_i(\theta, n_i)} \leq \frac{-\theta}{\sigma_i(\theta, n_i)} \right] \\
&\approx 1 - \Phi\left(\frac{-\theta}{\sigma_i(\theta, n_i)} \right)
\end{aligned}
$$

and where $\Phi(\cdot)$ denotes the standard normal cumulative distribution function. Hence

$$
\pi_i \approx 1 - \Phi\left(\frac{-\theta}{\sigma_i(\theta, n_i)} \right). \tag{16.8}
$$

When the n_i's are assumed to be equal (or approximated by an average sample size), π's coincide and result in the simplified likelihood. By looking at Eq. (16.8) we easily note how π_i depends on the sample size n_i through the standard deviation $\sigma_i(\theta, n_i)$. Thus if the n_i's are unequal, then the π_i's will also be unequal. Now let $z_1, z_2, \ldots, z_k$ denote the observed values of the random variables $Z_1, Z_2, \ldots, Z_k$. Then the likelihood function for θ can be written as follows:

$$
\begin{aligned}
&\prod_{i=1}^{k} \pi_i^{z_i} \left(1 - \pi_i\right)^{(1-z_i)} \\
&\approx \prod_{i=1}^{k} \left[1 - \Phi\left(\frac{-\theta}{\sigma_i(\theta, n_i)} \right) \right]^{z_i} \left[1 - \left\{ 1 - \Phi\left(\frac{-\theta}{\sigma_i(\theta, n_i)} \right) \right\} \right]^{(1-z_i)} \\
&= \prod_{i=1}^{k} \left[1 - \Phi\left(\frac{-\theta}{\sigma_i(\theta, n_i)} \right) \right]^{z_i} \left[\Phi\left(\frac{-\theta}{\sigma_i(\theta, n_i)} \right) \right]^{(1-z_i)}.
\end{aligned}
$$

Using the approximate likelihood $L(\theta)$ defined as

$$L(\theta) = \prod_{i=1}^{k} \left[1 - \Phi\left(\frac{-\theta}{\sigma_i(\theta, n_i)}\right)\right]^{z_i} \left[\Phi\left(\frac{-\theta}{\sigma_i(\theta, n_i)}\right)\right]^{(1-z_i)}, \qquad (16.9)$$

we can then obtain the maximum likelihood estimate of θ.

Example 16.4. To illustrate this procedure we revisit the data in Example 16.3 and displayed in Table 16.2. Let us pretend that $r_1, r_2, \ldots, r_k$ are not observed; instead we observe $Z_1, Z_2, \ldots, Z_k$, where

$$Z_i = \begin{cases} 1, & r_i > 0, \\ 0, & r_i \leq 0. \end{cases}$$

We then use the likelihood function defined in Eq. (16.9) to draw inference upon ρ based on $Z_1, Z_2, \ldots, Z_k$. Using the expression for $L(\theta)$ given in Eq. (16.9) the likelihood function for ρ can be written as

$$L(\rho) = \prod_{i=1}^{k} \left[1 - \Phi\left(\frac{-\rho}{\sigma_i(\rho, n_i)}\right)\right]^{z_i} \left[\Phi\left(\frac{-\rho}{\sigma_i(\rho, n_i)}\right)\right]^{(1-z_i)}, \qquad (16.10)$$

where

$$\sigma_i^2(\rho, n_i) \approx \frac{(1 - \rho^2)^2}{n_i - 1}. \qquad (16.11)$$

Using a numeric optimization routine we find that for this example $L(\rho)$ is maximized when $\rho = 0.2064$, which is the maximum likelihood estimate of ρ. It is interesting to note that this estimate of ρ differs considerably from the earlier value 0.264.

An alternative way to perform the analysis in this example is instead of taking $\theta = \rho$ we take $\theta = \rho^* = \frac{1}{2} \ln \{(1 + \rho)/(1 - \rho)\}$. Then we let $T_i = r_i^* = \frac{1}{2} \ln \{(1 + r_i)/(1 - r_i)\}$. Note that $\frac{1}{2} \ln \{(1 + r_i)/(1 - r_i)\}$ is the well-known variance-stabilizing transformation of r_i. Since $r_i^* > 0 \Leftrightarrow r_i > 0$, we observe that

$$Z_i = \begin{cases} 1, & r_i^* > 0 \\ 0, & r_i^* \leq 0 \end{cases} = \begin{cases} 1, & r_i > 0 \\ 0, & r_i \leq 0 \end{cases}.$$

Following the general expression (16.9), we can then write down the following likelihood function for ρ^*:

$$L(\rho^*) = \prod_{i=1}^{k} \left[1 - \Phi\left(\frac{-\rho^*}{\sigma_i^*(\rho^*, n_i)}\right)\right]^{z_i} \left[\Phi\left(\frac{-\rho^*}{\sigma_i^*(\rho^*, n_i)}\right)\right]^{(1-z_i)},$$

where

$$\sigma_i^*(\rho^*, n_i) \approx \sqrt{\frac{1}{n_i - 3}}$$

and where $z_1, z_2, \ldots, z_k$ denote the observed values of $Z_1, Z_2, \ldots, Z_k$. Using a numeric optimization routine we find that for this example $L(\rho^*)$ is maximized when $\rho^* =$

0.2718, implying $\hat{\rho} = 0.2653$. It is rather interesting to observe the stern dissimilarity between the two estimates of ρ (namely, 0.2064 and 0.2653), obtained by using two approaches based on r and r^*, and the rather strange similarity between the two values (0.264 and 0.265), obtained by using the exact likelihood based on r^* and the approximate likelihood based on r and an average sample size! One wonders if this remarkable difference vanishes when the sample sizes are large, and here is our finding. Keeping the observed values of Z_i's the same, and just changing the sample sizes of the available studies, we have considered three scenarios and in each case applied the exact method based on r and r^*.

Case (i): $n_1 = 55, n_2 = 60, n_3 = 65, \ldots, n_{20} = 150$. Here we find that

$$\hat{\rho}_{\text{MLE}}(r) = 0.1158 \quad \text{and} \quad \hat{\rho}_{\text{MLE}}(r^*) = 0.1315.$$

Case (ii): $n_1 = 505, n_2 = 510, n_3 = 515, \ldots, n_{20} = 600$. Here we find that

$$\hat{\rho}_{\text{MLE}}(r) = 0.0520 \quad \text{and} \quad \hat{\rho}_{\text{MLE}}(r^*) = 0.0549.$$

Case (iii): $n_1 = 1005, n_2 = 1010, n_3 = 1015, \ldots, n_{20} = 1100$. In this case of extreme large sample sizes, we find that

$$\hat{\rho}_{\text{MLE}}(r) = 0.0381 \quad \text{and} \quad \hat{\rho}_{\text{MLE}}(r^*) = 0.0397.$$

Looking at the results above it appears that for large sample sizes the methods of analysis based on r and r^* give nearly the same results.

We conclude this chapter with the observation that although the procedures described above provide quick estimates of an overall effect size along with its estimated standard error, their uses are quite limited due to the requirement of large sample sizes. For details, we refer to Hedges and Olkin (1985).

CHAPTER 17

COMPUTATIONAL ASPECTS

In this chapter, we consider various computational aspects of the meta-analytical methods discussed in this book. First, we describe some methods of extracting summary statistics from a set of publications relevant for a meta-analysis study. Then, we indicate how to conduct meta-analysis using existing statistical softwares. Fortunately, several commercial and freely available meta-analysis softwares are now available. An overview of these available softwares is given by Sterne, Egger, and Sutton (2001). Here, we only consider the general and commonly used statistical softwares SAS and R and indicate how these softwares can be used in applying the methods described in various previous chapters.

17.1 EXTRACTING SUMMARY STATISTICS

Usually, the different publications do not deliver the same precise information on the results of trials. The ideal situation would be if each publication reports the estimate of the effect size, say $\hat{\theta}$, and its estimated standard error, say $\hat{\sigma}(\hat{\theta})$. Whereas one can expect that $\hat{\theta}$ will in general be reported, the information on the precision of this estimate is often given indirectly.

Statistical Meta-Analysis with Applications. By Joachim Hartung, Guido Knapp, Bimal K. Sinha   **213**
Copyright © 2008 John Wiley & Sons, Inc.

Consider the situation in which $\hat{\theta}$ and a $100(1 - \alpha)\%$ confidence interval, say $[\hat{\theta}_L; \hat{\theta}_U]$, are reported. Assuming that the confidence interval is based on (approximate) normality, that is,

$$[\hat{\theta}_L; \hat{\theta}_U] = [\hat{\theta} \pm \hat{\sigma}(\hat{\theta}) \, z_{\alpha/2}], \tag{17.1}$$

we can extract the information on the estimated standard error by

$$\hat{\sigma}(\hat{\theta}) = \frac{\hat{\theta}_U - \hat{\theta}_L}{2 \, z_{\alpha/2}}. \tag{17.2}$$

In case only the estimate of the effect size in combination with a one-sided P-value is reported, we can proceed as follows. Assuming that the calculation of the P-value is based on the (approximate) normal test statistic $\hat{\theta}/\hat{\sigma}(\hat{\theta})$ and large values of the test statistic are in favor of the alternative, that is,

$$P = \Pr\left(N(0,1) > \frac{\hat{\theta}}{\hat{\sigma}(\hat{\theta})} \mid H_0\right), \tag{17.3}$$

then we can extract the standard error as

$$\hat{\sigma}(\hat{\theta}) = \frac{\hat{\theta}}{z_{1-P}}. \tag{17.4}$$

Given a two-sided P-value and the effect size estimate $\hat{\theta}$, the standard error can be computed as

$$\hat{\sigma}(\hat{\theta}) = \frac{|\hat{\theta}|}{z_{1-P/2}} \tag{17.5}$$

since in this case

$$P = 2 \Pr\left(N(0,1) > \frac{|\hat{\theta}|}{\hat{\sigma}(\hat{\theta})} \mid H_0\right). \tag{17.6}$$

17.2   COMBINING TESTS

In Chapter 3, we presented various methods of combining tests via a combination of P-values. Given the P-values of the component tests, the methods can be easily programmed using functions for the cdf and quantiles of beta, chi-square, normal, and t distributions. Table 17.1 contains a summary of the syntax of the necessary functions in both software packages.

As an example of the use of R code, let us consider the five P-values from Examples 3.1 to 3.5, that is, 0.015, 0.077, 0.025, 0.045, 0.079. We calculate the combined test statistics and combined P-values of Tippett's, Stouffer's (inverse normal), and Fisher's methods in the following. In contrast to the examples in Chapter 3, we do not calculate the critical values but provide the P-values of the combined tests. Given

Table 17.1   Probability and quantile functions in R and SAS

Distribution	R function	SAS function
Beta	pbeta(x, a, b)	cdf('beta', x, a, b)
	qbeta(prob, a, b)	quantile('beta', x, a, b)
χ^2	pchisq(x, df)	cdf('chisquare', x, df)
	qchisq(prob, df)	quantile('chisquare', prob, df)
Normal	pnorm(x, mean, sd)	cdf('normal', x, mean, sd)
	qnorm(prob, mean, sd)	quantile('normal', prob, mean, sd)
t	pt(x,df)	cdf('t', x)
	qt(prob,df)	quantile('t', prob)

a significance level of $\alpha = 0.05$, Tippett's test fails to reject H_0, whereas the other two combined tests reject H_0.

R code for combined test statistics:

```
> # Data
> pvalues  <- c(0.015, 0.077, 0.025, 0.045, 0.079)
> # Number of trials
> k        <- length(pvalues)
> # Test statistics
> (tippett  <- min(pvalues))
[1] 0.015
> (stouffer <- sum(qnorm(pvalues)) / sqrt(k))
[1] -3.874134
> (fisher   <- sum(-2 * log(pvalues)))
[1] 32.18387
> # Alternative calculation of Fisher's method
> (fisher.2  <- sum(qchisq(1 - pvalues, 2)))
[1] 32.18387
> # P-values of the three tests}
> (pv.tippett  <- pbeta(tippett, 1, k))
[1] 0.0727835
> (pv.stouffer <- pnorm(stouffer))
[1] 5.350234e-05
> (pv.fisher  <- 1 - pchisq(fisher, 2*k))
[1] 0.0003731391
```

17.3   GENERALIZED *P*-VALUES

In Chapters 5 to 7 we used the notion of generalized *P*-values for exact inference in some nonstandard testing problems. The determination of a generalized *P*-value can often easily be done using Monte Carlo simulation. As an example the R code presented below shows how the generalized P-value can be computed in the homogeneity testing problem in Example 6.4.

```
# Below we input the data
k <- 4
y1 <- c(21.4, 13.5, 21.1, 13.3, 18.9, 19.2, 18.3)
y2 <- c(27.3, 22.3, 16.9, 11.3, 26.3, 19.8, 16.2, 25.4)
y3 <- c(18.7, 19.1, 16.4, 15.9, 18.7, 20.1, 17.8)
y4 <- c(19.9, 19.3, 18.7, 20.3, 22.8, 20.8, 20.9, 23.6, 21.2)
# Computing the means
y1_bar <- mean(y1)
y2_bar <- mean(y2)
y3_bar <- mean(y3)
y4_bar <- mean(y4)
# Computing the variances
s1 <- var(y1)
s2 <- var(y2)
s3 <- var(y3)
s4 <- var(y4)
# Defining the sample sizes
n1 <- length(y1)
n2 <- length(y2)
n3 <- length(y3)
n4 <- length(y4)
# Below we run the simulation which computes an approximate value
# of the generalized P-value.
set.seed(20080129)
numSims <- 1000000
U  <- rchisq(n=numSims, df=(k-1))
V1 <- rchisq(n=numSims, df=(n1-1))
V2 <- rchisq(n=numSims, df=(n2-1))
V3 <- rchisq(n=numSims, df=(n3-1))
V4 <- rchisq(n=numSims, df=(n4-1))
b1 <- ( n1 / ((n1-1)*s1)) * V1
b2 <- ( n2 / ((n2-1)*s2)) * V2
b3 <- ( n3 / ((n3-1)*s3)) * V3
b4 <- ( n4 / ((n4-1)*s4)) * V4
c1 <- b1*y1_bar + b2*y2_bar + b3*y3_bar + b4*y4_bar
c2 <- b1 + b2 + b3 + b4
term1 <- b1*(y1_bar - c1/c2)^2
term2 <- b2*(y2_bar - c1/c2)^2
term3 <- b3*(y3_bar - c1/c2)^2
term4 <- b4*(y4_bar - c1/c2)^2
( GPValue <- mean(U > (term1 + term2 + term3 + term4)) )
[1] 0.021089
```

17.4 COMBINING EFFECT SIZES

The general results for combining effect sizes described in Chapters 4 and 7 can be obtained by statistical software using weighted least-squares regression. Often, the general method described in Chapter 4 (fixed effects model) or in Chapter 7 (random effects model) is referred to as the generic inverse variance method.

Recall that the overall effect size is estimated by

$$\hat{\theta} = \frac{\sum_{i=1}^{k} \hat{w}_i \, \hat{\theta}_i}{\sum_{i=1}^{k} \hat{w}_i} \tag{17.7}$$

given k studies with $\hat{\theta}_i$ the study-specific effect size estimate and $\hat{w}_i$ appropriate nonnegative weights. In the fixed effects model, the weight $\hat{w}_i = 1/\hat{\sigma}^2(\hat{\theta}_i)$ is the inverse of the within-study variance, and in the random effects model, the weight $\hat{w}_i = 1/[\hat{\sigma}_a^2 + \hat{\sigma}^2(\hat{\theta}_i)]$ is the inverse of the sum of between-study and within-study variance. The standard $100(1 - \alpha)\%$ confidence interval for the overall effect size is then computed as

$$\hat{\theta} \pm (\sum_{i=1}^{k} \hat{w}_i)^{-1/2} \, z_{1-\alpha/2}. \tag{17.8}$$

Whitehead (2002) shows the use of SAS PROC GLM for fitting a weighted least-squares regression. For k trials, the observed responses are the study estimates, say $\hat{\theta}_i$, $i = 1, \ldots, k$, and there are no explanatory variables, only a constant term. The weights are the inverse of the estimated variances, say $w_i = 1/\hat{\sigma}^2(\hat{\theta}_i)$. The estimated intercept of this weighted least-squares regression is the estimate of the common effect size. However, as Whitehead (2002) noted, the standard error and the test statistics displayed for the intercept parameter are incorrect for the required model, because the model assumption is $\sigma^2(\hat{\theta}) = \sigma^2/w_i$, where σ^2 is to be estimated from the data, instead of being equal to 1. This will also be the case for other statistical packages.

Van Houwelingen, Arends, and Stijnen (2002) show the use of SAS PROC MIXED for fitting a weighted least-squares regression. Moreover, they show how to use SAS PROC MIXED for the meta-analysis in the random effects model, that is, how to implement the standard method from Section 7.3. However, in the random effects model, SAS PROC MIXED computes (restricted) maximum likelihood estimates of the between-trial variance. Other estimates of the between-trial variance, like the DerSimonian-Laird estimate, are not available. Van Houwelingen, Arends, and Stijnen (2002) also discuss advanced methods in meta-analysis like multivariate meta-analysis and meta-regression and the implementation of these methods in SAS PROC MIXED. A SAS example program is given below.

There are two R packages available in which several meta-analysis methods have been implemented. The packages rmeta and meta provide methods for simple fixed and random effects meta-analysis for two-sample comparisons and cumulative meta-analyses and compute summaries and tests for association and heterogeneity. In both packages, functions are implemented for conducting a random effects model meta-analysis with the DerSimonian-Laird estimate as the choice of estimate of between-study variance. More or less, the functions of both packages are identical. Additionally, in rmeta, combining binary data via the Mantel-Haenszel method is possible, whereas meta provides tests for funnel plot asymmetry or, equivalently, for publication bias. Both packages provide standard graphics for meta-analysis described below and an R example program is given below as well.

17.4.1   Graphics

A graphical representation of the results of a meta-analysis is the confidence interval plot, sometimes also referred as a forest plot. The confidence interval plot displays a study-specific estimate and corresponding $100(1 - \alpha)\%$ confidence interval for each study as well as the meta-analytical estimate of the common effect size and corresponding $100(1 - \alpha)\%$ confidence interval. The two above-mentioned R packages provide functions for drawing confidence interval plots. Also funnel plots (see Chapter 13) for detecting or assessing publication bias can be drawn in both packages.

17.4.2   Sample program in R

Let us demonstrate the use of some functions of the R package meta in this section. We analyze a data set with continuous outcome using the functions *metagen* and *metacont*. The function *metagen* can be generally applied to all types of data when estimates of the effect size and corresponding estimated standard errors are given.

As an example we consider the dentifrice data set from Section 18.3. Part of the R code for the data set is given below:

```
> # Data
> # NaF
> n.naf    <-  c( 134,  175, ...,  679)
> mean.naf <-  c(5.96, 4.74, ..., 3.88)
> std.naf  <-  c(4.24, 4.64, ..., 4.85)
> # SMFP
> n.smfp    <-  c( 113,  151, ...,  673)
> mean.smfp <-  c(6.82, 5.07, ..., 4.37)
> std.smfp  <-  c(4.72, 5.38, ..., 5.37)
```

The parameter of interest here is the difference between normal means. In the programming code below, we first compute the treatment differences NaF − SMFP with corresponding estimated standard errors:

```
> # Calculation of effect size estimates and standard errors
> meandiff  <-  mean.naf - mean.smfp
> std.error <-  sqrt(std.naf**2 / n.naf + std.smfp**2 / n.smfp)
```

Using the R package meta and the function *metagen* we obtain the following output:

```
> # Loading package meta
> library(meta)
> # Generic function for meta-analysis
> # requires effect size estimates and standard errors
> dentifrice <- metagen(meandiff, std.error)
> print(dentifrice)
```

```
                      95%-CI %W(fixed) %W(random)
1 -0.86  [-1.9882;  0.2682]      2.58       2.58
2 -0.33  [-1.4295;  0.7695]      2.71       2.71
3 -0.47  [-1.1575;  0.2175]      6.94       6.94
4 -0.50  [-0.9922; -0.0078]     13.53      13.53
5  0.28  [-0.7792;  1.3392]      2.92       2.92
6 -0.04  [-0.5793;  0.4993]     11.27      11.27
7 -0.80  [-2.3340;  0.7340]      1.39       1.39
8 -0.19  [-0.4523;  0.0723]     47.65      47.65
9 -0.49  [-1.0356;  0.0556]     11.01      11.01
```

```
Number of trials combined: 9
                              95%-CI       z  p.value
Fixed effects model  -0.2833 [-0.4644; -0.1023] -3.0671   0.0022
Random effects model -0.2833 [-0.4644; -0.1023] -3.0671   0.0022
```

```
Quantifying heterogeneity:
tau^2 = 0; H = 1 [1; 1.38]; I^2 = 0% [0%; 47.7%]
```

```
Test of heterogeneity:
   Q d.f.  p.value
5.38    8   0.7162
```

```
Method: Inverse variance method
```

First the study-specific estimates together with corresponding 95% confidence interval are reported, indicating here that only in study 4 do we observe a significant result whereas all the other confidence intervals include the value zero. Moreover, the weight each trial contributes to the overall estimate is given for the fixed effects as well as for the random effects model. In this example, the estimate of the between-study variance is zero, called here $\tau^2 = 0$, so that the analyses in the fixed effects and random effects models are identical, hence the weights are identical, too. The overall estimate is given here as -0.2833 with 95% confidence interval $[-0.4644, -0.1023]$. The P value for the test that the overall effect size is zero is 0.0022. So, for any convenient significance level, we reject the null hypothesis that there is no effect. Note that the confidence interval as well as the P-value is calculated using the standard large-sample test from Chapter 4. The test of heterogeneity is the large-sample test of homogeneity described in Chapter 4, also called Cochran's homogeneity test; see also Chapter 6.

Alternatively, we can use the function *metacont* for analyzing the dentifrice data set. Using the programming code below, we obtain the same output. The function *metacont* can handle the parameters difference of means (called weighted mean difference here) and standardized difference of means. Moreover, one can directly use the observed summary statistics; no prior calculation of the effect size and its standard error is required.

```
> # Function for meta-analysis of continuous data
> # option sm = "WMD": weighted mean difference
> # option sm = "SMD": standardized mean difference
> dent.alternate <- metacont(n.naf, mean.naf, std.naf,
                         n.smfp, mean.smfp, std.smfp, sm ="WMD")
> print(dent.alternate)
```

We omit the repeated presentation of the known output.

Finally, let us consider the graphical representation of the meta-analysis using the confidence interval plot. The programming code below forces us to show the result for the fixed effects as well as for the random effects model.

```
> # Confidence interval plot
> plot(dentifrice, comb.f = TRUE, comb.r=TRUE)
```

The confidence interval plot is displayed in Figure 17.1. Presented are the point estimates of the trials with corresponding 95% confidence intervals as well as the meta-analysis results. The size of the shown point estimates is proportional to the precision of the estimates.

17.4.3   Sample program in SAS

Van Houwelingen, Arends, and Stijnen (2002) presented some advanced methods of meta-analysis and also provided a sample SAS program for carrying out fixed effects and random effects meta-analysis as well as meta-regression. Here we report their programs with some comments. The example data set is the vaccination example on the prevention of tuberculosis, which we also already used in our meta-regression chapter; see also Section 18.8. For illustration purposes we consider the log odds ratio as the parameter of interest. Possible covariates that may explain the heterogeneity between the trials are latitude, year of study, and type of allocation. The coding of the type of allocation is as follows: $1 =$ random, $2 =$ alternate, and $3 =$ systematic. First, we consider the SAS data step. From the data, we calculate the log odds ratio with corresponding variance and define the weight variable as the inverse of the variance.

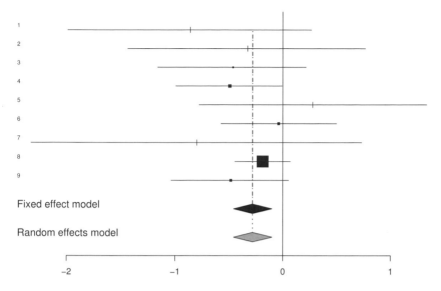

Figure 17.1 Confidence interval plot for dentifrice data

```
DATA bcg;
INPUT trial vd vwd nvd nvwd latitude year allocation;
logor = log(vd/vwd) - log(nvd/nvwd);
est    = 1/vd + 1/vwd + 1/nvd + 1/nvwd;
weight = 1/est;
DATALINES;
 1    4    119    11      128  44  48  1
 2    6    300    29      274  55  49  1
 3    3    228    11      209  42  60  1
 4   62  13536   248    12619  52  77  1
 5   33   5036    47     5761  13  73  2
 6  180   1361   372     1079  44  53  2
 7    8   2537    10      619  19  73  1
 8  505  87886   499    87892  13  80  1
 9   29   7470    45     7232  27  68  1
10   17   1699    65     1600  42  61  3
11  186  50448   141    27197  18  74  3
12    5   2493     3     2338  33  69  3
13   27  16886    29    17825  33  76  3
;
RUN;
```

In the fixed effects analysis, referring to the programming code below, it is important that the variable of the variances is called *est*, since the variances are assumed to be known. The weighted regression analysis model is only an intercept model.

```
PROC MIXED METHOD=ml DATA=bcg;
CLASS trial;                    * trial' classification variable;
MODEL logor = / S CL;           * intercept only model;
REPEATED / GROUP = trial;       * each trial has own variance;
* parmsdata option reads the variable est from data set BCG
  and the within-trial variances are kept constant;
PARMS / PARMSDATA = bcg  EQCONS = 1 to 13; RUN;
```

A part of the output is presented below. The common log odds ratio estimated is -0.4361 with 95% confidence interval $[-0.5282, -0.3441]$.

```
                  Solution for Fixed Effects
                Standard
   Estimate      Error  DF  t Value    Lower      Upper
   -0.4361      0.04227  12   -10.32   -0.5282    -0.3441
```

The confidence interval provided by SAS PROC MIXED as above is based on the t distribution rather than on the standard normal distribution. To mimic the standard normal distribution, we can force SAS PROC MIXED to use a t distribution with a large number of degrees of freedom; this is done in the alternative program below with DDF=1000. Note that the variable intercept has to be a self-made intercept variable equal to 1.

```
* Alternative in PROC MIXED;
* Normality approximation because of DDF =1000;
PROC MIXED METHOD = ml DATA=bcg;
CLASS trial;
MODEL logor = intercept / S CL NOINT DDF = 1000;
REPEATED / GROUP = trial;
PARMS / PARMSDATA = bcg EQCONS = 1 to 13; RUN;
```

The 95% confidence interval for the common log odds ratio is now $[-0.5191, -0.3532]$.

```
                  Solution for Fixed Effects
                Standard
   Estimate      Error  DF   t Value    Lower     Upper
   -0.4361      0.04227  1000   -10.32   -0.5191   -0.3532
```

For the random effects model we have to specify that there is an additional variation between the trials and this is done in the RANDOM statement below. We choose the maximum likelihood method for estimating the between-trial variance; alternatively one can use restricted maximum likelihood.

```
PROC MIXED CL METHOD=ml DATA=bcg;
CLASS trial;
MODEL logor = / S CL;
*  trial is specified as random effect;
RANDOM int / SUBJECT = trial S;
```

```
REPEATED / GROUP = trial;
* defining grid value for between trial variances,
  followed by the 13 within-trial variance which are
  assumed known and must be kept fixed;
PARMS (0.01 to 2.00 by 0.01) (0.35712)
(0.20813)(0.43341)(0.02031)(0.05195)
(0.00991)(0.22701)(0.00401)(0.05698)
(0.07542)(0.01253)(0.53416)(0.07164)
/ EQCONS = 2 to 14; RUN;
```

Part of the output is given below. The estimate of the between-trial variability is 0.3025 with large-sample 95% confidence interval $[0.1350, 1.1810]$, clearly indicating that heterogeneity between the trials is present. The overall estimate of the log odds ratio is -0.7420 with 95% confidence interval $[-1.1297, -0.3542]$, where the confidence interval uses again the critical value from the t distribution with 12 df.

```
            Covariance Parameter Estimates
    Subject  Group   Estimate   Lower      Upper
    trial            0.3025     0.1350     1.1810
```

```
            Solution for Fixed Effects
            Standard
Estimate    Error      DF   t Value   Lower     Upper
-0.7420     0.1780     12   -4.17     -1.1297   -0.3542
```

Finally, we can add explanatory variables into the model, for example, the covariate latitude in the example below:

```
PROC MIXED CL METHOD=ml DATA=bcg;
CLASS trial;
* Latitude is explanatory variable;
MODEL logor = latitude / S CL;
RANDOM int / SUBJECT = trial S;
REPEATED / GROUP = trial;
PARMS (0.01 to 2.00 by 0.01) (0.35712)
(0.20813)(0.43341)(0.02031)(0.05195)
(0.00991)(0.22701)(0.00401)(0.05698)
(0.07542)(0.01253)(0.53416)(0.07164)
/eqcons = 2 to 14;
RUN;
```

Summarizing the essential results, we obtain an estimate of the between-trial variability of 0.00393 showing that the explanatory variable latitude explains a large amount of the heterogeneity. The estimated intercept of the regression line is 0.3711 and the slope parameter is -0.03272, indicating the vaccine is more effective the larger the distance of the study population from the equator.

CHAPTER 18

DATA SETS

In this chapter we have put together the main data sets which have been used throughout the book for illustrating various meta-analysis techniques. The first two data sets are taken from the field of education, the other ones from biometry and epidemiology. The reader should note that, in addition to these main data sets, we have also provided meta-analysis of many other data sets in different chapters.

18.1 VALIDITY STUDIES

Cohen (1983) reviewed studies of the validity of student ratings of instructors. The studies were usually conducted in multisection courses in which the sections had different instructors but all sections used a common final examination. The index of validity was a correlation coefficient (a partial correlation coefficient, controlling for a measure of student ability) between the section mean instructor ratings and the section mean examination score. Thus, the effective sample size was the number of sections. Table 18.1 gives the effect size (product moment correlation coefficient) and a summary of each study with a sample size of 10 or greater.

Statistical Meta-Analysis with Applications. By Joachim Hartung, Guido Knapp, Bimal K. Sinha
Copyright © 2008 John Wiley & Sons, Inc. **225**

Table 18.1   Validity studies correlating student ratings of the instructor with student achievement

Study	Sample	n	r
Bolton et al. (1979)	General psychology	10	0.68
Bryson (1974)	College algebra	20	0.56
Centra (1977)[1]	General biology	13	0.23
Centra (1977)[2]	General psychology	22	0.64
Crooks and Smock (1974)	General physics	28	0.49
Doyle and Crichton (1978)	Introductory communications	12	−0.04
Doyle and Whitely (1974)	Beginning French	12	0.49
Elliot (1950)	General chemistry	36	0.33
Ellis and Richard (1977)	General psychology	19	0.58
Frey, Leonard, and Beatty (1975)	Introductory calculus	12	0.18
Greenwood et al. (1976)	Analytic geometry and calculus	36	−0.11
Hoffman (1978)	Introductory math	75	0.27
McKeachie et al. (1971)	General psychology	33	0.26
Marsh et al. (1956)	Aircraft mechanics	121	0.40
Remmer et al. (1949)	General chemistry	37	0.49
Sullivan and Skanes (1974)[1]	First-year science	14	0.51
Sullivan and Skanes (1974)[2]	Introductory psychology	40	0.40
Sullivan and Skanes (1974)[3]	First-year math	16	0.34
Sullivan and Skanes (1974)[4]	First-year biology	14	0.42
Wherry (1952)	Introductory psychology	20	0.16

Note: See Cohen (1983) for the references cited.

18.2   EFFECTS OF TEACHER EXPECTANCE ON PUPIL IQ

Raudenbush (1984) reviewed randomized experiments of the effects of teacher expectancy on pupil IQ (see also Raudenbush and Bryk, 1985). The experiments usually involve the researcher administering a test to a sample of students. A randomly selected portion of the students (the treatment group) are identified to their teachers as "likely to experience substantial intellectual growth." All students are tested again, and the standardized difference between the mean treatment group and that of the other students is the effect size. The theory underlying the treatment is that the identification of students as showing promise of exceptional growth changes teacher expectations about those students, which may turn affect outcomes such as intelligence (possibly through intermediate variables). Raudenbush (1984) proposed that an important characteristic of studies that was likely to be related to effect size was the amount of contact that teachers had with the students prior to the attempt to change expectations. He reasoned that teachers who had more contact would have already formed more stable expectations of students—expectations that would prove more difficult to change via the experimental treatment. A summary of the studies and their effect sizes is given in Table 18.2. The effect size is the standardized difference between the means of the expectancy group and the control group on an intelligence test. Positive values of the effect size imply a higher mean score for the experimental (high-expectancy) group.

Table 18.2   Studies of the effects of teacher expectancy on pupil IQ

Study	Estimated weeks of teacher-student contact prior to expectancy induction	d	Standard error
Rosenthal et al. (1974)	2	0.03	0.125
Conn et al. (1968)	21	0.12	0.147
Jose and Cody (1971)	19	−0.14	0.167
Pellegrini and Hicks (1972)[1]	0	1.18	0.373
Pellegrini and Hicks (1972)[2]	0	0.26	0.369
Evans and Rosenthal (1968)	3	−0.06	0.103
Fiedler et al. (1971)	17	−0.02	0.103
Claiborn (1969)	24	−0.32	0.220
Kester (1969)	0	0.27	0.164
Maxwell (1970)	1	0.80	0.251
Carter (1970)	0	0.54	0.302
Flowers (1966)	0	0.18	0.223
Keshock (1970)	1	−0.02	0.289
Henrikson (1970)	2	0.23	0.290
Fine (1972)	17	−0.18	0.159
Greiger (1970)	5	−0.06	0.167
Rosenthal and Jacobsen (1968)	1	0.30	0.139
Fleming and Anttonen (1971)	2	0.07	0.094
Ginsburg (1970)	7	−0.07	0.174

Note: See Raudenbush (1984) for the references cites.

18.3 DENTIFRICE DATA

The data set is taken from Abrams and Sanso (1998) and concerns a previously published meta-analysis which was conducted of all randomized controlled trials comparing sodium monofluorophosphate (SMFP) to sodium fluoride (NaF) dentifrices (toothpastes) in the prevention of caries; see Johnson (1993). The outcome in each trial was the change from baseline in the decayed missing (due to caries) filled surface (DMFS) dental index at three years follow-up. Of 12 studies identified as meeting the inclusion criteria, 9 considered a straight comparison of NaF and SMFP. Table 18.3 displays the data from these 9 studies in terms of mean change in DMFS index for each treatment.

Table 18.3 Randomized evidence comparing NaF with SMFP dentrifices in terms of differences from baseline in DMFS dental index

Study	N	NaF Mean	SD	N	SMFP Mean	SD
1	134	5.96	4.24	113	6.82	4.72
2	175	4.74	4.64	151	5.07	5.38
3	137	2.04	2.59	140	2.51	3.22
4	184	2.70	2.32	179	3.20	2.46
5	174	6.09	4.86	169	5.81	5.14
6	754	4.72	5.33	736	4.76	5.29
7	209	10.10	8.10	209	10.90	7.90
8	1151	2.82	3.05	1122	3.01	3.32
9	679	3.88	4.85	673	4.37	5.37

18.4 EFFECTIVENESS OF AMLODIPINE ON WORK CAPACITY

The following data set is taken from Li, Shi, and Roth (1994). A drug called amlodipine has been developed for the treatment of angina. To test its effectiveness, several randomized controlled trials have compared the changes in work capacity for patients who received either the drug or a placebo. The change in work capacity for each patient is the ratio of the exercise time after the patient receives the intervention (drug or placebo) to before the patient receives the intervention. The logarithms of the observed changes are assumed to be normally distributed. Table 18.4 contains the results of eight trials. Reported are sample size, observed sample mean, and observed sample variance for treatment and control group.

Table 18.4 Randomized controlled trials on the effectiveness of amlodipine for the treatment of angina

Protocol	Amlodipine 10 mg (E)			Placebo (C)		
	n_{Ei}	$\bar{x}_{Ei}$	s^2_{Ei}	n_{Ci}	$\bar{x}_{Ci}$	s^2_{Ci}
154	46	0.2316	0.2254	48	−0.0027	0.0007
156	30	0.2811	0.1441	26	0.0270	0.1139
157	75	0.1894	0.1981	72	0.0443	0.4972
162A	12	0.0930	0.1389	12	0.2277	0.0488
163	32	0.1622	0.0961	34	0.0056	0.0955
166	31	0.1837	0.1246	31	0.0943	0.1734
303A	27	0.6612	0.7060	27	−0.0057	0.9891
306	46	0.1366	0.1211	47	−0.0057	0.1291

18.5   EFFECTIVENESS OF CISAPRIDE ON THE TREATMENT OF NONULCER DYSPEPSIA

Nonulcer dyspepsia is characterized by a variety of upper abdominal symptoms in the absence of an organic disease. Due to the high frequency of these symptoms an empirical probative therapy of nonulcer dyspepsia without prior diagnostic procedures has been recommended for the management of these patients. For this empirical therapy either acid blocking substances such as histamine H_2-receptor antagonists or gastroprokinetics such as cisapride or domperidone have been suggested.

A major problem in treatment studies of nonulcer dyspepsia is the relatively high and variable rate of placebo responders. The reason for this variability is unclear, but based on this placebo response rate, it becomes difficult to draw valid conclusions on the treatment recommendations. This highly variable response rate can be overcome if available clinical studies are put together and evaluated with appropriate statistical methods in a meta-analysis. Only those placebo-controlled studies were included which used similar criteria for "treatment success" and which documented their results sufficiently for a possible reanalysis.

The data displayed in Table 18.5 are taken from Hartung and Knapp (2001b) where the references for the original studies are given. Reported here are the number of successes and the number of patients in the treatment group as well as in the control group.

Table 18.5   Placebo-controlled trials on the effect of cisapride in the treatment of nonulcer dyspepsia

	Cisapride		Placebo	
Study	No. of successes	Sample size	No. of successes	Sample size
Creytens (1984)	15	16	9	16
Milo (1984)	12	16	1	16
Francois and De Nutte (1986)	29	34	18	34
Deruyttere et al. (1987)	42	56	31	56
Hannon (1987)	14	22	6	22
Roesch (1987)	44	54	17	55
De Nutte et al. (1989)	14	17	7	15
Hausken and Bestad (1992)	29	58	23	58
Chung (1993)	10	14	3	15
Van Outryve et al. (1993)	17	26	6	27
Al-Quorain. Larbi, and Al-Shedoki (1995)	38	44	12	45
Kellow et al. (1995)	19	29	22	30
Yeoh et al. (1997)	21	38	19	38

Note: See Hartung and Knapp (2001b) for the references cited.

18.6   SECOND-HAND SMOKING

The effect of exposure to environmental tobacco smoke on lung cancer risk is a topic of considerable public health importance. By 1991, there were 19 case-control studies of lung cancer in which information on exposure to environmental tobacco smoke was available in addition to information on active smoking. The strong effect of active cigarette smoking on lung cancer made it impossible to separate the effect of active smoking from other sources of environmental tobacco smoke in smokers, and the question of an effect of environmental tobacco smoke on lung cancer risk had to be addressed using lung cancer cases in nonsmokers. The possibility of confounding due to occupational exposure made it desirable to restrict analysis to women. As shown in Table 18.6 taken from Pettiti (1994), the number of cases of lung cancer in women who never smoked cigarettes was small in each of the 19 case-control studies. Fifteen studies found an estimated relative risk greater than 1; 3 found an estimated relative risk less than 1; 1 study found essentially no increase or decrease in estimated relative risk.

In a meta-analysis of these data by scientists at the U.S. Environmental Protection Agency (EPA 1990), the relative risk of lung cancer in women exposed to environmental tobacco smoke was estimated to be 1.42 with 95% confidence limits of 1.24 and 1.63. This information was the basis for a decision by an advisory committee of the EPA to designate environmental tobacco smoke as a carcinogen.

18.7   EFFECTIVENESS OF MISOPROSTOL IN PREVENTING GASTROINTESTINAL DAMAGE

Thirteen controlled trials were undertaken to investigate whether concurrent treatment with the synthetic prostaglandin misoprostol would prevent or at least reduce the degree of gastrointestinal damage without reducing the anti-inflammatory effect of nonsteroidal anti-inflammatory drugs (NSAIDs). Patients suffering from arthritis are often prescribed NSAIDs. In the trials, different scoring systems were used to assess the extent of gastrointestinal damage. The number of categories ranges from two up to five. The data with the different classification schemes are put together in Table 18.7. For a more detailed description of the trials refer to Whitehead and Jones (1994) Since the number of categories are not identical for all the trials, the definition of the categories may differ from trial to trial. But classification category 1 in Table 18.7 always stands for the best category in each trial, category 2 for the second best, and so on.

18.8   PREVENTION OF TUBERCULOSIS

The data set taken from van Houwelingen, Arends, and Stijnen (2002) consists of randomized controlled trials of a vaccine, Bacillus Calmette-Guérin (BCG), for the prevention of tuberculosis (TB). This vaccine has been in use outside the United States since 1921 for routine vaccination at birth in many countries worldwide, yet debate

Table 18.6 For 19 case-control studies, number of cases of lung cancer in women who did not actively smoke cigarettes and estimated relative risk of lung cancer in relation exposure to environmental tobacco smoke

	Number of cases	Estimated relative risk (95% confidence interval)
Akiba, Kato, and Blot (1986)	94	1.52 (0.88 – 2.63)
Brownson et al. (1987)	19	1.52 (0.39 – 5.99)
Buffler et al. (1984)	41	0.81 (0.34 – 1.90)
Chan et al. (1979)	84	0.75 (0.43 – 1.30)
Correa et al. (1983)	22	2.07 (0.82 – 5.25)
Gao et al. (1978)	246	1.19 (0.82 – 1.73)
Garfinkel, Auerbach, and Joubert (1985)	134	1.31 (0.87 – 1.98)
Geng, Liang, and Zhang (1988)	54	2.16 (1.08 – 4.29)
Humble, Samet, and Pathak (1987)	20	2.34 (0.81 – 6.75)
Inoue and Hirayama (1988)	22	2.55 (0.74 – 8.78)
Kabat and Wynder (1984)	24	0.79 (0.25 – 2.45)
Koo et al. (1987)	86	1.55 (0.90 – 2.67)
Lam et al. (1987)	199	1.65 (1.16 – 2.35)
Lam (1985)	60	2.01 (1.09 – 3.71)
Lee, Chamberlain, and Alderson (1986)	32	1.03 (0.41 – 2.55)
Pershagen, Hrubec, and Svensson (1987)	67	1.28 (0.76 – 2.15)
Svensson, Pershagen, and Klominek (1988)	34	1.26 (0.57 – 2.82)
Trichopoulos, Kalandidi, and Sparros (1983)	62	2.13 (1.19 – 3.83)
Wu et al. (1985)	28	1.41 (0.54 – 3.67)

Note: See United States Environmental Protection Agency (1990) for the references cited.

over its efficacy continues. The data presented in Table 18.8 consist of the sample size and the number of cases of tuberculosis. Furthermore some covariates are available that might explain the heterogeneity among studies: geographic latitude of the place where the study was done, year of publication, and method of treatment allocation (random, alternate, or systematic). Latitude is one of several factors historically suspected as associated with true vaccine efficacy because the distance of each trial from the equator may serve as a surrogate for the presence of environmental mycobacteria that provide a certain level of natural immunity against TB.

Table 18.7 Controlled randomized trials of misoprostol by endoscopic classification

Study	Treatment	Endoscopic classification				
		1	2	3	4	5
Lanza et al. (1988)[1]	Misoprostol	21	2	4	2	0
	Placebo	2	2	4	9	13
Jiranenk et al. (1989)	Misoprostol	17	8	3	2	0
	Placebo	0	3	4	10	13
Lanza et al. (1989)	Misoprostol	20	4	6	0	0
	Placebo	8	4	9	4	5
Lanza (1987)	Misoprostol	20	4	6	0	0
	Placebo	0	2	5	5	17
Lanza et al. (1988)[2]	Misoprostol	1	4	5	0	0
	Placebo	0	0	0	4	6
Bardhan et al. (1991)	Misoprostol	93	5	3	1	1
	Placebo	85	10	10	4	5
Saggiori and Vaiani (1988)	Misoprostol	61	12	0		
	Placebo	49	28	3		
Delmas et al. (1988)	Misoprostol	45	1	0		
	Placebo	65	6	3		
Graham, Agrawal, and Roth (1988)	Misoprostol	138	1			
	Placebo	121	17			
Agrawal, Stromatt, and Brown (1990)	Misoprostol	126	2			
	Placebo	110	21			
Elliot et al. (1990)	Misoprostol	30	1	1		
	Placebo	20	11	7		
Searle & Co.	Misoprostol	56	12	8	0	
	Placebo	50	15	12	5	
Searle & Co.	Misoprostol	12	3	1	0	
	Placebo	11	5	2	3	

Note: See Whitehead and Jones (1994) for the references cited.

Table 18.8 Data on 13 trials on the prevention of tuberculosis

Trial	Vaccinated		Not vaccinated		Latitude	Year	Allocation
	Disease	No disease	Disease	No disease			
1	4	119	11	128	44	1948	Random
2	6	300	29	274	55	1949	Random
3	3	228	11	209	42	1960	Random
4	62	13536	248	12619	52	1977	Random
5	33	5036	47	5761	13	1973	Alternate
6	180	1361	372	1079	44	1953	Alternate
7	8	2537	10	619	19	1973	Random
8	505	87886	499	87892	13	1980	Random
9	29	7470	45	7232	27*	1968	Random
10	17	1699	65	1600	42	1961	Systematic
11	186	50448	414	27197	18	1974	Systematic
12	5	2493	3	2338	33	1969	Systematic
13	27	16886	29	17825	33	1976	Systematic

*This was actually a negative number; we used the absolute value in the analysis

REFERENCES

Chapters in which the references are cited are shown in parentheses.

Abrams, K. R., Lambert, P. C., Sanso, B., Shaw, C., and Marteau, T. M. (2000). Meta-analysis of heterogeneously reported study results: A Bayesian approach. In *Meta-Analysis in Medicine and Health Policy*, D. Stangl and D. A. Berry (Eds.). New York: Marcel Dekker. (12)

Abrams, K. and Sanso, B. (1998). Approximate Bayesian inference for random effects meta-analysis. *Statistics in Medicine*, 17, 201–218. (4, 18)

Agresti, A. (1980). Generalized odds ratio for ordinal data. *Biometrics*, 36, 59–67. (9)

Allescher, H.-D., Böckenhoff, A., Knapp, G., Wienbeck, M., and Hartung, J. (2001). Treatment of non-ulcer dyspepsia: a meta-analysis on placebo-controlled prospective studies. *Scandinavian Journal of Gastroenterology*, 36, 934–941. (1, 9)

Ananda, M. M. A. and Weerahandi, S. (1997). Two-way anova with unequal cell frequencies and unequal variances. *Statistica Sinica*, 7, 631–646. (6)

Anderson, T. W. (1984). *An Introduction to Multivariate Statistical Analysis*. New York: Wiley. (11)

Antiplatelet Trialists' Collaboration (1988). Secondary prevention of vascular disease by prolonged antiplatelet treatment. *British Medical Journal*, 296, 320–332. (1)

Argac, D., Makambi, K. H., and Hartung, J. (2001). A note on testing the nullity of the between group variance in the one-way random effects model under variance heterogeneity. *Journal of Applied Statistics*, 28, 215–222. (7)

Asiribo, O. and Gurland, J. (1990). Coping with variance heterogeneity. *Communications in Statistics – Theory and Methods*, 19, 4029–4048. (6)

Bashore, T. R., Osman, A., and Heffley, E. F. (1989). Mental slowing in elderly persons: a cognitive psychophysiological analysis. *Psychology & Aging*, 4, 235–244. (10)

Becker, B. J. (1990). Coaching for the scholastic aptitude test: further synthesis appraisal. *Review of Educational Research*, 60, 373–417. (1, 11)

Becker, B. J. (1994). Combining significance levels. In *The Handbook of Research Synthesis*, H. Cooper and L. V. Hedges (Eds.). New York: Russell Sage Foundation. (3)

Becker, B. J. (2000). Multivariate meta-analysis. In *Handbook of Applied Statistics and Mathematical Modeling*, H. E. A. Tinsley and S. G. Brown (Eds.) San Diego: Academic Press. (11)

Begg, C. B. (1994). Publication bias. In *The Handbook of Research Synthesis*, H. Cooper and L.V. Hedges (Eds.). New York: Russell Sage Foundation. (13)

Begg, C. B. and Mazumdar, M. (1994). Operating characteristics of a rank correlation test for publication bias. *Biometrics*, 50, 1088–1101. (13)

Begg, C. B. and Pilote L. (1991). A model for incorporating historical controls into a meta-analysis. *Biometrics*, 47, 899–906. (10)

Berger, J. O. (1980). *Statistical Decision Theory and Bayesian Analysis* (2nd ed.). Berlin: Springer. (5)

Berger, J. O. (1985). *Statistical Decision Theory and Bayesian Analysis*. New York: Springer. (12)

Berkey, C. S., Anderson, J. J., and Hoaglin, D. C. (1996). Multiple-outcome meta-analysis of clinical trials. *Statistics in Medicine*, 15, 537–557. (11)

Berkey, C. S., Hoaglin, D. C., Antezak-Bouckoms, A., Mosteller, F., and Colditz, G. A. (1998). Meta-analysis of multiple outcomes by regression with random effects. *Statistics in Medicine*, 17, 2537–2550. (11, 12)

Berkey, C. S., Hoaglin, D. C., Mosteller, F., and Colditz, G. A. (1995). A random effects regression model for meta-analysis. *Statistics in Medicine*, 14, 395–411. (10, 11, 12)

Berlin, J. A. and Antman, E. M. (1994). Advantages and limitations of meta-analytic regressions of clinical trials data. *Online Journal of Current Clinical Trials*, Doc No 134. (10)

Bernardo, J. M. and Smith, A. F. (1993). *Bayesian Theory*. Chichester: Wiley. (12)

Berry, S. C. (2000). Meta-analysis versus large trials: Resolving the controversy. In *Meta-Analysis in Medicine and Health Policy*, D. Stangl and D. A. Berry (Eds.). New York: Marcel Dekker. (1, 12)

Bhattacharya, C. G. (1980). Estimation of a common mean and recovery of interblock information. *Annals of Statistics*, 8, 205–211. (5)

Biggerstaff, B. J. and Tweedie, R. L. (1997). Incorporating variability in estimates of heterogeneity in the random effects model in meta-analysis. *Statistics in Medicine* 16, 753–768. (7)

Birge, R. T. (1932). The calculation of errors by the method of least squares. *Physical Review*, 40, 207–227. (1)

Birnbaum, A. (1954). Combining independent tests of significance. *Journal of the American Statistical Association*, 49, 559–575. (3)

Bishop, Y. M. M., Fienberg, S. E., and Holland, P. W. (1975). *Discrete Multivariate Analysis: Theory and Practice*. Cambridge, MA: MIT Press. (2)

Boardman, T. J. (1974). Confidence intervals for variance components – A comparative Monte Carlo study. *Biometrics*, 30, 251–262. (7)

Brophy, J. and Joseph, L. (2000). A Bayesian meta-analysis of randomized mega-trials for the choice of thrombolytic agent in acute myocardial infarction. In: *Meta-Analysis in Medicine and Health Policy*, D. Stangl and D. A. Berry (Eds.). New York: Marcel Dekker. (1, 12)

Brown, L. D. and Cohen, A. (1974). Point and confidence estimation of a common mean and recovery of interblock information. *Annals of Statistics*, 2, 963–976. (5)

Brown, M. B. and Forsythe, A. B. (1974). The small sample behavior of some statistics which test the equality of several means. *Technometrics*, 16, 129–132. (6)

Burdick, R. K. and Eickman, J. (1986). Confidence intervals on the among group variance component in the unbalanced one-fold nested design. *Journal of Statistical Computation and Simulation*, 26, 205–219. (7)

Burdick, R. K. and Graybill, F. A. (1992). *Confidence Intervals on Variance Components*. New York: Marcel Dekker. (7)

Burdick, R. K., Maqsood, F., and Graybill, F. A. (1986). Confidence intervals on the intraclass correlation in the unbalanced one-way classification. *Communications in Statistics – Theory and Methods*, 15, 3353–3378. (7)

Chiu, C. W. T. (1997). *Synthesizing multiple outcome measures with missing data: A sensitivity analysis on the effect of metacognitive reading intervention.* Unpublished manuscript, Department of Counseling, Educational Psychology, and Special Education, Michigan State University, East Lansing, MI. (11)

Churchill, G. A., Ford, N. M., Hartley, S. W., and Walker, O. C. (1985). The determinants of salesperson performance: a meta-analysis. *Journal of Marketing Research*, 22, 103–118. (1)

Cochran, W. G. (1937). Problems arising in the analysis of a series of similar experiments. *Journal of the Royal Statistical Society (Supplement)*, 4, 102–118. (1, 4, 6)

Cochran, W. G. (1954). The combination of estimates from different experiments. *Biometrics*, 10, 101–129. (7, 9)

Cohen, A. and Sackrowitz, H. B. (1974). On estimating the common mean of two normal distributions. *Annals of Statistics*, 2, 1274–1282. (5)

Cohen, A. and Sackrowitz, H. B. (1984). Testing hypotheses about the common mean of normal distributions. *Journal of Statistical Planning and Inference*, 9, 207–227. (5, 8)

Cohen, A., and Sackrowitz, H. B. (1989). Exact tests that recover inter-block information in balanced incomplete block designs. *Journal of the American Statistical Association*, 84, 556–559. (1, 14)

Cohen, J. (1969). *Statistical Power Analysis for the Behavioral Sciences*. New York: Academic Press. (2)

Cohen, J. (1977). *Statistical Power Analysis for the Behavioral Sciences* (rev. ed.). New York: Academic Press. (2)

Cohen, J. (1988). *Statistical Power Analysis for the Behavioral Sciences* (2nd ed.). Hillsdale, NJ: Erlbaum. (2)

Cohen, P. A. (1983). Comment on "A selective review of the validity of student ratings of teaching." *Journal of Higher Education*, 54, 449–458. (13, 16, 18)

Colditz, G. A., Brewer, F. B., Berkey, C. S., Wilson, E. M., Burdick, E., Fineberg, H. V., and Mosteller, F. (1994). Efficacy of BCG vaccine in the prevention of tuberculosis. *Journal of the American Medical Association* 271, 698–702. (10)

Collins, R., Gray, R., Godwin, J., and Peto, R. (1987). Avoidances of large biases and large random errors in the assessment of moderate treatment effects: The need for systematic overviews. *Statistics in Medicine*, 6, 245–250. (13)

Cooper, H. and Hedges, L. V. (1994). *The Handbook of Research Synthesis*. New York: Russell Sage Foundation. (Preface, 1, 16)

Das, R. and Sinha, B. K. (1987). Robust optimum invariant unbiased tests for variance components. *Proceedings of 2nd International Tampere Conference in Statistics*, University of Tampere, Finland. (7)

Dasgupta, A. and Sinha, B. K. (2006). On some statistical aspects of combining gallup poll results. Technical Report, Department of Mathematics and Statistics, University of Maryland, Baltimore County. (1, 15)

DerSimonian, R. and Laird, N. M. (1983). Evaluating the effect of coaching on SAT scores: a meta-analysis. *Harvard Educational Review*, 53, 1–15. (1)

DerSimonian, R. and Laird, N. M. (1986). Meta-analysis in clinical trials. *Controlled Clinical Trials*, 7, 177–188. (7, 8)

Dominici, F. and Parmigiani, G. (2000). Combining studies with continuous and dichotomous responses: A latent variables approach. In: *Meta-Analysis in Medicine and Health Policy*, D. Stangl and D. A. Berry (Eds.). New York: Marcel Dekker. (1, 12)

Draper, D., Gaver, D. P., Jr. , Goel, P. K., Greenhouse, J. B., Hedges, L. V., Morris, C. N., Tucker, J. R., and Waternaux, C. M. (1992). *Combining Information: Statistical Issues and Opportunities for Research.* American Statistical Association, National Academy Press, Washington, D.C. (3)

DuMouchel, W. and Normand, S. L. (2000). Computer-modeling and graphical strategies for meta-analysis. In: *Meta-Analysis in Medicine and Health Policy*, D. Stangl and D. A. Berry (Eds.). New York: Marcel Dekker. (12)

Eberhardt, K. R., Reeve, C. P., and Spiegelman, C. H. (1989). A minimax approach to combining means, with practical examples. *Chemometrics and Intelligent Laboratory Systems*, 5, 129–148. (4, 5, 6)

Egger, M., Davey Smith, G., Schneider, M., and Minder, C. (1997). Bias in meta-analysis detected by a simple, graphical test. *British Medical Journal*, 315, 629–634. (13)

Fairweather, W. R. (1972). A method of obtaining an exact confidence interval for the common mean of several normal populations. *Applied Statistics*, 21, 229–233. (5, 8)

Farley, J. U. and Lehmann, D. R. (1986). *Meta-Analysis in Marketing: Generalization of Response Models*. Lexington, MA: Lexington Books. (1)

Farley, J. U. and Lehmann, D. R. (2001). The important role of meta-analysis in international research in marketing. *International Marketing Review*, 18, 70–79. (1)

Farley, J. U., Lehmann, D. R., and Sawyer, A. (1995). Empirical marketing generalization using meta-analysis. *Marketing Science*, 14, G36–G46. (1)

Feingold, M. (1985). A test statistic for combined intra- and inter-block estimates. *Journal of Statistical Planning and Inference*, 12, 103–114. (1, 14)

Feingold, M. (1988). A more powerful test for incomplete block designs. *Communications in Statistics – Theory and Methods*, 17, 3107–3119. (1, 14)

Fisher, R. A. (1932). *Statistical Methods for Research Workers* (4th ed.) London: Oliver and Boyd. (1, 3, 5, 14)

Fleiss, J. L. (1994). Measures of effect size for categorical data. In: *The Handbook of Research Synthesis*, H. Cooper and L. V. Hedges (Eds.). New York: Russell Sage Foundation. (2)

Gamage, J. and Weerahandi, S. (1998). Size performance of some tests in one-way anova. *Communications in Statistics – Simulation and Computation*, 27, 625–640. (6)

Gart, J. J. and Zweifel, J. R. (1967). On the bias of various estimators of the logit and its variance with application to quantal bioassay. *Biometrika*, 54, 181–187. (9)

Gauss, C. F. (1809). *Theoria motus corporum coelestium in sectionis conicis solem ambientum.* Hamburg: Perthes and Besser. (1)

Gelman, A., Carlin, J. B., Stern, H. S., and Rubin, D. B. (2004). *Bayesian Data Analysis.* Boca Raton, FL: Chapman & Hall/CRC Press. (5)

George, E. O. (1977). Combining independent one-sided and two-sided statistical tests – Some theory and applications. Doctoral dissertation, University of Rochester. (3, 5)

Givens, G. H., Smith, D. D., and Tweedie, R. L. (1997). Publication bias in meta-analysis: A Bayesian data-augmentation approach to account for issues exemplified in the passive smoking debate. *Statistical Science*, 12, 221–247. (13)

Glass, G. V. (1976). Primary, secondary, and meta-analysis. *Educational Researcher*, 5, 3–8. (Preface, 1)

Glass, G. V., McGaw, B., and Smith, M. L. (1981). *Meta-Analysis in Social Research.* Beverly Hills, CA: Sage. (1, 2)

Gleser, L. J. and Olkin, I. (1994). Stochastically dependent effect sizes. In *The Handbook of Research Synthesis*, H. Cooper and L. V. Hedges (Eds.). New York: Russell Sage Foundation. (11)

Graybill, F. A. (1976). *Theory and Application of the Linear Model.* North Scituate, MA: Duxbury Press. (7, 11)

Graybill, F. A. and Deal, R. B. (1959). Combining unbiased estimators. *Biometrics*, 15, 543–550. (5)

Greenhouse, J. B. and Iyengar, S. (1994). Sensitivity analysis and diagnostics. In *The Handbook of Research Synthesis*, H. Cooper and L. V. Hedges (Eds.). New York: Russell Sage Foundation. (11)

Greenland, S. (1994). A critical look at some popular meta-analytical methods. *American Journal of Epidemiology*, 140, 290–296. (10)

Greenwald, R., Hedges, L. V., and Laine, R. D. (1996). The effect of school resources on student-achievement. *Review of Educational Research*, 66, 361–396. (11)

Griffiths, W. and Judge, G. (1992). Testing and estimating location vectors when the error covariance matrix is unknown. *Journal of Econometrics*, 54, 121–138. (6)

Haff, L. R. (1979). An identity for the Wishart distribution with applications. *Journal of Multivariate Analysis*, 9, 531–544. (5)

Haldane, J. B. S. (1955). The estimation and significance of the logarithm of a ratio of frequencies. *Annals of Human Genetics*, 20, 309–311. (9)

Hardy, R. J. and Thompson, S. G. (1996). A likelihood approach to meta-analysis with random effects. *Statistics in Medicine* 15, 619–629. (7)

Hartung, J. (1981). Nonnegative minimum biased invariant estimation in variance component models. *Annals of Statistics*, 9, 278–292. (7)

Hartung, J. (1999a). A note on combining dependent tests of significance. *Biometrical Journal*, 41, 849–855. (3)

Hartung, J. (1999b). An alternative method for meta-analysis. *Biometrical Journal*, 41, 901–916. (7, 8, 9)

Hartung, J. and Argac, D. (2002). Generalizing the Welch test to nonzero hypotheses on the variance component in the one-way random effects model under variance heterogeneity. *Statistics*, 36, 89–99. (7)

Hartung, J., Argac, D., and Makambi, K. H. (2002). Small sample properties of tests on homogeneity in one-way anova and meta-analysis. *Statistical Papers*, 43, 197–235. (6, 8)

Hartung, J., Böckenhoff, A., and Knapp, G. (2003). Generalized Cochran–Wald statistics in combining of experiments. *Journal of Statistical Planning and Inference*, 113, 215–237. (7)

Hartung, J. and Knapp, G. (2000). Confidence intervals for the between group variance in the unbalanced one-way random effects model of analysis of variance. *Journal of Statistical Computation and Simulation 65*, 4, 311–324. (7)

Hartung, J. and Knapp, G. (2001a). On tests of the overall treatment effect in the meta-analysis with normally distributed responses. *Statistics in Medicine*, 20, 1771–1782. (7, 8)

Hartung, J.and Knapp, G. (2001b) A refined method for the meta-analysis of controlled clinical trials with binary outcome. *Statistics in Medicine*, 20, 3875–3889. (7, 8, 9, 18)

Hartung, J. and Knapp, G. (2004). Improved tests of homogeneity in randomized controlled multi-center trials with binary outcome. *Far East Journal of Theoretical Statistics*, 13, 101–126. (9)

Hartung, J. and Knapp, G. (2005a). On confidence intervals for the among-group variance in the one-way random effects model with unequal error variances. *Journal of Statistical Planning and Inference*, 127, 157–177. (7, 8, 9)

Hartung, J. and Knapp, G. (2005b). Models for combining results of different experiments: retrospective and prospective. *American Journal of Mathematical and Management Sciences*, 25, 149–188. (10)

Hartung, J. and Makambi, K. H. (2002). Positive estimation of the between-study variance in meta-analysis. *South African Statistical Journal*, 36, 55–76. (7)

Hartung, J., Makambi, K. H., and Argac, D. (2001). An extended ANOVA F-test with applications to the heterogeneity problem in meta-analysis. *Biometrical Journal*, 43, 135–146. (7)

Hedges, L. V. (1981). Distribution theory for Glass's estimator of effect size and related estimators. *Journal of Educational Statistics*, 6, 107–128. (2)

Hedges, L. V. (1982). Estimating effect size from a series of independent experiments. *Psychological Bulletin*, 92, 490–499. (2)

Hedges, L. V. (1994). Fixed effects models. In: *The Handbook of Research Synthesis*, H. Cooper and L.V. Hedges (Eds.). New York: Russell Sage Foundation. (1)

Hedges, L. V., Gurevitch, J., and Curtis, P. S. (1999). The meta-analysis of response ratios in experimental ecology. *Ecology* 80, 1150–1156. (8)

Hedges, L. V. and Olkin, I. (1985). *Statistical Methods for Meta-Analysis*. Boston: Academic Press. (Preface, 1, 2, 3, 4, 11, 16)

Heine, B. (1993). Nonnegative estimation of variance components in an unbalanced one-way random effects model. *Communications in Statistics – Theory and Methods*, 22, 2351–2371. (7)

Higgins, J. P. T. and Thompson, S. G. (2004). Controlling the risk of spurious findings from meta-regression. *Statistics in Medicine*, 23, 1663–1682. (10)

Hunter, J. E., Schmidt, F. L., and Jackson, G. B. (1982). *Meta-analysis: Cumulating Research Finding across Studies*. Beverly Hills, CA: Sage. (1)

Iyengar, S. and Greenhouse, J. B. (1988). Selection models and the file drawer problem. *Statistical Science*, 3, 109–135. (13)

Iyer, H., Wang, J. M., and Mathew, T. (2004). Models and confidence intervals for true values in interlaboratory trials. *Journal of the American Statistical Association*, 99, 1060–1071. (7)

Johnson, M. (1993). Comparative efficacy of NaF and SMFP dentifrices in caries prevention: a meta-analysis overview. *Caries Research*, 27, 328–336. (1, 18)

Johnson, N. L. and Kotz, S. (1970). *Distributions in Statistics: Continuous Univariate Distributions*. New York: Wiley. (11)

Jones, D. R. (1992). Meta-analysis of observational epidemiological studies: a review. *Journal of the Royal Society of Medicine*, 85, 165–168. (10)

Jordan, S. M. and Krishnamoorthy, K. (1996). Exact confidence intervals for the common mean of several normal populations. *Biometrics*, 52, 77–86. (5, 8)

Kalaian, H. and Becker, B. J. (1986). The effects of coaching on Scholastic Aptitude Test performance: A multivariate meta-analysis approach. Paper presented at the annual meeting of the American Educational Research Association, San Francisco. (11)

Kempthorne, O., Mukhopadhyay, N., Sen, P. K., and Zacks, S. (1991). Research–How to do it: A panel discussion. *Statistical Science*, 6, 149–162. (5)

Khatri, C. G. and Shah, K. R. (1974). Estimation of location parameters from two linear models under normality. *Communications in Statistics*, 3, 647–663. (5)

Khuri, A. I., Mathew, T., and Sinha, B. K. (1998). *Statistical Tests for Mixed Linear Models*. New York: Wiley. (5, 6, 7, 14)

Kim, J. P. (1998). Meta-analysis of equivalence of computerized and pencil-and-paper testing for ability measures. Unpublished manuscript, Department of Counseling, Educational Psychology, and Special Education, Michigan State University, East Lansing, MI. (11)

Knapp, G. and Hartung, J. (2003). Improved tests for a random effects meta-regression with a single covariate. *Statistics in Medicine*, 22, 2693–2710. (10)

Kubokawa, T. (1990). Minimax estimation of common coefficients of several regression models under quadratic loss. *Journal of Statistical Planning and Inference*, 24, 337–345. (5)

LaMotte, L.R. (1973). On nonnegative quadratic unbiased estimation of variance components. *Journal of the American Statistical Association*, 68, 728–730. (7)

Larose, D.T. (2000). A Bayesian meta-analysis of the relationship between duration of estrogen exposure and occurrence of endometrial cancer. In: *Meta-Analysis in Medicine and Health Policy*, D. Stangl and D. A. Berry (Eds.). New York: Marcel Dekker. (12)

Legendre, A. M. (1805). *Nouvelles méthodes pour la détermination des orbites des comètes*. Paris: Courcier. (1)

Lentner, M. and Bishop, T. (1986). *Experimental Design and Analysis*. Blacksburg, VA: Valley Book. (14)

Li, X. (2000). Statistical Issues in Environmental Problems. Ph.D. dissertation, University of Maryland, Baltimore County, MD. (1)

Li, X., Nussbaum, B., and Sinha, B. K. (2000). A statistical analysis of hillsdale lake data. *Calcutta Statistical Association Bulletin*, 50, 293–305. (1)

Li, Y., Shi, L., and Roth, H. D. (1994). The bias of the commonly-used estimate of variance in meta-analysis. *Communications in Statistics – Theory and Methods*, 23, 1063-1085. (18)

Li, Z. and Begg, C. B. (1994). Random effects models for combining results from controlled and uncontrolled studies in a meta-analysis. *Journal of the American Statistical Association*, 89, 1523–1527. (10)

Liang, K. Y. and Self, S. G. (1985). Test for homogeneity of odds ratio when the data are sparse. *Biometrika*, 72, 353–358. (9)

Light, R .J. and Pillemer, D. B. (1984). *Summing up: The Science of Reviewing Research*. Cambridge, MA: Harvard University Press. (13)

Lipsitz, S. R., Dear, K. B. G., Laird, N. M., and Molenberghs, G. (1998). Tests for homogeneity of the risk difference when data are sparse. *Biometrics*, 54, 148–160. (9)

Little, R. J. A, and Rubin, D. B. (1987). Statistical Analysis with Missing Data. New York: Wiley. (11)

Lodish, L. M., Abraham, M., Kalmenson, S., Livelsberger, J., Lubetkin, B., Richardson, B., and Stevens, M. E. (1995). How T.V. advertising works: a meta-analysis of 389 real world split cable T.V. advertising experiments. *Journal of Marketing Research*, 32, 125–139. (1)

Makambi, K. H. (2003). Weighted inverse chi-square method for correlated significance tests. *Journal of Applied Statistics*, 30, 225–234. (3)

Mandel, J. and Paule, R. C. (1970). Interlaboratory evaluation of a material with unequal number of replicates. *Analytical Chemistry*, 42, 1194–1197. (7, 8)

Mantel, N. and Haenszel, W. (1959). Statistical aspects of the analysis of data from retrospective studies of disease. *Journal of the National Cancer Institute*, 22, 719–748. (12)

Marden, J. I. (1991). Sensitive and sturdy p-values. *The Annals of Statistics*, 19, 918–934. (3)

Mathew, T., Sinha, B. K., and Zhou, L. (1993). Some statistical procedures for combining independent tests. *Journal of the American Statistical Association*, 88, 912–919. (1, 14)

McCullagh, P. (1980). Regression models for ordinal data. *Journal of the Royal Statistical Society, Series B*, 42, 109–142. (9, 14)

Mehrotra, D. V. (1997). Improving the Brown-Forsythe solution to the generalized Behrens-Fisher problem. *Communications in Statistics – Simulation and Computation*, 26, 1139–1145. (6)

Mehta, J. S. and Gurland, J. (1969). Combination of unbiased estimates of the mean which consider inequality of unknown variances. *Journal of the American Statistical Association*, 64, 1042–1055. (5)

Meier, P. (1953). Variance of a weighted mean. *Biometrics*, 9, 59–73. (4, 5, 6, 8)

Mitra, P. K. and Sinha, B. K. (2007). On some aspects of estimation of a common mean of two independent normal populations. *Journal of Statistical Planning and Inference* 137, 184–193. (5)

Montgomery, D. (1991). *Design and Analysis of Experiments* (3rd ed.). New York: Wiley. (5)

Mosteller, F. and Bush, R. (1954). Selected quantitative techniques. In *Handbook of Social Psychology: Theory and Method*, Vol. 1, G. Lindsey (Ed.). Cambridge, MA: Addison-Wesley. (1, 3)

Nair, K. A. (1980). Distribution of an estimator of the common mean of two normal populations. *Annals of Statistics*, 8, 212–216. (5)

Norwood, T. E. and Hinkelmann, K. (1977). Estimating the common mean of several normal populations. *Annals of Statistics*, 5, 1047–1050. (5)

Patil, G. P. and Rao, C. R. (1977). The weighted distributions: A survey of their applications. In *Applications of Statistics*, Krishnaiah (Ed.). Amsterdam: North-Holland. (13)

Pauler, D. K. and Wakefield, J. (2000). Modeling and implementation issues in Bayesian meta-analysis. In: *Meta-Analysis in Medicine and Health Policy*, D. Stangl and D. A. Berry (Eds.). New York: Marcel Dekker. (1, 12)

Pearson, K. (1904). Report on certain enteric fever inoculation statistics. *British Medical Journal*, 2, 1243–1246. (1)

Pearson, K. (1933). On a method of determining whether a sample of given size n supposed to have been drawn from a parent population having a known probability integral has probably been drawn at random. *Biometrika*, 25, 379–410. (3)

Petitti, D. B. (1994). *Meta-Analysis, Decision Analysis, and Cost-Effectiveness Analysis.* New York: Oxford University Press. (18)

Pettigrew, H. M., Gart, J. J., and Thomas, D. G. (1986). The bias and higher cumulants of the logarithm of a binomial variate. *Biometrika*, 73, 425–435. (9)

Piggott, T. D. (1994). Methods for handling missing data in research synthesis. In: *The Handbook of Research Synthesis*, H. Cooper and L. V. Hedges (Eds.). New York: Russell Sage Foundation. (11)

Rao, C. R. (1947). General methods of analysis for incomplete block designs. *Journal of the American Statistical Association*, 42, 541–561. (1, 14)

Rao, C. R. (1972). Estimation of variance and covariance components in linear models. *Journal of the American Statistical Association*, 67, 122–115. (7)

Rao, C. R. (1973). *Linear Statistical Inference and Its Applications.* New York: Wiley. (1, 2, 5, 15)

Rao, P. S. R. S, Kaplan, J., and Cochran, W. G. (1981). Estimators for the one-way random effects model with unequal error variances. *Journal of the American Statistical Association*, 76, 89–97. (7)

Raudenbush, S. W. (1984). Magnitude of teacher expectancy effects on pupil IQ as a function of the credibility of expectancy induction: A synthesis of findings from 18 experiments. *Journal of Educational Psychology*, 76, 85–97. (18)

Raudenbush, S. W., Becker, B. J., and Kalaian, H. (1988). Modeling multivariate effect sizes. *Psychological Bulletin*, 103, 111–120. (11)

Raudenbush, S. W. and Bryk, A. S. (1985). Empirical Bayes meta-analysis. *Journal of Educational Statistics*, 10, 75–98. (13, 16, 18)

Riley, R. D., Abrams, K. R., Lambert, P. C., Sutton, A. J., and Thompson, J. R. (2007a). An evaluation of bivariate random-effects meta-analysis for the joint synthesis of two correlated outcomes. *Statistics in Medicine*, 26, 78–97. (11, 12)

Riley, R. D., Abrams, K. R., Lambert, P. C., Sutton, A. J., and Thompson, J. R. (2007b). Bivariate random-effects meta-analysis and the estimation of between-study correlation. *BMC Medical Research Methodology*, 7:3, 1471–2288/7/3. (11)

Riley, R. D., Heney, D., Jones, D. R., Sutton, A. J., Lambert, P. C., Abrams, K. R., Young, B., and Wailoo, A. J. (2004). A systematic review of molecular and biological tumor markers in neuroblastoma. *Clinical Cancer Research*, 10, 4–12. (11)

Rohatgi, V. K. (1976). *An Introduction to Probability Theory and Mathematical Statistics.* New York: Wiley. (1)

Rosenthal, R. (1978). Combining results of independent studies. *Psychological Bulletin*, 85, 185–193. (3)

Rosenthal, R. (1979). The "file drawer problem" and tolerance for null results. *Psychological Bulletin*, 86, 638–641. (13)

Rosenthal, R. (1984). *Meta-Analytic Procedures for Social Research.* Beverly Hills, CA: Sage. (1)

Rosenthal, R. (1994). Parametric measures of effect size. In: *The Handbook of Research Synthesis*, H. Cooper and L. V. Hedges (Eds.). New York: Russell Sage Foundation. (4)

Rosenthal, R. and Rubin, D. B. (1986). Meta-analytical procedures for combining studies with multiple effect sizes. *Psychological Bulletin*, 99, 400–406. (11)

Rubin, D. B. (1981). Estimation in parallel randomized experiments. *Journal of Educational Statistics*, 6, 337–401. (1)

Rukhin, A. L. (2007). Conservative confidence intervals based on weighted means statistics. *Statistics & Probability Letters*, 77, 853–861. (5)

Rukhin, A. L., Biggerstaff, B. J., and Vangel, M. G. (2000). Restricted maximum likelihood estimation of a common mean and the Mandel-Paule algorithm. *Journal of Statistical Planning & Inference*, 83, 319–330. (7)

Rukhin, A. L. and Vangel, M. G. (1998). Estimation of a common mean and weighted mean statistics. *Journal of the American Statistical Association*, 93, 303–309. (7)

Ryan, E. D., Blakeslee, T., and Furst, D. M. (1986). Mental practice and motor skill learning: an indirect test of the neuromuscular feedback hypothesis. *International Journal of Sport Psychology*, 17, 60–70. (1, 11)

Satterthwaite, F. E. (1946). An approximate distribution of estimates of variance components. *Biometrics Bulletin*, 2, 110–114. (8)

Searle, S. R. (1971). *Linear Models*. New York: Wiley. (11)

Searle, S. R., Casella, G., and McCulloch, C. E. (1992). *Variance Components*. New York: Wiley. (7)

Sethuraman, R. (1995). A meta-analysis of national brand and store brand cross-promotional price elasticities. *Marketing Letters*, 6, 275–286. (1)

Shah, K. R. (1975). Analysis of block designs. *Gujarat Statistical Review*, 2, 1–11. (14)

Shah, K. R. (1992). Recovery of inter-block information: an update. *Journal of Statistical Planning and Inference*, 30, 163–172. (14)

Shinozaki, N. (1978). A note on estimating the common mean of k normal populations and the Stein Problem. *Communications in Statistics A*, 7, 1421–1432. (5)

Sidik, K. and Jonkman, J. N. (2002). A simple confidence interval for meta-analysis. *Statistics in Medicine* 21, 3153–3159. (7)

Sinha, B. K. (1979). Is the maximum likelihood estimate of the common mean of several normal populations admissible? *Sankhyā*, B, 40, 192–196. (5)

Sinha, B. K. (1985). Unbiased estimation of the variance of the Graybill-Deal estimator of the common mean of several normal distributions. *Canadian Journal of Statistics*, 13, 243–247. (5)

Sinha, B. K. and Mouqadem, O. (1982). Estimation of the common mean of two univariate normal populations. *Communications in Statistics – Theory and Methods*, 11, 1603–1614. (5)

Sinha, B. K., O'Brien, R., and Smith, W. (1991). A statistical procedure to evaluate cleanup standards. *Journal of Chemometrics*, 5, 249–261. (1)

Sinha, B. K. and Sinha, B. K. (1995). An application of bivariate exponential models and related inference. *Journal of Statistical Planning and Inference*, 44, 181–191. (1)

Skinner, J. B. (1991). On combining studies. *Drug Information Journal*, 25, 395–403. (5)

Smith, T. C., Spiegelhalter, D. J., and Thomas, A. (1995). Bayesian approaches to random-effects meta-analysis: a comparative study. *Statistics in Medicine*, 14, 2685–2699. (9)

Snedecor, G. W. and Cochran, W. G. (1967). *Statistical Methods* (6th ed.). Ames, IA: The Iowa State University Press. (7)

Steinkamp, M. W. and Maehr, M. L. (1983). Affect, ability and science achievement: A quantitative synthesis of correlation research. *Review of Educational Research*, 53, 369–396. (11)

Sterne, J. A. C., Egger, M., and Sutton, A. J. (2001). Meta-analysis software. In: *Systematic Reviews in Health Care: Meta-Analysis in Context* (2nd ed.), M. Egger, G. D. Smith, and D. G Altman (Eds.). London: BMJ Books. (17)

Stigler, S. M. (1986). *The History of Statistics – The Measurement of Uncertainty before 1900*. Cambridge, MA: Harvard University Press. (1)

Stouffer, S. A., Suchman, E. A., DeVinney, L. C., Star, S. A., and Williams, R. M., Jr. (1949). *The American Soldier, Volume I. Adjustment during Army Life.* Princeton, NJ: Princeton University Press. (3, 5, 13)

Tellis, G. J. (1988). The price elasticity of selective demand: a meta-analysis of econometric models of sales. *Journal of Marketing Research*, 25, 331–341. (1)

Thomas, J. D. and Hultquist, R. A. (1978). Interval estimation for the unbalanced case of the one-way random effects model. *Annals of Statistics*, 6, 582–587. (7)

Thursby, J. G. (1992). A comparison of several exact and approximate tests for structural shift under heteroscedasticity. *Journal of Econometrics*, 53, 363–386. (6)

Timm, N. H. (1975). *Multivariate Analysis with Applications in Education and Psychology.* Belmont, CA: Brooks/Cole. (11)

Timm, N. H. (1999). A note on testing for multivariate effect sizes. *Journal of Educational and Behavioral Statistics*, 24, 132–145. (11)

Tippett, L. H. C. (1931). *The Methods of Statistics.* London: Williams & Norgate. (1, 3, 5)

Tsui, K. and Weerahandi, S. (1989). Generalized p-values in significance testing of hypotheses in the presence of nuisance parameters. *Journal of the American Statistical Association*, 84, 602–607. (6,7)

Tukey, J.W. (1951). Components in regression. *Biometrics*, 7, 33–69. (7)

United States Environmental Protection Agency (1990). *Health Effects of Passive Smoking: Assessment of Lung Cancer in Adults and Respiratory Disorders in Children.* US EPA Publication NO. EPA-600-90-006A, Washington DC. (18)

Van Houwelingen, H. C., Arends, L. R., and Stijnen, T. (2002). Advanced methods in meta-analysis: multivariate approach and meta-regression. *Statistics in Medicine*, 21, 589–624. (10, 17, 18)

Verbeke, G. and Molenberghs, G. (1997). *Linear Mixed Models in Practice.* New York: Springer. (7)

Viechtbauer, W. (2007). Confidence intervals for the amount of heterogeneity in meta-analysis. *Statistics in Medicine*, 26, 37–52. (7, 8, 9)

Wald, A. (1940). A note on the analysis of variance with unequal class frequencies. *Annals of Mathematical Statistics*, 11, 96–100. (7)

Wang, C. M. (1990). On the lower bound of confidence coefficients for a confidence interval on variance components. *Biometrics*, 46, 187–192. (7)

Warn, D. E., Thompson, S. G., and Spiegelhalter, D. J. (2002). Bayesian random effects meta-analysis of trials with binary outcomes: methods for the absolute risk difference and relative risk scales. *Statistics in Medicine*, 21, 1601–1623. (9)

Weerahandi, S. (1993). Generalized confidence intervals. *Journal of the American Statistical Association*, 88, 899–905. (7)

Weerahandi, S. (1995). *Exact Statistical Methods for Data Analysis.* New York: Springer. (6, 7)

Weerahandi, S. (2004). *Generalized Inference in Repeated Measures.* New York: Wiley. (6)

Welch, B. L. (1951). On the comparison of several mean values: an alternative approach. *Biometrika*, 38, 330–336. (6)

White, H. D. (1994). Scientific communication and literature retrieval. In *The Handbook of Research Synthesis*, H. Cooper and L.V. Hedges (Eds.). New York: Russell Sage Foundation. (1)

Whitehead, A. (2002). *Meta-Analysis of Controlled Clinical Trials.* Chichester: Wiley. (1, 17)

Whitehead, A. and Jones, N. M. B. (1994). A meta-analysis of clinical trials involving different classifications of response into ordered categories. *Statistics in Medicine*, 13, 2503–2515. (9)

Whitehead, A., Omar, R. Z., Higgins, J. P. T., Savaluny, E., Turner, R. M., and Thompson, S. G. (2001). Meta-analysis of ordinal outcomes using individual patient data. *Statistics in Medicine*, 20, 2243–2260. (9)

Wilkinson, B. (1951). A statistical consideration in psychological research. *Psychological Bulletin*, 48, 156–158. (3)

Williams, J. S. (1962). A confidence interval for variance components. *Biometrika*, 49, 278–281. (7)

Witte, S. and Victor, N. (2004). Some problems with the investigation of noninferiority in meta-analysis. *Methods of Information in Medicine*, 43, 470–474. (10)

Woolf, B. (1955). On estimating the relation between blood group and disease. *Annals of Human Genetics*, 19, 251–253. (2)

Yates, F. (1939). The recovery of inter-block information in varietal trials arranged in three dimensional lattice. *Annals of Eugenics*, 9, 136–156. (1, 14)

Yates, F. (1940). The recovery of inter-block information in balanced incomplete block designs. *Annals of Eugenics*, 10, 317–325. (1, 14)

Yates, F. and Cochran, W. G. (1938). The analysis of groups of experiments. *Journal of Agricultural Science*, 28, 556–580. (1)

Yu, P., Sun, Y., and Sinha, B. K. (2002). Estimation of the common mean of a bivariate normal population. *Annals of the Institute of Statistical Mathematics*, 54, 861–878. (1, 5)

Zacks, S. (1966). Unbiased estimation of the common mean of the two normal distributions based on small samples of equal size. *Journal of American Statistical Association*, 61, 467–476. (5)

Zacks, S. (1970). Bayes and fiducial equivariant estimators of the common mean of two populations. *Annals of Mathematical Statistics*, 41, 59–69. (5)

Zhang, Z. (1992). Recovery tests in BIBD's with very small degrees of freedom for inter-block errors. *Statistics and Probability Letters*, 15, 197–202. (14)

Zhou, L. and Mathew, T. (1993). Combining independent tests in linear models. *Journal of the American Statistical Association*, 88, 650–655. (1, 14)

INDEX

WILEY SERIES IN PROBABILITY AND STATISTICS
ESTABLISHED BY WALTER A. SHEWHART AND SAMUEL S. WILKS

Editors: *David J. Balding, Noel A. C. Cressie, Garrett M. Fitzmaurice, Iain M. Johnstone, Geert Molenberghs, David W. Scott, Adrian F. M. Smith, Ruey S. Tsay, Sanford Weisberg*
Editors Emeriti: *Vic Barnett, J. Stuart Hunter, Jozef L. Teugels*

The *Wiley Series in Probability and Statistics* is well established and authoritative. It covers many topics of current research interest in both pure and applied statistics and probability theory. Written by leading statisticians and institutions, the titles span both state-of-the-art developments in the field and classical methods.

Reflecting the wide range of current research in statistics, the series encompasses applied, methodological and theoretical statistics, ranging from applications and new techniques made possible by advances in computerized practice to rigorous treatment of theoretical approaches.

This series provides essential and invaluable reading for all statisticians, whether in academia, industry, government, or research.

*Now available in a lower priced paperback edition in the Wiley Classics Library.
†Now available in a lower priced paperback edition in the Wiley–Interscience Paperback Series.

BELSLEY · Conditioning Diagnostics: Collinearity and Weak Data in Regression
† BELSLEY, KUH, and WELSCH · Regression Diagnostics: Identifying Influential
  Data and Sources of Collinearity
BENDAT and PIERSOL · Random Data: Analysis and Measurement Procedures,
  Third Edition
BERRY, CHALONER, and GEWEKE · Bayesian Analysis in Statistics and
  Econometrics: Essays in Honor of Arnold Zellner
BERNARDO and SMITH · Bayesian Theory
BHAT and MILLER · Elements of Applied Stochastic Processes, *Third Edition*
BHATTACHARYA and WAYMIRE · Stochastic Processes with Applications
BILLINGSLEY · Convergence of Probability Measures, *Second Edition*
BILLINGSLEY · Probability and Measure, *Third Edition*
BIRKES and DODGE · Alternative Methods of Regression
BISWAS, DATTA, FINE, and SEGAL · Statistical Advances in the Biomedical Sciences:
  Clinical Trials, Epidemiology, Survival Analysis, and Bioinformatics
BLISCHKE AND MURTHY (editors) · Case Studies in Reliability and Maintenance
BLISCHKE AND MURTHY · Reliability: Modeling, Prediction, and Optimization
BLOOMFIELD · Fourier Analysis of Time Series: An Introduction, *Second Edition*
BOLLEN · Structural Equations with Latent Variables
BOLLEN and CURRAN · Latent Curve Models: A Structural Equation Perspective
BOROVKOV · Ergodicity and Stability of Stochastic Processes
BOULEAU · Numerical Methods for Stochastic Processes
BOX · Bayesian Inference in Statistical Analysis
BOX · R. A. Fisher, the Life of a Scientist
BOX and DRAPER · Response Surfaces, Mixtures, and Ridge Analyses, *Second Edition*
* BOX and DRAPER · Evolutionary Operation: A Statistical Method for Process
  Improvement
BOX and FRIENDS · Improving Almost Anything, *Revised Edition*
BOX, HUNTER, and HUNTER · Statistics for Experimenters: Design, Innovation,
  and Discovery, *Second Editon*
BOX, JENKINS, and REINSEL · Time Series Analysis: Forcasting and Control, *Fourth
  Edition*
BOX and LUCEÑO · Statistical Control by Monitoring and Feedback Adjustment
BRANDIMARTE · Numerical Methods in Finance: A MATLAB-Based Introduction
† BROWN and HOLLANDER · Statistics: A Biomedical Introduction
BRUNNER, DOMHOF, and LANGER · Nonparametric Analysis of Longitudinal Data in
  Factorial Experiments
BUCKLEW · Large Deviation Techniques in Decision, Simulation, and Estimation
CAIROLI and DALANG · Sequential Stochastic Optimization
CASTILLO, HADI, BALAKRISHNAN, and SARABIA · Extreme Value and Related
  Models with Applications in Engineering and Science
CHAN · Time Series: Applications to Finance
CHARALAMBIDES · Combinatorial Methods in Discrete Distributions
CHATTERJEE and HADI · Regression Analysis by Example, *Fourth Edition*
CHATTERJEE and HADI · Sensitivity Analysis in Linear Regression
CHERNICK · Bootstrap Methods: A Guide for Practitioners and Researchers,
  Second Edition
CHERNICK and FRIIS · Introductory Biostatistics for the Health Sciences
CHILÈS and DELFINER · Geostatistics: Modeling Spatial Uncertainty
CHOW and LIU · Design and Analysis of Clinical Trials: Concepts and Methodologies,
  Second Edition
CLARKE · Linear Models: The Theory and Application of Analysis of Variance
CLARKE and DISNEY · Probability and Random Processes: A First Course with
  Applications, *Second Edition*

*Now available in a lower priced paperback edition in the Wiley Classics Library.
†Now available in a lower priced paperback edition in the Wiley–Interscience Paperback Series.

*Now available in a lower priced paperback edition in the Wiley Classics Library.
†Now available in a lower priced paperback edition in the Wiley–Interscience Paperback Series.

---

*Now available in a lower priced paperback edition in the Wiley Classics Library.
†Now available in a lower priced paperback edition in the Wiley–Interscience Paperback Series.

*Now available in a lower priced paperback edition in the Wiley Classics Library.
†Now available in a lower priced paperback edition in the Wiley–Interscience Paperback Series.

LACHIN · Biostatistical Methods: The Assessment of Relative Risks

LAD · Operational Subjective Statistical Methods: A Mathematical, Philosophical, and Historical Introduction

LAMPERTI · Probability: A Survey of the Mathematical Theory, *Second Edition*

LANGE, RYAN, BILLARD, BRILLINGER, CONQUEST, and GREENHOUSE · Case Studies in Biometry

LARSON · Introduction to Probability Theory and Statistical Inference, *Third Edition*

LAWLESS · Statistical Models and Methods for Lifetime Data, *Second Edition*

LAWSON · Statistical Methods in Spatial Epidemiology

LE · Applied Categorical Data Analysis

LE · Applied Survival Analysis

LEE and WANG · Statistical Methods for Survival Data Analysis, *Third Edition*

LePAGE and BILLARD · Exploring the Limits of Bootstrap

LEYLAND and GOLDSTEIN (editors) · Multilevel Modelling of Health Statistics

LIAO · Statistical Group Comparison

LINDVALL · Lectures on the Coupling Method

LIN · Introductory Stochastic Analysis for Finance and Insurance

LINHART and ZUCCHINI · Model Selection

LITTLE and RUBIN · Statistical Analysis with Missing Data, *Second Edition*

LLOYD · The Statistical Analysis of Categorical Data

LOWEN and TEICH · Fractal-Based Point Processes

MAGNUS and NEUDECKER · Matrix Differential Calculus with Applications in Statistics and Econometrics, *Revised Edition*

MALLER and ZHOU · Survival Analysis with Long Term Survivors

MALLOWS · Design, Data, and Analysis by Some Friends of Cuthbert Daniel

MANN, SCHAFER, and SINGPURWALLA · Methods for Statistical Analysis of Reliability and Life Data

MANTON, WOODBURY, and TOLLEY · Statistical Applications Using Fuzzy Sets

MARCHETTE · Random Graphs for Statistical Pattern Recognition

MARDIA and JUPP · Directional Statistics

MASON, GUNST, and HESS · Statistical Design and Analysis of Experiments with Applications to Engineering and Science, *Second Edition*

McCULLOCH, SEARLE, and NEUHAUS · Generalized, Linear, and Mixed Models, *Second Edition*

McFADDEN · Management of Data in Clinical Trials, *Second Edition*

* McLACHLAN · Discriminant Analysis and Statistical Pattern Recognition

McLACHLAN, DO, and AMBROISE · Analyzing Microarray Gene Expression Data

McLACHLAN and KRISHNAN · The EM Algorithm and Extensions, *Second Edition*

McLACHLAN and PEEL · Finite Mixture Models

McNEIL · Epidemiological Research Methods

MEEKER and ESCOBAR · Statistical Methods for Reliability Data

MEERSCHAERT and SCHEFFLER · Limit Distributions for Sums of Independent Random Vectors: Heavy Tails in Theory and Practice

MICKEY, DUNN, and CLARK · Applied Statistics: Analysis of Variance and Regression, *Third Edition*

* MILLER · Survival Analysis, *Second Edition*

MONTGOMERY, JENNINGS, and KULAHCI · Introduction to Time Series Analysis and Forecasting

MONTGOMERY, PECK, and VINING · Introduction to Linear Regression Analysis, *Fourth Edition*

MORGENTHALER and TUKEY · Configural Polysampling: A Route to Practical Robustness

MUIRHEAD · Aspects of Multivariate Statistical Theory

---

*Now available in a lower priced paperback edition in the Wiley Classics Library.

†Now available in a lower priced paperback edition in the Wiley–Interscience Paperback Series.

*Now available in a lower priced paperback edition in the Wiley Classics Library.

†Now available in a lower priced paperback edition in the Wiley–Interscience Paperback Series.

RYAN · Modern Experimental Design
RYAN · Modern Regression Methods
RYAN · Statistical Methods for Quality Improvement, *Second Edition*
SALEH · Theory of Preliminary Test and Stein-Type Estimation with Applications
* SCHEFFE · The Analysis of Variance
SCHIMEK · Smoothing and Regression: Approaches, Computation, and Application
SCHOTT · Matrix Analysis for Statistics, *Second Edition*
SCHOUTENS · Levy Processes in Finance: Pricing Financial Derivatives
SCHUSS · Theory and Applications of Stochastic Differential Equations
SCOTT · Multivariate Density Estimation: Theory, Practice, and Visualization
† SEARLE · Linear Models for Unbalanced Data
† SEARLE · Matrix Algebra Useful for Statistics
† SEARLE, CASELLA, and McCULLOCH · Variance Components
SEARLE and WILLETT · Matrix Algebra for Applied Economics
SEBER · A Matrix Handbook For Statisticians
† SEBER · Multivariate Observations
SEBER and LEE · Linear Regression Analysis, *Second Edition*
† SEBER and WILD · Nonlinear Regression
SENNOTT · Stochastic Dynamic Programming and the Control of Queueing Systems
* SERFLING · Approximation Theorems of Mathematical Statistics
SHAFER and VOVK · Probability and Finance: It's Only a Game!
SILVAPULLE and SEN · Constrained Statistical Inference: Inequality, Order, and Shape
    Restrictions
SMALL and McLEISH · Hilbert Space Methods in Probability and Statistical Inference
SRIVASTAVA · Methods of Multivariate Statistics
STAPLETON · Linear Statistical Models
STAPLETON · Models for Probability and Statistical Inference: Theory and Applications
STAUDTE and SHEATHER · Robust Estimation and Testing
STOYAN, KENDALL, and MECKE · Stochastic Geometry and Its Applications, *Second
    Edition*
STOYAN and STOYAN · Fractals, Random Shapes and Point Fields: Methods of
    Geometrical Statistics
STREET and BURGESS · The Construction of Optimal Stated Choice Experiments:
    Theory and Methods
STYAN · The Collected Papers of T. W. Anderson: 1943–1985
SUTTON, ABRAMS, JONES, SHELDON, and SONG · Methods for Meta-Analysis in
    Medical Research
TAKEZAWA · Introduction to Nonparametric Regression
TANAKA · Time Series Analysis: Nonstationary and Noninvertible Distribution Theory
THOMPSON · Empirical Model Building
THOMPSON · Sampling, *Second Edition*
THOMPSON · Simulation: A Modeler's Approach
THOMPSON and SEBER · Adaptive Sampling
THOMPSON, WILLIAMS, and FINDLAY · Models for Investors in Real World Markets
TIAO, BISGAARD, HILL, PEÑA, and STIGLER (editors) · Box on Quality and
    Discovery: with Design, Control, and Robustness
TIERNEY · LISP-STAT: An Object-Oriented Environment for Statistical Computing
    and Dynamic Graphics
TSAY · Analysis of Financial Time Series, *Second Edition*
UPTON and FINGLETON · Spatial Data Analysis by Example, Volume II:
    Categorical and Directional Data
† VAN BELLE · Statistical Rules of Thumb, *Second Edition*
VAN BELLE, FISHER, HEAGERTY, and LUMLEY · Biostatistics: A Methodology for
    the Health Sciences, *Second Edition*

*Now available in a lower priced paperback edition in the Wiley Classics Library.

†Now available in a lower priced paperback edition in the Wiley–Interscience Paperback Series.